Shifting Boundaries of Public Health

Rochester Studies in Medical History

Senior Editor: Theodore M. Brown
Professor of History and Preventive Medicine
University of Rochester

ISSN 1526–2715

Shifting Boundaries of Public Health

Europe in the Twentieth Century

Edited by
Susan Gross Solomon,
Lion Murard, and Patrick Zylberman

UNIVERSITY OF ROCHESTER PRESS

First published 2008
Reprinted in paperback 2013

University of Rochester Press
668 Mt. Hope Avenue, Rochester, NY 14620, USA
www.urpress.com
and Boydell & Brewer Limited
PO Box 9, Woodbridge, Suffolk IP12 3DF, UK
www.boydellandbrewer.com

ISSN: 1526-2715
hardcover ISBN: 978-1-58046-283-9
paperback ISBN: 978-1-58046-455-0

Library of Congress Cataloging-in-Publication Data
    Shifting boundaries of public health : Europe in the twentieth century / edited
by Susan Gross Solomon, Lion Murard, and Patrick Zylberman.
        p. ; cm.—(Rochester studies in medical history, ISSN 1526–2715 ; v. 12)
    Includes bibliographical references and index.
    ISBN-13: 978-1-58046–283–9 (hardcover : alk. paper)
    ISBN-10: 1-58046–283–9
    1. Public health—Europe—History—20th century. I. Solomon, Susan Gross. II.
Murard, Lion. III. Zylberman, Patrick. IV. Series. [DNLM: 1. History, 20th Century—Europe—Essays. 2. Public Health—history—Europe—Essays. WA 11 GA1
S555 2008]
    RA483.S55 2008
    362.1094—dc22

                                                                            2008005776

A catalogue record for this title is available from the British Library.

This publication is printed on acid-free paper.
Printed in the United States of America

Contents

Part Four: Navigating between International and Local

Preface

This volume of essays grew out of a spirited debate among the editors in a Viennese coffee house in December 2002. We were attending "Social Medicine in European Perspective," a symposium hosted by the Department of the History of Medicine, Medical University of Vienna. With the new millennium not yet two years old, conversation turned to the story of public health in Europe in the century that had just closed. As we traded accounts of the century's high and low points, we were struck by how much our interpretations depended on the vantage point from which the story was being told. Rather than privileging public health on the international, national, or local level, we decided to produce a volume that would foreground the shifting boundaries between these levels in the making of policy, the design of structures and instruments, and the refinement of expertise in European public health.

We invited leading historians of public health in twentieth-century Europe to contribute "think pieces" on a series of "hot-button" issues: the ways national and transnational institutions interacted to shaped definitions of and solutions to public health problems; the extent to which transnational communities of experts on public health took account of "localisms" and to which local experts drew on international expertise; and the degree to which public health policy makers and scientists accommodated new understandings of the sites of health and disease. Among the most pleasurable aspects of the editorial process was the give-and-take with contributors, occasioned sometimes (but not always) by the proverbial "red pencil."

The volume was prepared during our own version of "shifting boundaries." In April 2004, Patrick Zylberman and Lion Murard traveled to Toronto to participate in "Real Socialism and the Second World," a conference supported by the Connaught Foundation, University of Toronto. In late August 2004, with the support of the Institut National de la Santé et de la Recherche Médicale (INSERM, Paris), the Ministry of Foreign Affairs (France), Associated Medical Services, Inc. (Canada) and the consulate general of France (Toronto), Zylberman and Murard returned to Toronto for a three-week stay at the Munk Centre for International Studies, University of Toronto. Susan Gross Solomon went to Paris in May 2005 (as visiting professor, École des Hautes Études en Sciences Sociales); in May 2006 (to conduct research supported by Associated Medical Services, Inc.); and in May and June 2007 (as a participant on the Canadian Institute for Health Research [CIHR]–Centre National de la Recherche Scientifique [CNRS] faculty exchange, based at the Centre d'Études des Mondes Russe, Caucasien et Centre-Européen, École des Hautes Études en Sciences Sociales, Paris). These "Atlantic crossings" facilitated the dynamics of scientific collaboration and the juxtaposition of perspectives that makes intellectual work exciting.

In the process of bringing the project to fruition, we accumulated a series of additional debts, which it our pleasure to acknowledge in print. Funding from Associated Medical Services, Inc.; the Connaught Fund, University of Toronto (for the collaborative project "Real Socialism and the 'Second World'"); and the Faculty of Arts and Science, University of Toronto supported research, travel, communication among the editors, and the technical editing of the manuscript. The Centre de Recherche Médecine, Science, Santé et Société (CERMES, Paris) assisted in the production of the index. To the institutions and individuals who provided not only generous material but also collegial support, we are very grateful.

Invaluable intellectual and editorial assistance was offered by Janet Hyer (Munk Centre for International Studies, University of Toronto), who used her celebrated "eagle eye" not only to edit, but also to improve the text, and created the index. Special thanks to Ted Brown, general editor of Rochester Studies in Medical History, for his encouragement early on in the process; to the two anonymous readers for the press, who made excellent suggestions; and to Suzanne Guiod and Katie Hurley, for guiding the manuscript from submission to completion.

A word on the cover: concern over the fluidity of Europe's borders ran across the political spectrum, as evidenced in the map published by Les Editions de L'Ordre national, the publisher of a French right-wing, nationalist journal, *L'Ordre national*, which came out bimonthly from early 1938 to the end of 1939.

Introduction

Susan Gross Solomon, Lion Murard, and Patrick Zylberman

The twentieth century dawned auspiciously. Path-breaking developments were occurring in many fields of arts and culture.[1] It had been nearly three decades since a major European war. There was little reason to predict that, alongside the great advances in thought and sensibility, the new century in Europe would bear witness to unprecedented carnage carried out by the "gardening state"[2] in the service of one or another ideology[3] or vision of modernity.[4] But before the century had come to an end, on both national and international levels, a variety of political structures (liberal democratic, authoritarian, totalitarian)[5] would be essayed in the name of expanding and circumscribing the reach of politics.[6] The twentieth century, termed by Hobsbawm an "age of extremes," has left a legacy that defies neat categorization and continues to fuel heated debates.[7]

Public health was deeply implicated in the mixed record of the century. The advances in science made possible almost unimaginable progress in the conquest of contagious disease,[8] while new ways of thinking about social citizenship and economic progress bolstered the view that the health of the body politic was the concern of the state.[9] At the same time, public health (and medicine) played a seminal role in a range of ruthless and heinous human experiments—all in the effort to construct societal utopias.[10]

With belief in the link between the structure and substance of policy making widespread, new organizations for making health policy were created. After 1918, some states established centralized governmental structures; simultaneously, international structures were formed (and then reformed) with mandates to collect information, refine policies, and enforce norms across nations.[11] The new structures raised new questions. Could progress be made if individual nations were allowed to follow their own interests? Did international health structures guarantee benign and progressive health policy? And how could the agendas of individual nations be harmonized with the responsibilities of international agencies?

According to conventional wisdom, the promotion of health and that of international cooperation reinforced each other. After World War I, in international forums, health was seen as an instrument of reconciliation between hostile societies and states. A half century later, the Alma Ata conference (1978), convened in the heady belief in "convergence" that was part of the "thaw" in East-West relations, provided a demonstration effect of what the WHO's regional committee for Europe called Equity in Care.[12] The provision of food, housing, social insurance, paid holidays, cooperatives, leisure activities, education, and especially public health—taken together—would reduce the scope of politics, or so ran the thinking. And yet, for all the high hopes, international institutions proved susceptible to politics. As Jean-Claude Favez has shown, the close relations between the International Red Cross and conservative figures in Germany and Switzerland led to sins of omission in the late 1930s and forties.[13]

For their part, states were often loathe to surrender their hard-won control over matters of health. As early as 1848, public health was conceived by revolutionaries in France and Germany, as it was later by the architects of state medicine in Great Britain, as the responsibility (and the prerogative) of the nation-state. In carrying out that responsibility, the state often came into conflict with the jurisdiction of the localities and, far more seriously, with the rights of the individual. As recently as the beginning of the twentieth century, grounding its arguments in the new bacteriological concepts, the Board of Health of New York City had no qualms about locking up for life a thirty-seven-year-old Irish cook ("Typhoid" Mary Mallon) accused of infecting thirty-two people.[14] The American case was far from the most egregious. Certain totalitarian states treated health as an instrument (or even as a weapon) of state power.[15] But then, so did some democratic regimes, the Scandinavians being the most remarkable in this regard.[16]

Capturing the essence of public health in the twentieth century is no easy matter. The story could be told from the vantage point of national or international health. Each narrative has its own chronology, emphasizing some decades, downplaying others; each has its own "defining moments," its own set of heroes and antiheroes.

Rather than adopt either narrative to the exclusion of the other, the essays in *Shifting Boundaries of Public Health* explore an issue that spans both—namely, the connection between health and place in the twentieth century. In the last quarter century or so, "place" has emerged as a key concept in a range of fields—anthropology, literature, history, geography, to name but a few.[17] In the literature on both national and international public health in the twentieth century, references to place run like a red thread. For the last two hundred years at least, if not indeed longer, military commanders, travelers, local physicians, and researchers—each in their own way—have puzzled over why it was that certain diseases occurred in some locales not others, in some natural environments not others, among some populations not others, and in some states not others.

Among physicians, particularly military physicians and those engaged in expeditionary hygiene, there was a long-standing interest in the connection between disease and location (whether defined by climate, physical environment, topographic features, or flora).[18] The "geographical temper" among physicians, usually traced to the work of Leonhard Ludwig Finke in the late eighteenth century, reached its height in the mid-nineteenth century, after which point it experienced a precipitous decline.[19] As geographically oriented physicians sought to situate or locate disease in a place, they drew on a range of allied fields—climatology (A. Haviland, E. Huntington), soil science (M. v. Pettenkofer, F. F. Clemow), hygiene and preventive medicine (A. Proust), and history (A. Hirsch, K. Sudhoff, G. Sticker[20])—to name but a few. The interest of physicians in the sites of disease spurred advances in the conceptualization and representational strategies of cartography: by the late nineteenth century, even statisticians and demographers were taking note of disease maps.[21]

The first half of the twentieth century saw a broader notion of the "site" of disease. Even before World War I, place was no longer defined exclusively by geographic markers: for some writers, location included features of the social/ethnographic environment such as race or population.[22] Furthermore, as sanitary science began to disappear from the public health agenda in the early twentieth century, physicians began to identify disease as occurring not in a specific locale, but in the spaces between bodies; this insight increased interest in the sociology of health.[23]

The twentieth century has brought with it signal changes in the way students of health and disease think about location. We have moved from understanding "place" exclusively as the site of disease to including under this rubric sites of responsibility (governmental or nongovernmental structures, expert groups, or knowledge systems) for dealing with the problems of health and disease.[24] Then, too, we have moved from conceiving of "place" as fixed to including movement within and across borders (geographic, institutional, or disciplinary) that are themselves impermanent and porous.[25] The new approaches not only shape our agendas for the new century, but also provoke us to reflect on the role of "place" in the histories of public health written during the century that has just closed.

Politics as Place

In the second half of the twentieth century, scholars have begun to look at the disease-prevention strategies that nations adopt as a choice not simply of medical techniques, but of political values and commitments.[26] With that new awareness, scholars focused their attention, or more accurately, refocused it, on the seat of political choices about health. The interconnection of the state and public health was a theme with pedigree. Mid-nineteenth-century reformers such as Chadwick in England, Virchow in Germany, and Villermé in France had argued strenuously that public health and welfare should be part of state-craft. In the 1920s and 1930s, many of the "large" figures writing about the history of public health—both historians (René Sand, Sir Arthur Newsholme, George Rosen, Henry Sigerist)[27] and activist-reformers (John Kingsbury, John Ryle, Andrija Štampar)[28] alike—insisted on the fundamentally political character of developments in public health.

But among historians of public health, engagement with the problems of public health and the state was slow in developing. In all likelihood, a mix of factors conspired: historians of public health were captured by the enthusiasm of their profession for the questions raised by social history;[29] equally, if not more, important, the association of health and politics was tainted by the misuse of medicine for political ends under National Socialism.[30]

There were, of course, notable exceptions to the disregard of the state. The link between health and politics figured prominently in the 1948 Fielding Garrison Lecture delivered by the historian Erwin Ackerknecht, based at the time at the University of Wisconsin.[31] Ackerknecht argued that the approach to prevention that a nation chose was a function of the political character of the regime: authoritarian governments favored the cordon sanitaire and quarantine, whereas liberal governments inclined toward sanitationist policies.[32] Formulated as it was in the wake of World War II, Ackerknecht's contention that a state's political character was a determining factor gained wide acceptance.

Ackerknecht's view had important implications for the way history of health was written. For much of the period from the 1950s through the 1970s, the power of the state over health (both for good and for ill) was seen as unfettered.[33] Only in the 1980s did historians begin to write about the formation of health policy as part of the political process, with all the push and pull that that implies.[34] In Dorothy Porter's history of public health from ancient to modern times, the state emerges as but one in a concatenation of forces (including classes, social structures, organizations, and pressure groups) that constrain or shape policy.[35] In his large study of a hundred years of preventive strategies adopted by European countries in the face of contagious disease, Peter Baldwin concluded that although "politics were certainly part of the story," the preventive strategy a state chose was conditioned in good measure by its "geoepidemiological location" (in relation to the currents of contagious disease and the topographical features that affected the efficacy of preventive strategies), by commercial interests, and by administrative capacity.[36] Having turned on its head the Ackerknecht argument of the impact of politics on prophylaxis, Baldwin closed with the thought that the factors shaping preventive strategies ultimately shaped a nation's political traditions.

Scholars interested in the complex links between health and politics are beginning once again to focus on regime type—to think in particular about the challenges that making policy for health poses for democratic governance and values. In his chapter, "Can There Be a Democratic Public Health? Fighting AIDS in the Industrialized World," Peter Baldwin suggests that a democracy confronted by infectious disease has a choice between two alternative strategies—the "individualized" strategy, in which each citizen acts as his or her own quarantine officer, and the "governmentalist" or communal strategy, which regulates behavior from above. For Baldwin, the strategies differ in their educative value for the citizen. Indeed, the choice a nation makes may well tell us more about its understanding of democracy than about its approach to epidemiology. But are both strategies equally open to a nation at all times? Writing from the vantage point of historical institutionalism,[37] scholars such as Ellen Immergut and Jacob Hacker have portrayed states as constrained by their previous choices, by the structure of the institutions administering public health, and by the rules of the decisional game.[38]

At the same time, scholars are questioning the role of the democratic state in making hard political choices. Dorothy Porter's chapter, "The Social Contract of Health in the Twentieth and Twenty-First Centuries: Individuals, Corporations, and the State," is a valedictory for the nineteenth-century social contract of health, which assigned responsibility to the state for the health of its citizens. With the growing focus on chronic disease characteristic of the twentieth century, the individual has been made responsible for making lifestyle choices that promote health. But Porter's study of how the United States handled the problem of obesity suggests that withdrawal of the state may galvanize collective actors. As the American government shows itself disinclined to rein in the large corporations profiting from unwise eating habits, the cudgels may be taken up by a vocal citizenry or by transnational agencies seeking to impose standards. Whatever the case, the impact of the state's diminished responsibility for health on its relationship with the citizenry will be felt.

Studies such as Porter's raise "big" political questions. There has been much talk about "bringing the state back in." But if the state is unable or disinclined to make the hard choices, what kinds of political controls can there be? What happens to democratic accountability?

Discussions of responsibility and accountability by scholars such as Porter and Baldwin expand our notion of the challenges facing health policy and provoke us to think about politics not just as the push and pull of interests or the conflict over divisible goods, but as the seat of strategies that must fit with core democratic values and procedures.

Emphasizing the political and social context in which health policy choices are made does not mean minimizing the role played by health sciences. Science, which has informed so much of diagnosis and treatment in health, is continually being revised. But can we—or should we—separate scientific innovations from their social and political contexts? To be sure, some recent works continue to privilege the internal history of biological or medical science, whereas others stress the social relations that accompany or underpin medical advances.[39] *Shifting Boundaries* goes beyond merely linking scientific programs and the social or political valuations that help promote or block them to insist that developments in public health were "interrelated and embedded" in the social and political concerns of twentieth-century health policy and health politics.[40]

Expertise and Place: The Geography of Public Health Advice

With the increasing mobility of diseases and of physicians who study and treat those diseases, questions about the relation between location and expertise became pressing. Is expertise developed in one place (sometimes called "local knowledge") specific to that location? Can knowledge in the field of public health be transnational, that is, placeless? If so, what might such knowledge look like?

In search of answers to these questions, a number of historians of internationalism in public health gravitated to the concept of "epistemic communities," introduced by P. M. Haas.[41] Appealing though it is, the concept of an epistemic community begs the question, for it begins with the assumption that there is a transnational community of experts and advisors. But is that community defined by its membership or by the advice it gives? Who decides who's in and who's out? Does the fact that the community is multinational in its composition guarantee that it is international? In his chapter "American Foundations and the Internationalizing of Public Health," Paul Weindling analyzes cohorts of academic advisers and program officers as key sources of the internationalism that corporate philanthropies such as the Rockefeller Foundation and the Milbank Memorial Fund deployed in the reconstruction of health activities in Europe between the two world wars. The foundations believed in the international transferability of American models, but they soon came to realize that American experts could profit from model schemes developed elsewhere. American philanthropies were marked by a dual flow of exchanges—between a cluster of foundations, which very often were partners thanks to the close relations between their trustees and officers, and between sources of innovation on both sides of the Atlantic.[42]

Those interested in the relation between the local and the translocal in public health knowledge might well get leverage from focusing on the "what" of expertise rather than on the "who."[43] The last half decade has seen some original thinking on the problem. In *Seeing Like a State*, James Scott begins from the insight that a state that wishes to redesign society must first make it "legible," a task that requires arranging the population, cat-egorizing it, measuring it, and mapping it.[44] The creation of a "readable" society invariably involves what Scott terms "thin simplification."[45] In the service of that simplification, by the late nineteenth century, if not indeed before, the spheres of human endeavor freest of contingency, guesswork, and context came to be seen as humanity's highest work. Scott sometimes characterizes local knowledge as a kind of trial and error—not unlike the Greek *metis*—that produced "practical solutions without benefit of scientific method." The elevation of the simplification necessary for social engineer-ing brings with it the denigration of practical ("nonscientific") knowledge of the local that favors complexity and contingency.

The connection Scott draws between the two kinds of knowing—scientific and nonscientific—is neither conceptually neat nor untroubled. As Scott himself allows, the two spheres are not mutually exclusive. "Generic formulas cannot supply the local knowledge that will allow the successful translation of the necessarily crude understandings to successful nuanced local applica-tions." Put even more strongly, "The more general the rules, the more they require translation to be locally successful."[46]

But how are the two kinds of knowledge to be connected? In his book on the relationship of laboratory and field in biology, Robert Kohler distinguishes two kinds of scientific knowledge: the "placeless" knowledge produced in the laboratory and the knowledge produced in the field, which is a respecter of place.[47] In Kohler's view, the challenge for modern science is to make knowl-edge that is locally produced "placeless" and therefore generally acceptable. In contrast, in his analysis of critical demography, Simon Szreter and his col-leagues insist that the task confronting policy science is to make knowledge that is centrally produced relevant to the locale. The problem with the reli-ance on knowledge that presents as "quasi-universal validity, neutral of con-text ideology" is that it is, by definition, invalid as a practical guide to action in a specific locale. Yet, explains Szreter, public policy (including health policy) is all about devising strategies to deal with conditions in specific places.[48]

To what extent does public health knowledge display the tension between generic (placeless) knowledge and local knowledge (rooted in place) in the sense that Scott described? Scott included public health among the instances of "thin simplification" projects through which the state expands its control over society.[49] But the issue that bedevils public health is not how to integrate two different kinds of knowledge (scientific and nonscientific), but rather how to devise knowledge-based policies that are both placeless in range and respecters of place.

In his chapter, "A Transatlantic Dispute: The Etiology of Malaria and the Redesign of the Mediterranean Landscape," Patrick Zylberman contrasts two approaches to dealing with malaria. The League of Nations Malaria Commis-sion saw malaria as a "social" disease linked to underdevelopment, whereas

American malariologists, wedded to the ecological approach, believed malaria to be a "local" disease, contingent on insect and human geography. Proponents of the two approaches differed in their conceptions of the "local." According to Lewis Hackett, the head of the Rockefeller Foundation's experimental station in Rome and one of the leading advocates of the ecological view, each paludal village was its own norm. This flew in the face of the view that a universal strategy for dealing with malaria could be found. The debate was inherently political, but malaria defied ready-made schemes.

The difficulty of framing science-based policies that are useful for a range of disparate cases has often been underrated—if not totally ignored—by policy makers, at both the international and local levels. For example, over the course of the century, leading international philanthropies involved in public health (the Rockefeller Foundation, the Milbank Memorial Foundation) and international health agencies (the League of Nations Health Organization, the World Health Organization) were engaged on a routine basis in applying public health yardsticks (templates, indicators) and proffering advice produced in New York or Geneva to a wide variety of countries whose specific features had not been factored into the generalized schemes. Could such a template transcend the place of its origin and attain translocal applicability?

In "A Matter of 'Reach': Fact-Finding in Public Health in the Wake of World War I," Susan Solomon contrasts two early twentieth-century approaches to public health fact-finding. The first, introduced by American foundations in Europe, deployed a single template to survey public health across nations; the second, honed by the Russian Commissariat of Public Health for use in "Western" capitals, used "representatives" embedded in different countries to collect information on the public health priorities of their host countries. Each approach had limitations. Because the American templates treated the political context of nations as "background information" divorced from the structure and goals of public health, they were useful only for countries whose "background" was "Western" (i.e., similar to America's). The country-by-country approach deployed by the Soviet government hinged on the acuity and the networks of the "representatives." Whether either approach facilitated comparison across nations is an open question.

The problem of the general and the specific affected individual countries with no less force. In the department of Meurthe-et-Moselle, the French health statesman Jacques Parisot devised a prototype of public health cooperation among doctors, representatives of health insurance funds, medical associations, and officials of public health services. Efforts were made to treat the prototype as reproducible in other departments, but ironically the experiment had its greatest resonance outside France.

To treat the problem of placelessness and place in public health knowledge solely as one of epistemology would be to impoverish it. At its base, public health knowledge is what Theda Skocpol and Dieter Rueschemeyer would term "social knowledge"—that is, knowledge distinguished both by its object (society) and its purpose (social policy making).[50] Social knowledge was a creature of the emerging welfare state: it owed much to the belief that society develops in lawlike ways to which behavior and public policies can be made to conform[51] and to the reliance on scientific quantification that does not depend on personal contact among researchers (Theodore Porter's "trust in numbers").[52] Over the course of the twentieth century, the legitimacy and utility of social knowledge became increasingly accepted.

The relationship between social knowledge (analysis) and policy (action) is not a technical, but a political one. Although information can inform policy making, the choice of strategies to deal with health and disease is ultimately political.[53] In "Contested Spaces: Models of Public Health in Occupied Germany," Sabine Schleiermacher contrasts the public health systems created in the British and Soviet zones of occupation after World War II. The story reads like a laboratory experiment, albeit one "atop of a graveyard."[54] In both zones, key principles of prewar German public health remained—the commitment to social insurance, to preventive medicine, and to the tenet of social hygiene that social conditions affected health status. But on these principles the Soviet and British occupation authorities built radically different systems. The Soviets engaged in quite concerted denazification of the medical profession and annulled some of the National Socialist regulations (especially the odious "Law for the Prevention of Hereditarily Diseased Offspring"). In contrast, in the name of keeping politics out of their rebuilding, the British left some structures standing and some Nazi-era regulations in place.

The Question of Levels

In twentieth-century public health, the focus of innovation, initiative, and expertise oscillated dramatically between the local, the national, and the international levels. To complicate matters further for the historian, the very meaning of the terms "international" and "local" shifted over time.

For example, the three decades between the end of the 1880s and the end of the 1920s were years of what Eric Weil would have termed "inter-national" cooperation:[55] even the much-publicized gatherings at the Sanitary Conferences (the first held in Paris in 1851) and the creation of the Office international d'hygiène publique in Paris in 1907 were little more than the coming together of official representatives from a variety of countries.[56] Interaction was episodic and the circulation of ideas was rather limited. World War I was followed by an explosion of international activity, which, in contrast to that of the earlier period, was more regular and formalized. This activity was driven not by diplomats but by experts with strong scientific credentials, selected for their competence, not their nationality. These experts, who continued to represent their own nations, forged an esprit de corps, a professional language, and ongoing networks of exchange.[57] In many ways, Geneva was *the* address for public health experts. Although local- or municipal-level public health was often discussed at international gatherings, local developments were not the business of international organizations. To the extent that the "local" was affected at all by outside forces, it was through the travel and exchange of experts.[58]

The 1930s saw a marked rebalancing toward the local, which was almost universally recognized as the seat of innovation in public health. As Weindling points out in his chapter, philanthropies with global reach now chose to work with community-based health activities rather than with nation-states. International organizations, which had heretofore presented themselves as the avant-garde, now found themselves on the defensive, weighted down by bureaucracy and political obstacles. As Iris Borowy's chapter shows, an odd dynamic emerged: international organizations were maneuvering for "space" (read "function," funds, and visibility) while innovative policies and approaches were being honed elsewhere. Of course, in some dictatorships in the 1930s, local initiatives were blocked by political centralization and the insistence on control.[59]

In the wake of World War II, the truly "cosmopolitical" order of the twenties and early thirties crumbled. In public health, what collapsed was not only the international structures, but the very goal of creating a single "watchtower" for health around the world. Recall that at the beginning of the twenties, the medical director of the League of Nations Health Organization (LNHO) was referred to as "the general superintendent of the world."[60] In place of the original design, formulated to promote peace, myriad national regimes now emerged, often at odds with one other. The assertive and quarrelsome nation-states became the pillars on which newly created or reformed international organizations were forced to stand. But empires, often the proxies for nations, were fading.[61] On the ruins of those fading structures, as James Gillespie points out, new regional structures were growing, even as the World Health Organization was in the process of taking root. Within short order the new structures would uncouple the identification of "international" with "Europe."

The final decades of the twentieth century saw the retreat of the nation-state—whether because of incapacity or ideology—leaving to the localities the function (and the burden) of a range of public services.[62] Some observers have read this "delegation" as the empowerment of the local; others saw it as draining resources from the local level. At the same time that the local level was gaining in visibility, the international level became the seat of a staggering variety of agencies. In their struggle for place, some of the new international agencies attempted to capture terrain from the localities—or from one another—with uneven success and most often without input from the local. Indeed, international organizations routinely imposed programs on nation-states without hearing from the national (much less the local) experts.[63] Perhaps because of the plethora of new international organizations, the concept of international health governance came into its own at the very end of the century, when the World Health Assembly consented to reform the International Health Regulations.[64]

A review of the record of the twentieth century suggests that at a few moments—the last half of the 1920s, the late 1950s, and the brief "thaw" of the 1960s—international health organizations came close to functioning as the "brave new world" that their proponents and designers had hoped for. Yet even the rosiest moments saw counterpressure from the nation-states.

During the 1920s, despite their titles and inclusionary mandates, international organizations and scientific forums were not open to all. After World War I and the Bolshevik revolution, for example, German and Soviet public health researchers, like their colleagues in science, were excluded from most international scientific gatherings and—even worse—treated as pariahs.[65] To offset the consequences of isolation—lack of access to information, to cutting-edge work in their fields, to patient populations, and to resources—the Germans and Soviets engaged in a series of collaborative ventures, even as they bent every effort to reclaim their "place" in international public health and medicine. Historians of the German-Soviet interwar cooperation have focused on the impact of the bilateral relationship on the health policies of the two nations.[66] The impact of the German-Soviet relationship on international health is a story that remains to be told.

Even the Health Committee of the LNHO, the jewel in the international crown, was marked by ongoing internecine strife between those who pressed the League to develop into a primarily humanitarian organization and those, opposed to the development of a strong international health organization, who would have agreed with its British member that "the conception of a superepidemiologist at Geneva seems radically unsound."[67] In fact, the League remained an association of nations whose corporate solidarity was feeble. It was much less than an all-powerful superstate but much more than a mere international letterbox.

Indeed, following Pierre Hassner, we may question whether the "international" was anything more than a vast array of competitive/cooperative relations between nation-states or powers.[68] In his chapter, "Europe, America, and the Space of International Health," James Gillespie examines the reorientation of international health during and after World War II from Eurocentric concerns to a singled-minded focus on the developmental problems of the tropics. The often-forgotten Health Division of the United Nations Relief and Rehabilitation Administration (UNRRA) was the theater in which Europeans' suspicions that America intended to interfere in their colonial possessions and the U.S. Congress's cooler view of multilateral commitments were both played out. By a twist of fate, European nations, once the colonial masters, now became the protectors of the colonies. The legacy of the tensions in UNRRA was long: excluding UNRRA's successor, the World Health Organization, from "interference" in colonial affairs became the byword of the 1950s. But could technical advice in matters of health—which was welcomed—be so easily separated from political counsel?

To be sure, international activity did spur the entry into interstate relations not only of technical but of moral considerations, though states could not be compelled to comply; they could only be enjoined. The "international" materialized most often as local experiments or prototypes, for example, the health cooperatives in Serbia supported by the Milbank Memorial Fund (1920–1935) or the programs for malaria control in Italy (1923–51) and in the Balkans (in Yugoslavia, Albania, and Bulgaria, there were short-term programs between 1929 and 1937) operated by Rockefeller Foundation officers. But of course, these local prototypes could not be legitimately imposed on other states.

The struggle for terrain among the various levels of public health activity during the twentieth century has led some historians to reify these levels and to treat them as hermetically sealed from one another. In contrast, historians of colonialism are arguing for and writing histories that are "connected," intricate, and contradictory.[69] Yet in public health, no less than in other fields, evidence is ample that the borders among the international, national, and local levels are porous. In his chapter, "British Public Health and the Problem of Local Demographic Structures," Graham Mooney documents the shifting and uncertain role of demographic standardization on the local level. From the dawn of the twentieth century, notions of healthy and unhealthy places centered on what came to be considered the average rate of mortality. Mooney, himself a research assistant in the Liverpool Public Health Observatory in the mid-1990s (Liverpool was the birthplace of local public health services in the United Kingdom), problematizes the science of the local. Mortality rates were linked to geography, albeit in a complex relationship. But Mooney underscores that what is "local" exists conceptually only in relation to other locals or to the national. The science of the local thus appears as fundamentally negotiated knowledge between localized and nationalized conceptions.

How do we write the story of the porous borders among levels? Where, for example, do we situate health statesmen who claim to speak on behalf of this or that organization? The heroes of Iris Borowy's chapter, "Maneuvering for Space: International Health Work of the League of Nations during World War II," Raymond Gautier and Yves Biraud, were creatures of Geneva. Indeed, when the League of Nations Health Organization came unraveled, they had difficulty not only in finding a place for themselves, but in recasting their identities. But some of their colleagues, such as Ludwik Rajchman,[70] Jacques Parisot,[71] and René Sand, had multiple identities, presenting themselves as placeless experts while representing or speaking on behalf of places they knew well. Research suggests that these figures were often "playing on two tables,"[72] courting international patrons to advance domestic agendas,[73] or using local demonstrations to make a case in the global arena. What, we may ask, are the factors that made some experts see themselves and be seen as "above nations," whereas others were firmly tied to the boundaries of their states? How much of their status was a function of their training and how much of the places from which they hailed?

How much circulation of ideas was there between the levels? In his chapter, "Designs within Disorder: International Conferences on Rural Health Care and the Art of the Local, 1931–1939," Lion Murard scrutinizes the series of conferences sponsored by the League of Nations and the associated experiments carried out in Yugoslavia and Hebei Province in China. Murard documents the extraordinary record of a "contagion effect" between the local-level health demonstrations, with their focus on grassroots participation, in a variety of countries. Pilot projects inaugurated in Yugoslavia reverberated in China. Sometimes, the odyssey of the demonstrations produced new variations; at other times, merely replication. But as Murard's chapter makes clear, the spread of the pilot projects did not go from locale to locale. Ironically, the demonstrations—their goals, their successes, their failures—were refracted through institutions and discussion venues at the international level.

At critical junctures in the twentieth century, the local level was championed not only as the seat of innovation in public health, but also as a "school of democracy." For the guiding spirits behind the rural health conferences, self-government was the sine qua non for rural betterment. Although the twenties saw a strong push to spread or universalize the best approach (often equated with the "American model"), rural-life conferences pushed reliance on village-based expertise. That is not to say that participatory democracy was an unalloyed good. To public health researchers such as Lewis Hackett, local folk knowledge threatened to push out scientific expertise.[74] Moreover, in many locales, village-based expertise "sensitive to local folkways" skirted dangerously close to ethnonationalism and the politics of exclusion.[75] Half a century later, as Peter Baldwin points out, the seat of illiberalism had become popular opinion itself.[76]

Today, the attempt to locate or ground health policy in a particular place—whether geographic, social, or political—runs up against the pervasive assumption of deterritorialization, which underpins discussion in every arena of public policy. Whether the eclipse of territoriality reflects political realities or discursive practices is an open question.

Whatever the case, in the field of health policy today, there is a lively debate between proponents of two rival paradigms. Those who champion the older "quarantine model" stress the importance of national or local health borders; in its modern iteration, of course, "informational cordons" are replacing the physical isolation of (suspected) carriers and of the dangerously ill.[77] In contrast, spokesmen for the "emerging diseases worldview," which has become one of the key elements of WHO strategy, take as their starting point the idea that the world is in flux and that borders are porous and leaky. The emerging diseases worldview, which is clearly dominant today, starts from the observation that both health risks and the fight against them are not territorially bounded. Network has displaced territory as the relevant unit of analysis. As Joshua Lederberg put it in 1992, "There is nowhere in the world from which we are remote and no one from whom we are disconnected."[78]

The debate shows no signs of being resolved on the ground. Although most specialists in public health would readily admit that health borders do not correspond to political boundaries (the health borders were national in the case of "mad cow disease" but global in the case of avian flu), national borders do reemerge at the first symptom of a major epidemic. In 1995, Russian authorities fought cholera, typhoid, and Shigella dysentery with a quarantine and the forced isolation of suspected cases (with the help of the police and the army).[79] The 2001 outbreak of foot-and-mouth disease established quarantines in and out of Great Britain.

The 2003 campaign against SARS showed that under certain circumstances, the two "rival" paradigms could coexist. Although SARS was stamped out thanks to "medieval methods"—quarantine and isolation of the contaminated—success in bringing the epidemic under control depended on a global approach with real-time information sharing, coordinated by WHO, with significant input from nation-states and localities.[80]

Standing back from the details of the worldwide campaign against SARS, we note an assumption that was widespread in that most unusual of decades, the 1920s: namely, that empowering international health agencies did not necessarily preclude initiative and input from the national or local levels. The hardening of boundaries among the international, national, and the local was a creature of the post–World War II period. As David Fidler put it, the 1950s and the 1960s were the climax of the Westphalian order of public health.[81]

To be sure, both the present-day interests of international health agencies, states, and local political units and the relative power of the various protagonists differ profoundly from those of the 1920s. One of the pressing tasks for the twenty-first century will be to create a loosely structured framework in which the three levels of public health governance work together in a partnership whose boundaries shift as new challenges arise.

Notes

1. M. Eksteins, *Rites of Spring: The Great War and the Birth of the Modern Age* (Boston: Houghton Mifflin, 1989).

2. Z. Bauman, *Modernity and the Holocaust* (New York: Cornell University Press, 2000), 66–72.

3. A. Janos, *East Central Europe in the Modern World: The Politics of Borderland from Pre- to Post-Communism* (Stanford: Stanford University Press, 2000).

4. E. Hobsbawm, *Age of Extremes: The Short Twentieth Century,* 1914–1991 (London: M. Joseph, 1994); D. Diner, *Beyond the Conceivable: Studies on Germany, Nazism and the Holocaust* (Berkeley: University of California Press, 2000); R. Aron, "L'Aube de la civilisation universelle," in *Une histoire du XXe siècle,* ed. C. Bachelier, 787–808 (Paris: Plon, 1996); J. Herf, *Reactionary Modernism* (Cambridge: Cambridge University Press, 1984); R. Cooter, M. Harrison, and S. Sturdy, eds., *War, Medicine, and Modernity* (Stroud: Sutton, 1998).

5. M. Mazower, *Dark Continent: Europe's Twentieth Century* (Harmondsworth: Penguin, 1999).

6. C. Maier, ed., *Changing Boundaries of the Political: Essays on the Evolving Balance Between the State, Society, Public and Private in Europe* (Cambridge: Cambridge University Press, 1987); D. Held, *Democracy and the Global Order: From the Modern State to Cosmopolitan Governance* (Stanford: Stanford University Press, 1995).

7. C. Maier, "Consigning the Twentieth Century to History: Alternative Narratives for the Modern Era," *American Historical Review* 105 (2000): 807–31.

8. P. Baldwin, *Disease and Democracy: The Industrialized World Faces AIDS* (Berkeley: University of California Press, 2005).

9. D. Porter, *Health, Civilization and the State: A History of Public Health from Ancient Times to Modern Times* (London: Routledge, 1999); M. Harrison, *Disease and the Modern World: 1500 to the Present Day* (Cambridge: Polity, 2004).

10. P. Weindling, *Epidemics and Genocide in Eastern Europe,* 1890–1945 (Oxford: Oxford University Press, 2000); Mazower, *Dark Continent,* 76–103; S. Reverby, *Tuskegee's Truths: Rethinking the Tuskegee Syphilis Study* (Chapel Hill: University of North Carolina Press, 2000).

11. P. Weindling, *International Health Organizations and Movements* (Cambridge: Cambridge University Press, 1995); D. Porter, ed., *The History of Public Health and the Modern State* (Amsterdam: Rodopi, 1994).

12. S. Litsios, "The Long and Difficult Road to Alma Ata: A Personal Reflection," *International Journal of Health Services* 32 (2002): 709–32.

13. J. Favez, *The Red Cross and the Holocaust* (Cambridge: Cambridge University Press, 1999).

14. J. Walzer Leavitt, *Typhoid Mary, Captive to the Public's Health* (Boston: Beacon Press, 1996).

15. M. Burleigh and W. Wippermann, *The Racial State: Germany 1933–1945* (Cambridge: Cambridge University Press, 1991).

16. G. Broberg and N. Roll-Hansen, eds., *Eugenics and the Welfare State: Sterilization Policy in Denmark, Sweden, Norway, and Finland* (East Lansing: Michigan State University Press, 1996).

17. K. Schloegel, *Im Raum lessen wir die Zeit* (Munich: Carl Hanser Verlag, 2004); J. Agnew, *The Power of Place: Bringing Together Geographical and Sociological Imaginations* (Boston: Unwin Hyman, 1989); J. Agnew, *Geopolitics: Revisioning World Politics* (London: Routledge, 1998).

18. F. Barrett, *Disease and Geography: The History of an Idea* (Toronto: York University Press, 2000); M. Osborne, "The Geographical Imperative in Nineteenth-Century

French Medicine," in *Medical Geography in Historical Perspective*, ed. N. Rupke, 31–50 (London: Wellcome Institute for the History of Medicine, 2000); F. Garrison, "Medical Geography and Geographic Medicine," *Bulletin of the New York Academy of Medicine* 8, no. 10 (1932): 593–612.

19. For conflicting views of the decline of medical geography, see O. Amsterdamska, "Standardizing Epidemics: Infection, Inheritance, and Environment in Pre-War Experimental Epidemiology," in *Heredity and Infection: The History of Disease Transmission*, ed. J.-P. Gaudillière and I. Löwy, 135–79 (London: Routledge, 2001); M. Sorre, "Complexes pathogènes et géographie médicale," *Annales de Géographie* 42 (1933): 1–18.

20. F. Huisman and J. H. Warner, *Locating Medical History: The Stories and Their Meanings* (Baltimore and London: Johns Hopkins University Press, 2004).

21. F. Barrett, *Disease and Geography*, 469–523; N. Rupke and K. Wonders, "Humboldtian Representations in Medical Cartography," in *Medical History in Historical Perspective*, ed. N. Rupke, 163–77 (London: Wellcome Institute for the History of Medicine, 2000).

22. The multifactorial characterization of a location was endorsed by most physicians. See M. Grmek, "Géographie médicale et histoire des civilisations," *Annales ESC* 18 (1963): 1083. For the implications of the anthropological understanding of place, see M. Bassin, "Race Contra Space: The Conflict between German Geopolitik and National Socialism," *Political Geography Quarterly* 6 (1987): 115–34.

23. For this reading, see D. Armstrong, "Public Health Spaces and the Fabrication of Identity," *Sociology* 27 (1993): 393–410. For a variation by social geographers, see R. Kearns and A. Joseph, "Space in its Place: Developing the Link with Medical Geography," *Social Science and Medicine* 37 (1993): 711–17.

24. J.-P. Gaudillière, *Inventer la biomédecine. La France, l'Amérique et la production des savoirs du vivant (1945–1965)* (Paris: La Découverte, 2002; English translation forthcoming from Yale University Press, April 2008); S. Sturdy, ed., *Medicine, Health, and the Public Sphere in Britain, 1600–2000* (London: Routledge, 2002).

25. A. Bashford, ed., *Medicine at the Border: Disease, Globalization and Security, 1850 to the Present* (Basingstoke and New York: Palgrave, 2006); A. M. Kraut, *Silent Travelers: Germs, Genes, and the "Immigrant Menace"* (Baltimore: Johns Hopkins University Press, 1994).

26. P. Baldwin, *Contagion and the State in Europe 1830–1930* (Cambridge: Cambridge University Press, 1999), 11.

27. P. Zylberman, "René Sand," in *Dictionary of Medical Biography*, ed. W. F. Bynum and H. Bynum, 5:1104–5 (Westport, CT: Greenwood, 2007); P. Zylberman, "Fewer Parallels than Antitheses: René Sand and Andrija Štampar on Social Medicine (1919–1955)," *Social History of Medicine* 17 (2004): 1, 77–91; J. Eyler, *Sir Arthur Newsholme and State Medicine 1885–1935* (Cambridge: Cambridge University Press, 1997); E. Fee and Th. M. Brown, *Making Medical History: The Life and Times of Henry E. Sigerist* (Baltimore and London: Johns Hopkins University Press, 1997).

28. S. G. Solomon, "The Intermediary as Strategist: John A. Kingsbury, Soviet Socialized Medicine, and 1930s America" (unpublished manuscript); D. Porter, "John Ryle: Doctor of Revolution?" in *Doctors, Politics and Society: Historical Essays*, ed. D. Porter, 247–74 (Amsterdam: Rodopi, 1993).

29. Public health historians were also fascinated by the reigning Foucauldian and Marxist theories of the twentieth century; Porter, *Health Civilization and the State*, 3.

30. M. Burleigh, *Death and Deliverance: 'Euthanasia in Germany' c.* 1900–1945 (Cambridge: Cambridge University Press, 1994); G. Aly, P. Chroust, and C. Pross, *Cleansing the Fatherland: Nazi Medicine and Racial Hygiene* (Baltimore: Johns Hopkins University Press, 1994); G. Aly and S. Heim, *Architects of Annihilation: Auschwitz and the Logic of Destruction* (London: Phoenix, 2003); C. Browning, "Genocide and Public Health: German Doctors and Polish Jews 1939–1941," in *The Path to Genocide: Essays on Launching the Final Solution*, ed. C. Browning, 145–68 (Cambridge: Cambridge University Press, 1992).

31. See E. Ackerknecht, "Recollections of a Former Leipzig Student," *Journal of the History of Medicine and Allied Sciences* 13 (1958): 147–50.

32. E. Ackerknecht, "Anticontagionism between 1821 and 1867," *Bulletin of the History of Medicine* 22 (1948): 5.

33. For a benign view of the state, see G. Rosen, *From Medical Police to Social Medicine: Essays on the History of Health Care* (New York: Science History, 1974); at the other end of the spectrum, see M. Foucault, *Surveiller et punir: Naissance de la prison* (Paris: Gallimard, 1975).

34. S. Szreter, *Health and Wealth: Studies in History and Policy* (Rochester, NY: University of Rochester Press, 2005); D. Fox, *Health Policies, Health Politics: The British and American Experiences* (Princeton, NJ: Princeton University Press, 1986); D. Hirschfield, *The Lost Reform: The Campaign for Compulsory Health Insurance in the United States from 1932 to 1943* (Cambridge, MA: Harvard University Press, 1970); L. Jacobs, *The Health of Nations: Public Opinion and the Making of American and British Health Policy* (Cambridge: Cambridge University Press, 1993); A. Digby, "Medicine and the English State 1901–1948," in *The Boundaries of the State in Modern Britain*, ed. S. J. D. Green and R. C. Whiting, 213–30 (Cambridge: Cambridge University Press, 1996).

35. Porter, *Health, Civilisation, and the State.*

36. Baldwin, *Contagion and the State*, 550.

37. K. Thelen, "Historical Institutionalism in Comparative Politics," *Annual Review of Political Science* 2 (1999): 369–404; P. Pierson, "Increasing Returns, Path Dependence, and the Study of Politics," *American Political Science Review* 94 (2000): 251–67.

38. E. Immergut, "The Rules of the Game: The Logic of Health Policy-Making in France, Switzerland, and Sweden," in *Structuring Politics: Historical Institutionalism in Comparative Analysis*, ed. S. Steinmo, K. Thelen, and F. Longstreth, 57–89 (Cambridge: Cambridge University Press, 1992); E. Immergut, *Health Politics: Interests and Institutions in Western Europe* (Cambridge: Cambridge University Press, 1992); J. Hacker, *The Divided Welfare State: The Battle over Public and Private Social Benefits in the United States* (Cambridge: Cambridge University Press, 2002).

39. For a review of the current state of the internalist-externalist debate, see J. Ziman, *Real Science: What It Is, and What It Means* (Cambridge: Cambridge University Press, 2000).

40. H. Kamminga and A. Cunningham, eds., *The Science and Culture of Nutrition, 1840–1940* (Amsterdam and Atlanta: Rodopi, 1995), 2.

41. P. M. Haas, "Introduction [to Special Issue: Knowledge, Power, and International Policy Coordination]: Epistemic Communities and International Policy Coordination," *International Organization* 46 (1992): 1–35. For work that drew on this concept, see P. Weindling, "Introduction," in *International Health Organizations and*

Movements, 1918–1939, ed. P. Weindling (Cambridge: Cambridge University Press, 1995); M. D. Dubin, "The League of Nations Health Organization," in Weindling, *International Health,* 56–81 (Cambridge: Cambridge University Press, 1995); J. Farley, *To Cast Out Disease: A History of the International Health Division of the Rockefeller Foundation* 1913–1951 (Oxford: Oxford University Press, 2004).

42. D. Rogers, *Atlantic Crossings: Social Politics in a Progressive Age* (Cambridge, MA: Harvard University Press, 1998).

43. I. Katznelson, "Knowledge about What? Policy Intellectuals and the New Liberalism," in *States, Social Knowledge, and the Origins of Social Policies,* ed. D. Rueschemeyer and T. Skocpol, 17–47 (Princeton, NJ: Princeton University Press, 1996).

44. J. C. Scott, *Seeing Like a State: How Certain Schemes to Improve the Human Condition Have Failed* (New Haven: Yale University Press, 1998), 318.

45. The idea that demographic categories are political interventions animates I. Hacking, "Making Up People," in *Reconstructing Individualism,* ed. T. Heller, M. Sosna, and D. Wellberry, 222–36 (Stanford: Stanford University Press, 1986); S. Szreter, H. Sholkamy, and A. Dharmalingam, eds., *Categories and Contexts: Anthropological and Historical Studies in Critical Demography* (Oxford: Oxford University Press, 2004).

46. Scott, *Seeing Like a State,* 318.

47. R. Kohler, *Landscapes and Labscapes: Exploring the Lab-Field Border in Biology* (Chicago: University of Chicago Press, 2002).

48. S. Szreter, H. Sholkamy, and A. Dharmalingam, "Contextualizing Categories: Towards a Critical Reflexive Demography," in *Categories and Contexts: Anthropological and Historical Studies in Critical Demography,* ed. S. Szreter, H. Sholkamy, and A. Dharmalingam, 13 (Oxford: Oxford University Press, 2004).

49. Scott, *Seeing Like a State,* 191.

50. Rueschemeyer and Skocpol, *States, Social Knowledge, and the Origins of Modern Social Policies.*

51. A. Rabinbach, "Social Knowledge, Social Risk, and the Politics of Industrial Accidents in Germany and France," in *States, Social Knowledge, and the Origins of Modern Social Policies,* ed. D. Rueschemeyer and T. Skocpol, 48–89 (Princeton, NJ: Princeton University Press, 1996).

52. T. Porter, *Trust in Numbers: The Pursuit of Objectivity in Science and Public Life* (Princeton, NJ: Princeton University Press, 1995); G. Jorland, A. Opinel, and G. Weisz, eds., *Body Counts: Medical Quantification in Historical and Sociological Perspectives* (Montreal: McGill–Queen's University Press, 2005).

53. S. Szreter, "Economic Growth, Disruption, Deprivation, Disease, and Death: On the Importance of the Politics of Public Health for Development," in *Plagues and Politics: Infectious Disease and International Policy,* ed. A. Price-Smith, 104–5 (New York: Palgrave, 2001).

54. Thomas Masaryk as quoted in Mazower, *Dark Continent,* x.

55. E. Weil, *Philosophie politique* (Paris: Vrin, 1971), 225, 235.

56. N. Howard-Jones, *The Scientific Background of the International Sanitary Conferences* 1851–1938 (Geneva: World Health Organization, 1975); N. Howard-Jones, *International Public Health Between the Two World Wars: The Organizational Problems* (Geneva: World Health Organization, 1978); N. Goodman, *International Health Organizations and Their Work* (London: J. and A. Churchill, 1952).

57. I. Borowy and W. Gruner, *Facing Illness in Troubled Times: Health in Europe in the Interwar Years* 1918–1939 (Frankfurt am Main and Bern: Peter Lang, 2005); E. Rodríguez-Ocaña, ed., *The Politics of the Healthy Life: An International Perspective* (Sheffield: European Association for the History of Medicine and Health Publications, 2002).

58. E. Rodríguez-Ocaña, J. Bernabeu-Mestre, and J. L. Barona, "La Fundación Rockefeller y Espana 1914–1936: Un acuerdo para la modernización científica y sanitaria," in *Estudios de historia de las técnicas, la arqueologia industrial y las ciencias*, ed. J. L. García, J. M. Moreno, and G. Ruíz, 2:531–39 (Valladolid: Consejería de Educación y Cultura, 1998).

59. A. Labisch and F. Tennstedt, *Der Weg zum 'Gesetz über die Vereinheitlichung des Gesundheitswesens' vom 3. Juli 1934*, 2 vols. (Dusseldorf: Akademie für öffentliches Gesundheitswesen, 1985).

60. C. Broquet, "Le Bureau d'hygiene de la Sociéte des Nations," *Revue d'hygiene* 48 (1921): 131.

61. A. Hardy and L. Wilkinson, *Prevention and Cure: From Tropical Medicine to Global Public Health* (London: Kegan Paul, 2000); H. Tilley, "Ecologies of Complexity: Tropical Environments, African Trypanosomiasis, and the Science of Disease Control in British Colonial Africa 1900–1940," *Osiris* 19 (2004): 21–38; A. Bashford, *Imperial Hygiene: A Critical History of Colonialism, Nationalism, and Public Health* (London: Palgrave Macmillan, 2004); S. Watts, *Epidemics and History: Disease, Power, and Imperialism* (New Haven: Yale University Press, 1997).

62. Paradoxically, this was the moment when political scientists began to call for "bringing the state back in." P. Evans, D. Rueschemeyer, and T. Skocpol, eds., *Bringing the State Back In* (Cambridge: Cambridge University Press, 1985).

63. J. Siddiqi, *World Health and World Politics: The World Health Organization and the UN System* (London: Hurst, 1995).

64. D. Fidler, *SARS, Governance, and the Globalization of Disease* (London: Palgrave Macmillan, 2004).

65. B. Schroeder-Gudehus, "Pas de Locarno pour la science," *Relations internationales* 46 (1986): 173–94; B. Schroeder-Gudehus, "Internationale Wissenschaftsbeziehungen und auswärtige Kulturpolitik 1919–1933: Vom Boykott und Gegen-Boykott zu ihre Wiederaufnahme," in *Forschung im Spannungsfeld von Politik und Gesellschaft: Geschichte und Struktur der Kaiser-Wilhelm-/Max Planck Gesellschaft*, ed. R. Vierhaus and B. vom Brocke, 858–85 (Stuttgart: Deutsche Verlags-Anstalt, 1990); B. Schroeder-Gudehus, *Deutsche Wissenschaft und internationale Zusammenarbeit*, 1914–1928 (Geneva: Carrou, 1966); D. Kevles, "Into Hostile Camps: The Reorganization of International Science in World War I," *Isis* 62 (1971): 47–60. A notable exception to the exclusion of Germany and Russia was the Warsaw Conference of 1922, which representatives of both pariah nations attended. The exception was a function of the threat posed by epidemics.

66. S. G. Solomon, ed., *Doing Medicine Together: Germany and Russia Between the Wars* (Toronto: University of Toronto Press, 2006).

67. G. Buchanan to Th. Madsen, 27 July 1922, League of Nations Archives, Geneva, R 82obis, 12B/26216/11346.

68. P. Hassner, *La terreur et l'empire: La violence et la paix*, vol. 2 (Paris: Seuil, 2003), 69.

69. S. Subrahmanyam, "Connected Histories: Notes towards a Reconfiguration of Early Modern Eurasia," *Modern Asia Studies* 31 (1997): 735–62.

70. M. Balinska, *For the Good of Humanity: Ludwik Rajchman, Medical Statesman* (Budapest: Central European University Press, 1998).

71. L. Murard, "Health Policy Between the International and the Local: Jacques Parisot in Nancy and Geneva," in *Facing Illness in Troubled Times*, ed. I. Borowy and W. Gruner, 207–45 (Frankfurt am Main and Bern: Peter Lang, 2005).

72. R. Putnam, "Diplomacy and Domestic Politics: The Logic of the Two-Level Game," *International Organization* 42 (1988), 427–60.

73. For example, see N. Krementsov, *International Science between the Wars: The Case of Genetics* (London: Routledge, 2005).

74. G. Donelli and E. Serinaldi, *Dalla lotta alla malaria alla nascita dell'Istituto di Sanità Pubblica: Il ruolo della Rockefeller Foundation in Italia* 1922–1934 (Rome and Bari: Laterza, 2003).

75. P. Weindling and M. Turda, *"Blood and Homeland": Eugenics and Racial Nationalism in Central and Southeast Europe* 1900–1940 (Budapest: Central European University Press, 2006); M. Bucur, *Eugenics and Modernization in Interwar Romania* (Pittsburgh: University of Pittsburgh Press, 2002); P. Colla, *Per la Nazione e per la Razza: Citadini ed esclusi nel "modello svedese"* (Rome: Carocci, 2000).

76. Baldwin, *Disease and Democracy*, 202–26.

77. N. B. King, "Security, Disease, Commerce: Ideologies of Post-Colonial Global Health," *Social Studies of Science*, 32 (2002): 773.

78. J. Lederberg, R. E. Shope, and S. C. Oaks, Jr., *Emerging Infections: Microbial Threats to Health in the United States* (Washington, DC: National Academy Press, 1992), quoted in King, "Security, Disease, Commerce," 767.

79. See L. Garrett, *Betrayal of Trust: The Collapse of Global Health* (Oxford: Oxford University Press, 2000).

80. SARS is subsiding, but as unpredictably as it surfaced. K. Bradsher and L. K. Altmann, interview with Dr. Mark Ryan, WHO, *International Herald Tribune*, July 23, 2003, European edition.

81. Fidler, *SARS, Governance, and the Globalization of Disease*, 32–35.

Part One

Place as Politics

Chapter One

Can There Be a Democratic Public Health?

Fighting AIDS in the Industrialized World

Peter Baldwin

During the nineteenth century, the connection between politics and public health was clear.[1] In the heroic era of sanitary reform, reformers broke ground for new and, from a liberal point of view, drastic interventions. Private property rights were limited in the name of sanitary infrastructure. Individual behavior was curbed and controlled in the interest of public salubrity. The controversy over smallpox vaccination—a classic contest between individual and public goods—was one of the major political battles of the nineteenth century, though curiously forgotten now. The disputes over the Contagious Disease Acts during the 1880s laid the foundations for the women's movement, providing a dress rehearsal for disputes over suffrage a few years later.

In the intervening century, however, public health became a victim of its own success. It became taken for granted, a matter of everyday, uncontroversial political decision making. No longer were there Chadwicks, Virchows, Pasteurs, or Kochs—reformers and scientists whose exploits made them heroes. No longer were there controversies, except at the margins of politics, as with the decision on mass roundups and other measures against prostitutes during the two world wars. One exception to this rule was the grotesque inversion of public health by the Nazis. They exploited the rhetoric of public health to provide an aura of scientific respectability for hatred and genocide. Hitler portrayed himself as the Robert Koch of politics and the Jews as dangerous microorganisms to be exterminated. The Warsaw ghetto was walled off nominally as a typhus quarantine zone. And of course the supposed delousing showers in the death camps took this fiction to its extreme.[2] The other side of the spectrum provided only a pale echo of such conjunctions. Lenin worried about the petty bourgeois bacillus. In their sexual prurience, Eastern Bloc regimes often lambasted the decadent West over the epidemics of venereal disease that were the result of their allegedly extravagant sexual habits.[3] But generally for the First World, public health was no longer a concern.

Today, all this has changed dramatically. Public health is suddenly occupying the front pages again. Anthrax became a terrorist weapon after September 11, 2001. Military leaders worry that suicide fighters may infect themselves with smallpox, spreading it within the civilian population. Tuberculosis is transmitted in virulent forms that are resistant to antibiotics, and Directly Observed Therapy (whereby victims are required to take their medicine under official supervision) is mandated. The *Spectator* has spoken for the right wing of British opinion in worrying that immigration, in the form of diseased asylum seekers, will be deadlier than terrorism.[4] From the other side of the ideological spectrum, parents are beating the tom-toms of liberalist individualism. Fearing that triple vaccinations cause autism in their children, they are willing to abandon the collective solidarities of herd immunity. During the Sudden Acute Respiratory Syndrome (SARS) epidemic of 2003, the traditional artillery of public health, with its drastic impositions on individual freedoms, was wheeled out once again.

Public health first became a major political issue again during the early 1980s with the onset of the AIDS epidemic. Two themes suddenly burst onto the agenda. The first was the epidemiological interconnectedness of the world. The First World discovered that it no longer lived in isolation from the rest of humanity. That it had installed sewers and built hospitals did not spare it from afflictions that began elsewhere and were then imported via the mass peregrinations of modern life. AIDS was in all likelihood first imported to the United States by gay tourists to Haiti and the Dominican Republic. The developed world outsourced its unfulfilled sexual needs—both gay and straight—to the Third World, then harvested the epidemiological results. Other diseases that arose, or arose again, in the Third World were now also imported to the First along with increased transmigration: cholera from South America, horrifying hot-button sicknesses such as the Ebola, Marburg, and Lassa viruses from Africa. The developed nations discovered that they were in a position similar to that of the middle and upper classes during the nineteenth century, endangered by the poor.

Second among the themes raised by AIDS were the dangers posed to their own health by the habits of First World citizens themselves. We are now, of course, all victims of our own success. Obesity, cardiovascular disease, some cancers, and so forth, are the products of too many calories and too little motion, the toxic products of prosperity, and generally the lifestyles of the well-off and sedentary. That we are largely responsible for our own chronic diseases is well known. But even so, it is better to have problems such as these, rather than the acute epidemic diseases of the nineteenth century. The discovery of the 1980s was that our own habits, whether bad or not, could also worsen the situation when it came to transmissible disease.

Until surprisingly recently this realization was not a secret, but by the 1980s it had to be rediscovered. During the early 1900s, cholera was blamed on the nasty habits of the poor—overeating, filthiness, sexual immoderation, and the like. Even as late as the early twentieth century, syphilis was not regarded as a sexually transmitted disease, but as an ailment spread through everyday contacts. In Sweden, Russia, and the Balkans—especially in the countryside of these nations—syphilis was thought to spread through unfortunate rustic habits: indiscriminate sleeping together of family members and visitors, child minders sucking the penises of infants to quiet them, mothers chewing the food of their infants before spitting it into their mouths, everyone sharing household implements, and so on. Sexually transmitted diseases were, in this sense, conceptualized as a distinct group of ailments not because of our puritan fixation on sexual matters, but because, during the process of civilization, we gradually learned to avoid intimate bodily fluid contact with one another to the point where such diseases were finally spread only via sexual contact.[5]

This was the lesson the developed world relearned with the AIDS epidemic: that individual habits and customs contributed not only to chronic disease, but to contagion as well. The most generally noxious habit, shared by most, that poses epidemiological dangers is travel. With mass tourism, the airline and hospitality industries, and their spillover effects, travel is possibly the single largest industry in the world economy and one on which many nations increasingly depend. The economic consequences of restricting it, should that become even more necessary, would be devastating.

Certain more specific habits, however, also pose epidemiological dangers. AIDS was spread first, and in some nations foremost, through unprotected anal sex and intravenous needle sharing. Moreover, during the 1980s and early nineties, HIV infection rates ran parallel to those of epidemics of more conventional sexually transmitted diseases localized largely to the gay community. Gay sexual habits, in other words, were spreading not only AIDS, but the usual variety of STDs as well. In addition there were premonitory epidemics of intestinal ailments such as amebiasis and giardiasis among First World gays. These ailments were transmitted via the increasingly popular practices of fisting and rimming—and they were otherwise found only in the unsewered parts of the undeveloped world. Similar epidemics of disease were found also among intravenous-drug users. In other words, a group of First World citizens with above-average access to resources—gay males—had a disease profile similar to those of the urban underclass and the Third World. And it had this profile for reasons largely stemming from the chance introduction into its closed sexual circles of HIV, combined with the extraordinarily rapid and disastrous spread of the virus thanks to particular sexual habits, above all unprotected anal sex.

This raised a new and surprisingly political issue. Chronic diseases are of course private misfortunes, but also public problems. Insofar as they are public they tend to involve questions of distributing or redistributing the costs of illness and mortality. If I overeat and become obese and develop heart disease, I may incur costs that you have to pay as a member of a health insurance system. Some 90 percent of health costs are incurred by 20 percent of all insurance members. To the extent that disease is dependent on voluntary and avoidable decisions, it poses a major redistributive dilemma. But generally speaking, even if I overeat and incur costs that you have to pay, I do not damage you directly. When it became clear that our own habits also encouraged the spread of certain contagious diseases, however, each of us potentially became an immediate threat to our fellow citizens for reasons that we could control and possibly be held responsible for.

Contagious disease poses the political dilemma of reconciling the interests of the individual citizen with those of the community in the most immediate and unavoidable terms. Attempts to curtail epidemics raise—in the guise of public health—the most enduring political dilemma: how to align the individual's claim to autonomy and liberty with the community's concern with safety. How does the polity treat the patient who is both citizen and disease vector? How are individual rights and public goods pursued simultaneously? Public health is thus inherently, indeed unavoidably, political.

This is not a new claim. It is inherent in the argument put forth by Erwin Ackerknecht, the distinguished historian of medicine, in an unusually influential article: that different styles of public health corresponded to different political regimes. He distinguished quarantinism from sanitationism and correlated them with autocratic or conservative regimes and liberal democracies, respectively.[6] He characterized as quarantinist those regimes which sought to break chains of transmission via strict statutory interventions: quarantining travelers and goods, reporting the ill to the authorities and isolating them, tracing their contacts, disinfecting goods and houses, and in other ways violating the rights of the individual in the name of the public good. In contrast, sanitationist regimes sought to render healthy the immediate urban environment, allowing epidemics to gain no toehold. This, of course, involved major statutory interventions too, but mainly those of laying down infrastructure and violating the privacy of the domestic residence to ensure salubrious conditions. Such a view corresponded to a particular etiology of contagious illnesses as filth diseases. Once dirty conditions had been improved, according to this etiology, epidemics would largely disappear. Such a view fitted hand in glove with the desires of merchants for free trade, but also with a liberal democratic system that did not regiment or interfere with the individual.

Ackerknecht's view was, broadly, that sanitationism was the system adopted by liberal Britain during the nineteenth century, whereas quarantinism was preferred on the still largely autocratic Continent. Whatever one may say about this argument, if there is a causal relationship here, then it would have been most consistent during the nineteenth century, when political regimes really varied. But what about the modern era, the postwar period when all Western nations are liberal bourgeois democracies? Do they all share the same approach to public health? If so, what is it? What is democratic public health?

It is commonly argued that modern polities in the developed world share public health assumptions and tactics. These are based on the fundamental premise that epidemics of contagious disease are no longer a major issue. Legislation remains on the books that allows an old-fashioned, quarantinist approach, seeking to break chains of transmission. But such laws are notable above all for their disuse. Instead, the epidemiological sea change from contagious to chronic disease allowed a democratic, liberal, hands-off approach. Democratic public health has been based on self-restraint. It is one facet of social control in a democratic polity. Rather than having the state intervene from outside with a harsh hand, democratic citizens control their own behavior in a nominally voluntary way. Instead of statutory authority, we have governmentality. Such theories of democratic public health are based on the work of Max Weber, Norbert Elias, and Michel Foucault. Nikolas Rose is perhaps their most elaborate contemporary formulator, though not specifically in terms of public health. In his hands, voluntary self-restraint becomes the ethos on which democratic polities are possible. In his eyes, our freedom is not restricted by such social control; rather, it is made possible precisely through self-restraint.[7]

The onus of precaution thus was transferred to the increasingly well-to-do and educated citizens of emerging democracies. Appropriate habits became part of the conduct of good burghers. Citizens could take responsibility for their actions; indeed, the democratic ethos required them to do so. Controls shifted from the outward impositions of a predemocratic state to the internal restrictions each person put on his or her own behavior. Merely a subsidiary role was reserved for harsh measures to be imposed on those marginal people who could or would not conduct themselves appropriately. This was the ethos caricatured as the reign of the monogamous jogger.[8] Rather than the pest house, the quarantine station, mobile fumigation squads, and all the paraphernalia and impositions of the sanitary old regime, we now have James Fixx and Dr. Atkins, twelve-step programs and health clubs, designated drivers and condoms.

Those who refuse to be monogamous joggers are the new enemies of the people. Smokers, the overly carnivorous (but also the exclusively vegan, who are blamed for their children's nutritional deficiencies), the obese, drinkers of more than the occasional glass of Chablis, drug users, the promiscuous: these are the new social outcasts, violators of the ethos of democratic restraint. Bodily hygiene has become our religious tic. Health has become the morality of modern bourgeois society. Earlier, the imperative was to act in accord with the precepts of religion. Now the requirements of health and clean living are the codex, the bowels having replaced the soul as the source of the most potent anxieties. Those who long for the old regime of strict external control, combined with room for the indulgence of pleasurable bad habits, attack this ethos of behavioral autolimitation as "health fascism."[9] But in the main most of us have succumbed to teetotalling totalitarianism.

Take the antismoking campaign as an example. On the one hand are the massive attempts at mind control exercised by both the tobacco interests and their enemies. And on the other hand nonsmoking enforcement is among the most drastic of direct statutory incursions, forbidding behavior that a decade or so ago was socially acceptable. Tobacco smoking is now treated in the world's most liberalist societies—America's granola belt: Madison, Cambridge, Santa Monica, Berkeley, et al.—as it was in absolutist Prussia, with formal prohibitions in public, and sometimes in private too. This makes the example a bit ambiguous, of course, since antismoking campaigns combine informal control through education, advertisement, and attempts at public enlightenment with outright prohibition. It seems as though informal behavioral control is not trusted, so formal prohibitions are required as well. Given that smoking is inversely proportional to socioeconomic status, the antismoking campaign is perhaps the most overt, though wholly unacknowledged, act of class behavioral imposition since the antispitting campaigns of the late nineteenth century. If these campaigns have their desired effect, antismoking laws will become like antispitting ordinances, which were enforced a century ago, but no longer have to be. Almost no one, barring the occasional baseball player, spits in public. The same goes for antiurination laws, though these have come back into use as a means of controlling the homeless and vagrants. Will inhalation soon go the way of expectoration? Will ashtrays become quaint collector's items, like spittoons?

Democratic public health is thus something different from either of the two more traditional approaches, quarantinism and sanitationism. It does not involve massive public interventions into civil society. It relies instead on the accumulated effect of millions of individual decisions, out of which comes a public good. Just as collective decisions are the outcome of many individual ones in a democracy, so too public health has individualized its collective goods. The dilemma that we face now is how democratic public health, based on self-restraint in an era when most health problems are those of chronic disease, deals with new challenges of transmissible and epidemic ailments. The political analogy is what we do in circumstances when democratic decision making may in fact end democracy. May democracy defend its basic principles with undemocratic means? Are democratic forms of public health up to the challenge of resurgent contagious disease?

With certain diseases, there is no problem: we just roll out the inherited quarantinist measures. When cholera cases arrive in California on planes from Latin America, no one objects to quarantining or keeping them under surveillance. When hyperacute diseases such as Hanta, Marburg, or Ebola burn themselves out in horrifying swaths of destruction, few worry about the niceties of civil rights. With the SARS epidemic, the same proved true. In China, tens of thousands of people were quarantined, and the authorities threatened to execute anyone who deliberately spread the disease. Visitors to Singapore were passed through thermal scanners to detect the feverish. American authorities were granted powers to detain suspected victims against their will. In New York City, an arrival from Asia with symptoms who was detained involuntarily became, with one exception, the first nontubercular person in a quarter century to be compulsorily quarantined.[10]

But what about other diseases that are not spread quasi-involuntarily, through an offending cough or everyday contacts? What happens when transmissible disease is made epidemic in some measure by our own voluntary habits? That was the dilemma posed by AIDS. The disease spread most quickly and first became recognized as epidemic in very specific epidemiological ecological niches: among intravenous-drug users and especially in shooting galleries, and among gay males who practiced unprotected anal sex and especially when they did so in gay bathhouses. Just when the Eliasian civilizing process appeared to be nearing its highpoint, with Apollo ascendant, our Dionysian instincts became a problem again. Whether we craved the oblivion of the needle or the polymorphous *gesamtkörperliche* tactility of the bathhouses, the id was rattling the cage of the monogamous jogger. The fundamental public health dilemma posed by the early phases of the epidemic was brought into focus by disputes over shutting the bathhouses.

Gay males have challenged the heterosexual world in two fundamental ways. First, in the emotional economy of homosexuality, by being able to overcome the traditional male-female, active-passive dichotomy. Modern Western homosexuality differs from more traditional models of gayness in its role switching. Each partner takes both the penetrating and the penetrated roles. In traditional models, in contrast, one partner tends consistently to be the penetrated, the other the active. The former is generally considered homosexual. The active partner may not be thought of as homosexual and may live a completely conventional heterosexual life as well. Role switching has been celebrated by gay theorists as allowing male homosexuals to understand the mutuality of desire and fulfillment in a way impossible for either straights or lesbians. They see both sides of the act of love and understand both aspects of an emotional relationship. But role switching is also epidemiologically precisely what put gays at risk. In traditionally homosexual relationships, chains of infection would die out more quickly and harmlessly. An infected inserter might well infect the passive partner, but he in turn, so long as he remained passive, would be less likely to infect future partners. Those who switched roles, however, would have equal chances of passing the virus along to their next partner.[11]

Second, the gay world has challenged the heterosexual through its political economy. Gays have put to shame the fundamental Weberian-Freudian premise that there is a tradeoff between reason and instinct, a zero-sum distribution between energies going to different ends. Sublimation and the channeling of energies from pleasure to work, from instinct to reason— Western gays have put paid to such fundamental building blocks of the Protestant world view. They have shown the belief that sublimation is the key to worldly success to be a myth by combining above-average socioeconomic indicators with libidinous abandon, experimentation, and innovation on a scale and intensity undreamed of in the heterosexual imagination.

The debate that raged both within the gay communities of the Western world and between gays and public health officials over the closing of the bathhouses brought such considerations to a head. No one would think twice about shutting down a restaurant with a typhoid-infected cook. Why should bathhouses be allowed to stay open, when brothels were often illegal in the first place? That was the sort of logic advanced by public health officials and the gays who agreed with them.

On the other side stood those who argued that gay bathhouses were not just the equivalents of straight brothels. The bathhouses were not merely a bottleneck where transmission could be stopped. The baths were not like brothels—places where sex of the usual sort was consumed in unusual settings. They were the venue of sex without par in private, and thus emblematic of the gay world's rejection of received erotic values. Precisely the Dionysian erotic frenzy of the bathhouses, the anonymity and multiple coupling, was their point. Shutting them was therefore more than just a public health measure. Gay defenders of the baths argued that closing them attacked the heart of homosexual identity. It would be as though marriage had been forbidden in order to fight venereal disease, or like the attempt made by an enterprising rabbi in Posen during the 1832 cholera epidemic, who shut mikhvas to keep orthodox women impure after menstruation and thus incapable of relations with their husbands.[12]

What did the democratic style of public health do when faced with the AIDS epidemic? A large literature claims that AIDS was dealt with in precisely a democratic fashion.[13] When the epidemic broke out in the early 1980s, most nations had draconian laws on the books, inherited from the era when acute contagious disease was still a problem. These laws could have been applied and at first occasionally were. Nonetheless, most nations surprisingly quickly discovered that a disease such as this could not be handled in the usual way. It was at first transmitted primarily in situations of intimacy and often illegality, far from venues that the state could expect to control. Its first victims were members of social groups that were already stigmatized. To impose the heavy hand of traditional quarantinist remedies, so this argument went, such people and such behavior would have been driven even further into the epidemiological underground, thus defeating public health's own ambitions.

Instead, public health authorities developed a consensual model of prevention, educating high-risk groups about inherent dangers and encouraging them to undertake voluntary behavioral change. Such a new democratic approach to public health thus bespoke at least two changes. First was the peculiar nature of the new disease. There was as yet no cure and scarcely any treatment. Traditional public health tactics, which assumed a limited period of contagiousness or the possibility of treatment to justify identification and isolation of the infected, were thus of little avail. HIV's long latency period would have required an unfeasibly constant testing of all. Second, this approach testified to the political strength of some of the principal affected groups, above all gay males. The disease helped mobilize victims and potential victims, resulting in an unexpected concern paid to the wishes of the most victimized groups.

It would be easy to fall into a whiggish mode here. Saying that gays turned out to have surprising political clout and that their concerns left a mark on the public health measures adopted is not to take those things for granted— nor to underestimate the uphill battle it had been, and remains, for gays. Nor, of course, is it to turn away from the horrendous circumstances that gays faced as the initial victims, with their community devastated by the epidemic. It is rather to apply the logic of the commonplace observation that without the Holocaust, the state of Israel would have been unlikely to exist. Finding a silver lining does not minimize the horror of event.

In this case, an epidemic sparked political mobilization that went beyond the immediate problems of the disease. In that sense, AIDS was not like smallpox in the nineteenth century, when huge and turbulent resistance movements to vaccination arose in many European nations, especially Great Britain. These movements died out quickly, since there was no stable base for political mobilization beyond the possibility of being a victim of a particular disease.[14] A better analogy is the campaign against the Contagious Disease Acts in the late nineteenth century. In this case, women organized on the basis of their sex. They consciously joined in gendered solidarity across class lines to fight what they saw as a battle against the selfish sexual interest of men in having uninfected women available for commercial sex. All women, whether prostitutes or matrons, workers or middle class, had common interests as women in the face of a disease spread among them by men. The fight for suffrage drew heavily on these lessons. In this sense, an interest identity created in part by public health concerns lasted beyond its initial impetus.

The connection between AIDS and gay mobilization was similar. In some nations, especially the United States, but also somewhat in Germany, gay mobilization preceded the epidemic. In others, such as Britain and France, it was more of an outgrowth of the epidemic, or at least gained impetus by it. Nor were the results of gay mobilization the same everywhere. A somewhat consensual approach was the result in the United States, and also in the Netherlands, where gays were well organized. In Sweden, in contrast, where gays were also well organized, the outcome was nonetheless much more draconian. There was no one-to-one correspondence between gay mobilization and the tactics adopted. Yet it would be wrong to ignore or downplay the victories won by gay interests in a certain approach to public health.

One of the most widely accepted arguments of the AIDS literature is that out of this confluence of events—the peculiar nature of the disease and mobilization by directly affected groups of victims—emerged a new and successful form of public health adapted to modern democratic polities. Though widespread, this view deserves to be questioned. A few things are clear. First, nations responded with a much more varied palette of preventive techniques than is often realized.

For one thing, the timing of the response varied. It was more rapid in northern Europe, especially Scandinavia and the Netherlands, than in the United States or in the Mediterranean.[15] Some nations introduced many new laws to deal with the epidemic: Sweden, for example, and America, with a greater variety.[16] Other countries, such as Germany and Britain, passed almost nothing novel, relying instead on the existing armamentarium of precautions, however reinterpreted.[17] In more specific matters, the differences were also drastic. All American states required the reporting of AIDS and about half the reporting of seropositives. The Germans and the Dutch did not institute nominative notification of even full-blown cases. The Americans screened and excluded foreigners on the basis of serostatus, as did nations with which they generally did not compare themselves: Indonesia, China, South Africa and Japan, for example, not to mention the then-socialist nations of the Eastern Bloc.[18] In contrast, with a few exceptions, their European allies did not. The Swedes, otherwise among the most drastic interveners, were laissez-faire at the borders. The Americans required screening of certain civil servants, as did, to some extent, the Germans. The French and British shied away from any such measure. The military was screened in the United States, but, with a few exceptions such as French soldiers on duty in Africa, not in Europe. HIV screening was strictly anonymous in Germany; in Sweden anonymity was ruled out on principle. Testing, though voluntary, was considered much more important to preventive efforts in France and

Sweden than in Britain. In Austria, Sweden, Bavaria, and some North American states, prostitutes were screened and forbidden to work if infected; they were left alone in most other nations.

Contact tracing was required in Sweden and some American states, but in few other countries. Still considered an absolute in France, medical confidentiality was so strictly upheld that sometimes patients themselves were not told. In other nations, especially the Anglo-Saxon ones, concern with warning endangered third parties limited patients' privacy. Compared with the United States, all nations were laggards in terms of funding basic research, but many produced far franker and more effective public-education campaigns. Blinded seroprevalence studies were accepted without alarm in America, but hotly resisted in Britain, the Netherlands, and Germany. Transmissive behavior was criminalized and prosecuted in the United States and Germany, but largely ignored in Britain. Gay bathhouses were closed in some American cities, and in Sweden and Bavaria, yet left largely untouched in other American cities, as well as in France and the Netherlands.

To put the contrasts more pointedly: American soldiers were subject to one of the most draconian regimes of HIV surveillance anywhere. They were screened, obliged to follow rules of conduct to prevent transmission, required to inform their sexual partners and medical caregivers, and obliged to practice safe sex. Their spouses could be informed, their contacts traced; their sex partners could be identified, counseled, and tested without consent. They were, in other words, treated in much the same way as all Swedish citizens. Conversely, HIV-positive Dutch, non-Bavarian Germans, and French, other than being potentially excluded from private life insurance coverage and possibly sued for damages if they knowingly transmitted the disease, suffered few curtailments of their activities and rights.

Second among the points worth making about the public health response to the AIDS epidemic, the old bromide of how conservative governments took a stricter approach, whereas liberal ones were less draconian, simply does not hold. Reagan and Thatcher, though otherwise lumped together politically, presided over administrations that took quite different approaches, much more laissez-faire in the United Kingdom than in the United States. Even worse for this argument, those nations which took by far the strictest, most old-fashioned approach, were a very motley and unexpected crew: the liberalist United States, swinging from a Republican to Democratic president in mid-epidemic; Social Democratic Austria and Sweden (after the party's return to power in 1982 and except for the bourgeois interlude of 1991–94) and Christian Socialist Bavaria. Conversely, the most consistently consensual approach was taken in an equally polymorphous array of nations: Britain, shifting from Tory to Labour halfway through the epidemic; France, under the peculiarities of left-right cohabitation as of the mid-1980s; the Netherlands, moving from a center-right coalition to the Social Democrats in 1989.

It is, in other words, hard to spot any consistent political underpinnings of public health policy here.

Behind a common façade of democratic polities, stark differences remained in public health policies. To explain the variety of approaches to AIDS, we need something more than just the common democratic system shared by all Western nations, a system that ruled out of court the drastic impositions of old-fashioned public health. First of all, such impositions are very much still with us, as we discovered with the SARS epidemic. Second, some nations were happy to use them against AIDS even as others shied away. We also need something more than a simple politics of left and right, conservative and liberal, to make sense of how modern polities have acted in terms of public health.

Let us start with the question of a technical fix. Solving the problem of AIDS by finding a cure or vaccination would have been the politically easiest solution. Yet the interest of nations in this approach was not uniformly keen. The disparities in research spending were stark. The United States and, at a great remove, France provided the bulk of research funding on AIDS. In the 1980s, American research, measured in monetary terms, was one hundredfold that of the British, ten times per inhabitant that of the Swedes. In 1993, the French spent only 3 percent (2 percent in 1997) what the Americans did, but even this modest sum was a third more than what the British (their nearest competitors) spent and thrice what the Germans spent.[19] As one critic calculated, the French research budget for AIDS would have bought the construction of four kilometers of mountainous highway.[20] Why was the disparity among nations' interest in and willingness to fund a technical solution so great?

One reason was that a technical solution threatened to raise political and moral problems. Could one in this way sidestep the behavior associated with the spread of disease, which many found ethically and socially questionable? A very similar problem had gotten Guilbert de Préval expelled from the medical faculty of the University of Paris in 1772, when he claimed to have discovered a means of preventing syphilis. His detractors feared that, once this became known, libertinage would be given free rein. Such an approach had sent moralist observers of syphilis into frenzies of self-righteousness ever since. A cure, they worried, would lead to a spiritual syphilization more pernicious than the merely corporeal version.[21]

During this latest epidemic, such attitudes reemerged undaunted. A crash program for an AIDS vaccine, the neoconservative journalist Norman Podhoretz thundered, meant that in the name of compassion researchers would give "social sanction to what can only be described as brutish degradation." They would allow gays "to resume buggering each other by the hundreds with complete medical impunity."[22] The externalities of desire would be reduced to practically nil; allegedly immoral habits would be freed of their consequences. Social conservatives pinned their hopes for a socially regenerating effect from the epidemic precisely to the consequences it appeared to attach to immoral and illegal behaviors.

Such concerns with the lifestyle of infection were not monopolized by the socially conservative right. Less well known are the homosexuals who agreed that the liberties of the gay ghettos had perhaps been taken to an extreme. They argued that gays should seek to live more like their straight neighbors and could hardly be surprised if their excesses were attacked. Gabriel Rotello, Larry Kramer, and Philip Kayal gave voice to such ideas in the United States, as did Rosa von Praunheim in Germany. Randy Shilts, the author of the first popular history of the epidemic, *And the Band Played On*, was spat on by strangers in the Castro for arguing that gay sexual behavior was part of the problem. Even those who fancied themselves progressive, alert to the needs of the epidemic's victims and concerned with social reform, argued that curing AIDS, vaccinating against it, or even adopting the technical fix of condoms failed to address the fundamental problem raised by the conduct that spread the illness. Rather than advocating such narrow measures to avoid disease, they demanded broad social and sexual reform, including changes in behavior to eliminate IV drug use, promiscuity, and the anonymous anal sex at the root of the problem.[23] Curing the disease also threatened radicals of the left, who were convinced that AIDS had social causes or at least cofactors. Without changing society as a whole, they insisted, the epidemic could not be vanquished. "Without institutional change, the virus wins." A cure would solve the problem "while allowing the distribution of power and health to remain the same."[24]

Why did the United States and France in particular take a biomedical approach to the epidemic, hoping to find a technical fix, even though in some ways it held out the potentially most radical, or at least amoral, solution? Most obviously, both were among the hardest hit industrialized nations. But such pure functionalism is not enough of an answer. Other nations were happy to freeload on research done elsewhere and spent their money on social science investigations that allowed more effective internal targeting efforts, rather than biomedical research of interest to all humanity. Influential for the French choice was the cultural prediliction for seeing sexuality as an exclusively individual, personal, and private choice. The French regarded as illegitimate those intermediary social groups based on sexual identity—gays above all—that played important roles in the Anglo-Saxon, Dutch, and Scandinavian realms.[25] Biomedicine and a technical fix promised to sidestep such issues.

The Americans, in turn, put their money on biomedicine in hopes that it might gloss over gaps in their health insurance systems. Pouring greater resources into medical research than any other nation had been an American tradition since the 1930s. Besides the universalist goal of pursuing public goods, this approach had political payoffs as well. Voting for research funding was one way for American politicians to demonstrate their support for health, since other avenues of largesse—such as health insurance for all—were blocked. "Medical research," as Congressman Melvin Laird put it in 1960, "is the best kind of health insurance" the American people could have.[26] For countries with universal and effective health care systems, in contrast, the epidemic posed less of a political problem. So long as citizens were entitled to reasonable standards of care and as the problem did not mushroom out of control, a new illness was just another blip on the political radar. For these nations there was little political advantage to spending funds on biomedical research rather than, say, building hospices to ensure comfortable terminal care for the stricken. Even in France, the annual budget for indemnifying infected hemophiliacs was many times that for research; in America the proportions were reversed.[27] For the United States, in contrast, a new epidemic was much less digestible. It suffered from perennial problems of insurance coverage—and the disease struck precisely groups that were least provided for.

More generally, the Americans found a biomedical approach consistent with the values of a pluralistic democracy. It appealed especially to a polity fraught with multiculturalism—social, cultural, and sexual balkanization— and consequently unable to rely either on the cohesion of traditional European cultural homogeneity, or even any longer on the classic assimilationist ethos of Americanization. In a heterogeneous nation, with multiple moral and religious standards, even the act of disseminating consistent information was loaded with delicate issues in terms of what could be said to whom. Informal behavioral control was even less reliable.[28] Seeking biomedically to cure or avoid a stigmatized disease involved the least tinkering with civil society and its possibly mutually antagonistic proclivities. A biomedical approach thus promised to spare the United States vexing political choices. By intervening in nature, the country could dodge social interventions. The behavioral change that was unlikely to arise through informal social influence, and whose strict enforcement via rules and laws was difficult, could thus be avoided altogether.[29]

Once it comes, a biomedical cure will solve the public health problem once and for all. In the meantime, however, other smaller technical fixes played a role in the prevention of the epidemic, illustrating the individualization of prevention. All medical admissions to hospitals were now treated as though potentially infected, and universal barrier precautions were instituted. This avoided the need to test individual incoming patients and reserve such measures only for the infected. Also, of course, it avoided discrimination against those who appeared to come from high-risk groups. Instead of the authorities testing prisoners or the arrested, each suspect was to be treated as a potential source of danger whom medical personnel would approach gloved and masked.

Most obvious among the technical solutions was the advocacy of safe sex and in particular the use of condoms. This, too, was not the only way of dealing with the problem. In the Netherlands, for example, public health authorities at first sought to discourage anal sex among gays rather than insisting on condoms. They seemed to think that changing sexual behavior would be easier than encouraging the use of latex. In other nations it was widespread practice early in the epidemic to exhort gays to engage in non-penetrative sexual practices—what was felicitously known as outercourse. But in general, it must be said that public health officials showed breathtaking hubris in their belief that they could, by dint of sheer persuasion, convince gays to refocus their libidos from one orifice to another, or to none at all, and otherwise practice what could easily be seen as a new form of chastity. Attempts to reprogram sexual behavior without condoms did not work well. Gays wondered why such techniques were not recommended to heterosexuals. Long discussions ensued of whether penetration and what, in the unromantic vocabulary of social science, was called intercorporeal emission were fundamental parts of sex, or just window dressing.

As a result, the use of condoms became the basic preventive technique of the epidemic, the heart of safe sex. And here too, other techniques were, in theory, available. It would, for example, have been possible to enforce legal regulations on transmissive behavior, holding the infected, and those who suspected themselves of being infected, to very strict codes of conduct, and punishing them severely if they endangered others or actually transmitted disease.

This was largely the technique pursued in Sweden. Here, widespread testing identified seropositives. It was impossible to take a HIV test anonymously. Medical personnel revealed to the authorities the identities of all who tested positive. The authorities then imposed a very strict regimen of behavior: seropositives could have sex only with a single, constant partner who had been informed of their serostatus. They could, in any case, have only safe sex (mutual masturbation was allowed, but oral sex was considered highly risky, and condoms had to be worn throughout intercourse). They must not use drugs and certainly must not share needles. They had to inform attending medical personnel of their condition. If they ignored such prescriptions, they could be reported and isolated in a hospital for up to three months, extendable in half-year segments thereafter. Those who had had sex or shared needles with someone they knew to be infected were to regard themselves as infected. They too must be examined and follow the physician's prescriptions.

Seropositives in Sweden who failed to inform their partners before sex or to follow the prescribed medical regimen could be incarcerated. Swedish law did not even require evidence that disease had been deliberately transmitted. A mere suspicion that the infected would not follow the rules was enough. If an infected drug abuser, for example, said he would have unprotected sex, a court could jail him initially for three months.[30] Very few other nations attempted anything as draconian. Sweden's measure thus targeted the infected and those suspected of infection because of their lifestyle or their contacts with the infected.

In contrast to this focus on the infected, the dictates of universal safe sex were analogous to the idea that universal barrier precautions in hospitals made it unnecessary to test incoming patients or make decisions based on their apparent risk-group membership. The assumption was that any sexual partner, except perhaps the most intimate and trusted, could be a risk and that all should therefore protect themselves by means of condoms. In addition, people were urged to choose their sexual partners more carefully. Promiscuity, however that was defined, was discounted in favor of monogamy. This approach foisted an individualized technical and behavioral solution on all—high- and low-risk groups alike—with the goal of sparing certain especially endangered groups even further impositions.

In theory, the choice was between imposing legal strictures to forbid or control dangerous behavior, thereby sparing most citizens the need for individual precautions, and requiring all to throw up their own palisades against infection. As the German Society for Internal Medicine put it, why ask legions of uninfected citizens to change their behavior, rather than first and foremost seeking to change seropositives' conduct?[31] Whereas disease prevention had earlier been a public good, democratization and the obligations of modern citizenship increasingly privatized it. Public health now resulted from the interaction of millions of private decisions—in a kind of preventive Brownian motion—rather than the imposition of communal norms. All were required to take individual precautions to ensure that no one was ostracized. Rather than relying on publicly enforceable strictures that permitted a private unencumbrance of behavior, authorities called on each individual to curtail and adjust his or her behavior—not only to prevent transmission, but also to avoid being infected by those who did not conduct themselves as expected.

During the nineteenth century, when victims of smallpox and other diseases were forbidden to expose themselves in public, legal strictures sought to preserve the public's right to walk abroad without fear of infection. Similar measures could have been used against AIDS, but were tried and enforced in only some nations. The widespread assumption was that individual precautions such as using condoms or restricting sexual behavior were a small price to pay for avoiding measures that aimed instead to enforce monogamy, to impose widespread testing, and to punish endangerment or transmission. Whatever one may think of it, this assumption rests on a political, not a neutrally epidemiological, choice. Different nations with different political cultures met this decision in quite varied ways.

The logic of this new individualized, consensual, democratic public health mimicked that of American gun buffs who argue that, if all were armed, crime would decrease.[32] During the mid-nineteenth century, when it was gradually accepted that cholera spread via water, and not miasmatically or indiscriminately, it followed that people could avoid the disease by not drinking infected water. John Snow, who is famous for having identified the waterborne transmission of cholera in the Broad Street pump episode during the London epidemic of 1853, put it thus: "Every man may be his own quarantine officer and go about during an epidemic among the sick almost as if no epidemic were present."[33] So too, in the AIDS epidemic, everyone could be his or her own quarantine officer, taking the precautions required to avoid transmission. As Britain's chief rabbi, Immanuel Jakobovits, put it, it is like sending people into a contaminated atmosphere, but providing them with gas masks and protective clothing.[34]

The individualized solution was the one chosen by some democratic polities—at least those with no desire to impose restrictions on their citizens. It was also a victory for the minorities that were hardest hit by the epidemic and testified to the perhaps unexpected political prowess and organizational talents of gays, at least in certain nations. On the other hand, this victory also brought about the mainstreaming of those minorities. The bathhouse dispute showed that if gays claimed the right of democratic citizens not to have strictures imposed on them, then they must assume the responsibilities of democratic citizenship—and that meant an end to the baths. Democratic public health rested above all on self-abnegation. It was autonomously chosen and thus not an imposition. But it remained an abnegation and a sacrifice of habits that were now judged to be contrary to the public interest.

Informal, voluntarily adopted behavioral norms differed from regulations prescribing certain conduct on pain of legal punishment. But they were a form of control nonetheless. Self-imposed strictures meant the adoption of a code of conduct that claimed purely epidemiological justification, yet into which moral, ethical, and other normative evaluations easily crept. Breaking chains of transmission was key, but did this mean monogamy or at least sexual parsimony? Or would sporting a condom at the orgy suffice? Who decided what behavior was within the pale? Social conservatives argued that the epidemic provided the perfect reason to crack down on noxious behavior altogether, both drug abuse and sexual irregularity in all its forms. Gays, not surprisingly, feared that arguments for sexual parsimony were simply veiled attempts to roll back hard-won erotic freedoms. As a new ritual of heterosexuality and the nuclear family, HIV screening was suspect as another attempt designed to stigmatize gays. Gays attacked safe-sex campaigns, whatever their virtues, as cementing the distinction between "normal" heterosexual behavior and "deviant" gay practices.

The very self-contradictions of the problem shone through when the German Green Party warned against moralization and social control if advisors from very different backgrounds provided counseling on behavior modification for high-risk groups.[35] Their solution was to have self-help groups offer such services, rather than allowing, say, Catholic clergy to offer gays advice on the problematique of anonymous sex. But, of course, the dilemma was that either anonymous promiscuity was dangerous and to be avoided or it was not. Having fellow gays tell you not to go to the bathhouses was preferable to hearing it from Monsignor, if only because you were more likely to take their advice. The end effect remained the same: you were supposed to forgo the pleasures of the baths. If anything, gay counselors were imposing greater social control—however well-intentioned—than the church. Similar contradictions were inherent in the arguments for community-based, voluntarist approaches to the epidemic. These arguments assumed that behavioral norms characteristic of a specific subgroup might at one and the same time be epidemiologically safe, yet also differ from the standards of the general population.[36] Removing the doors from the bathhouse cubicles—creating a panopticon of promiscuity—was emblematic of the dilemma: the intent was to force gays to police themselves in the inner sanctum of their most daring transgression, enlisting their own shame to defeat practices that broke the fetters of heterosexual sex but left them vulnerable to infection. At heart, the problem was that, however gussied up in the rhetoric of (multi)cultural sensitivity, certain behaviors were toxic and in need of change.[37]

This shift of control from the outside impositions of an authoritarian state to the internal consensual behavior of governmentality particularly affected gays. Contemporary sexual freedom, such as it is, is based on assumptions of internal restraint that forbid certain behaviors that were formerly acceptable, or at least tolerated in the sense that they had to be outlawed rather than psychologically suppressed. For gays, who have been the primary motors of instinctual abandon in the culture of the late twentieth century, the implications were ambiguous. Resistance to self-restraint was not just risky behavior. It was not equivalent to the motorcycle rider who leaves the helmet at home, the driver who doesn't fasten the seatbelt. Rejecting safe sex, or remaining promiscuous, indicated a more fundamental refusal to enter into the web of mutually inflecting self-control on which modern democratic polities rest.

From this vantage, the efforts of the most "advanced" and liberal governments to include homosexuals in formulating and implementing policy to bring about behavioral change made gays police themselves. Whereas the old-fashioned approach of forbidding risky behavior and enforcing prohibitions by law sought to impose social norms on homosexuals (and other perceived miscreants) from without, governmentality made gays responsible for their own conduct. Either gays could cooperate with safer sex strategies, or face the consequences of a crackdown on their behavior: so ran the implicit bargain offered. The voluntary strategy did not, therefore, require less statutory imposition on the individual than the coercive approach, but a different and arguably more thoroughgoing kind. Gays could no longer be sexual outlaws (in John Rechy's romantic phrase), could no longer practice promiscuity as "the righteous form of revolution."[38]

In contrast, public health in the governmentalist mode may not have punished transgressions. But it sought to ensure healthy behavior by not only requiring all citizens to conduct themselves in much the same way, but also by requiring them to agree that this was only possible way to behave. The bourgeois habits of moderation, abstinence, and prudence became the conduct expected of all citizens. Self-restraint is the basic requirement of modern polities. One of the fundamental issues posed by the epidemic was whether behaviors such as promiscuity or IV drug use were compatible with democratic citizenship.

In terms of public health, the crucial political dilemma that the epidemic posed was whether to treat AIDS, and indeed all contagious disease, as a communal or an individual risk. If it was a communal risk, the solution was to restrict infected individuals sufficiently to render them harmless. If it was an individual risk, the strategy was to encourage everyone to take precautions rendering them resistant to infection, coupled with broad, but voluntary behavioral modification to reduce risk. Nations diverged in their tactics. Some places, such as Sweden, Bavaria, Austria, and the United States, tended to take a more communal approach than others, for example, France, Germany, and the United Kingdom. Despite common arguments that a new democratic form of public health spared the individual subordination to communal interests, no such policy was uniformly followed in the industrialized world. AIDS was dealt with quite differently in different nations.

Moreover, even the most consensual approach to AIDS may, in retrospect, turn out to have been an exception more than a sea change. Once the epidemic spread from gays to drug users, minorities, and others who were less able to mobilize on behalf of their civil rights, the old-fashioned approach regained favor. It did so too once medical treatments became more effective during the mid-1990s. As we have seen with SARS, as soon as a disease comes along that threatens everyone equally, and no identifiable group of vocal victims steps forward, communities show little political hesitation in clamping down.

In the developed world, AIDS has now gone from being an acute contagious disease to something more akin to a chronic disease such as cancer—managed, but not cured. In some senses, the seropositive has become emblematic for the human condition in this era of ever more unflinching knowledge of our own mortality. In a few years, once information about our genetic foibles becomes accurate and widespread, we will all know that we will likely die in a certain number of years of a specified cause. We will pass our lives in the shadow of that insight—much as seropositives do now.[39] All this goes beyond the question of the role of gays, who in this epidemic had the horrifying role of the miner's canary. The broader question concerns the extent to which public health solutions are inherently public goods and achievable only by communal means. In the era of governmentality, public health remains one clear area of statutory control where the average law-abiding citizen might expect to feel the iron fist through the velvet glove. AIDS has not changed that.

Notes

1. This article is based on my book, P. Baldwin, *Disease and Democracy: The Industrialized World Faces AIDS* (Berkeley and New York: University of California Press, 2005). I am grateful to audiences at the History and Economics Seminar at Trinity College, Cambridge; the Danish Medical History Society in Copenhagen; and the Center for European Studies at the University of Wisconsin, Madison, for comments and suggestions on earlier versions.

2. S. Friedländer, *Nazi Germany and the Jews*, vol. 1 (New York: HarperCollins, 1997), 100; M. Burleigh and W. Wippermann, *The Racial State: Germany 1933–1945* (Cambridge: Cambridge University Press, 1991), 107; M. Reich-Ranicki, *Mein Leben* (Stuttgart: Deutsche Verlags-Anstalt, 1999), 205–7; P. Weindling, *Epidemics and Genocide in Eastern Europe, 1890–1945* (Oxford: Oxford University Press, 2000), 273–74; R. Proctor, *The Nazi War on Cancer* (Princeton, NJ: Princeton University Press, 1999), 46.

3. J. C. Scott, *Seeing Like a State: How Certain Schemes to Improve the Human Condition Have Failed* (New Haven: Yale University Press, 1998), 155; N. Naimark, *The Russians in Germany: A History of the Soviet Zone of Occupation, 1945–1949* (Cambridge, MA: Belknap Press, 1995), 97.

4. A. Browne, "How the Government Endangers British Lives," *Spectator* 291 (2003): 12.

5. P. Baldwin, *Contagion and the State in Europe, 1830–1930* (Cambridge: Cambridge University Press, 1999), 410–12.

6. E. Ackerknecht, "Anticontagionism between 1821 and 1867," *Bulletin of the History of Medicine* 22 (1948): 562–93; E. Ackerknecht, *Medicine at the Paris Hospital 1794–1848* (Baltimore: Johns Hopkins Press, 1967), 156–57. Ackerknecht was following the cue given by Sigerist, who distinguished broadly between absolutist and liberal styles of public health. H. Sigerist, *Civilization and Disease* (Ithaca, NY: Cornell University Press, 1943), 91.

7. C. Jones and R. Porter, eds., *Reassessing Foucault: Power, Medicine and the Body* (London: Routledge, 1994); G. Burchell et al., eds., *The Foucault Effect: Studies in Governmentality* (Chicago: University of Chicago Press, 1991); J. Goudsblom, "Zivilisation, Ansteckungsangst und Hygiene: Betrachtungen über ein Aspekt des europäischen Zivilisationsprozesses," in *Materialen zu Norbert Elias' Zivilisationstheorie*, ed. P. Gleichmann et al. (Frankfurt: Suhrkamp, 1977); N. Rose, *Governing the Soul: The Shaping of the Private Self* (London: Free Association Books, 1999).

8. B. Turner, *The Body and Society: Explorations in Social Theory* (London: Sage Publications, 1996), 210.

9. S. Davies, *The Historical Origins of Health Fascism* (London: Forest, 1991).

10. L. K. Altman, "Public Health Fears Cause New York Officials to Detain Foreign Tourist," *New York Times*, April 28, 2003, 4; P. Shenon, "U.S. Approves Force in Detaining Possible SARS Carriers," *New York Times*, May 7, 2003, 3; N. Kristof, "Civil Liberties? If They're Really Sick, Lock 'Em Up," *International Herald Tribune*, May 3–4, 2003, 6.

11. M. Warner, *The Trouble with Normal: Sex, Politics and the Ethics of Queer Life* (New York: Free Press, 1999), 38; G. Stambolian, *Male Fantasies/Gay Realities* (New York: Sea Horse Press, 1984), 155; H. von Druten et al., "Homosexual Role Behavior and the Spread of HIV," in *AIDS in Europe: The Behavioural Aspect*, vol. 4, ed. D. Friedrich and W. Heckmann (Berlin: Edition Sigma, 1995), 259; M. Grmek, *History of AIDS: Emergence and Origin of a Modern Pandemic* (Princeton, NJ: Princeton University Press, 1990), 168–69; A. Coxon et al., "Sex Role Separation in Sexual Diaries of Homosexual Men," *AIDS* 7 (1993): 881; G. Rotello, *Sexual Ecology: AIDS and the Destiny of Gay Men* (New York: Dutton, 1997), 77–78; J. Carrier and J. R. Magana, "Use of Ethnosexual Data on Men of Mexican Origin for HIV/AIDS Prevention Programs," in *The Time of AIDS: Theory, Method, and Practice*, ed. G. Herdt and S. Lindenbaum, 252–56 (Newbury Park: Sage, 1992); J. Carrier, "Miguel: Sexual Life History of a Gay Mexican American," in *Gay Culture in America: Essays from the Field*, ed. G. Herdt (Boston: Beacon Press, 1992), 205–6; D. Mendelsohn, *The Elusive Embrace: Desire and the Riddle of Identity* (New York: Knopf, 1999), 73–74.

12. L. A. Gosse, *Rapport sur l'épidémie de choléra en Prusse, en Russie et en Pologne* (Geneva, 1833), 329–33.

13. See Baldwin, *Disease and Democracy*, 7–44, for references.

14. Baldwin, *Contagion and the State*, 244–354.

15. M. Pollak, *The Second Plague of Europe: AIDS Prevention and Sexual Transmission among Men in Western Europe* (Binghamton, NY: Haworth Press, 1994), 7–8.

16. W. Rubenstein, "Law and Empowerment: The Idea of Order in the Time of AIDS," *Yale Law Journal* 98 (1989): 986.

17. B. Schünemann, "Die Rechtsprobleme der AIDS-Eindämmung," in *Die Rechtsprobleme von AIDS*, ed. B. Schünemann and G. Pfeiffer (Baden-Baden: Nomos, 1988), 378; P. Wilson, "Colleague or Viral Vector? The Legal Construction of the HIV-Positive Worker," *Law and Policy* 16 (1994): 300–301.

18. L. Montagnier, *Vaincre le SIDA: Entretiens avec Pierre Bourget* (Paris: Cana, 1986), 148; 103rd Cong., 1st sess., *Congressional Record* (March 11, 1993), H 1204, H 1208; 103rd Cong., 1st sess., *Congressional Record* (February 18, 1993), 31763.

19. *Hansard Parliamentary Debates*, Sixth Series, vol. 144 (January 13, 1989), col. 1147; *Riksdagens Protokoll*, Bihang, 1985/86, Socialutskottets betänkande 1985/ 86:15, 10; J. Mann and D. Tarantola, eds., *AIDS in the World II* (New York: Oxford University Press, 1996), 203; M. Balter, "Europe: AIDS Research on a Budget," *Science* 280 (1998): 1856.

20. C. Martet, *Les combattants du sida* (Paris: Flammarion, 1993), 223.

21. E. Benabou, *La prostitution et la police des mœurs au XVIIIe siècle* (Paris: Perrin, 1987), 426; N. Himes, *Medical History of Contraception* (New York: Schocken Books, 1970), 188–202; J. Donzelot, *The Policing of Families* (New York: Pantheon, 1979), 172; E. Jeanselme, *Traité de la syphilis*, vol. 1 (Paris: Doin, 1931), 378.

22. M. Closen et al., *AIDS: Cases and Materials* (Houston: John Marshall, 1989), 182; 99th Cong., 1st sess., *Congressional Record* (October 1, 1985), vol. 131, E4296.

23. P. Kayal, *Bearing Witness: Gay Men's Health Crisis and the Politics of AIDS* (Boulder: Westview Press, 1993), 53–54, 92–95; Rotello, *Sexual Ecology*, 109, 186–202; P. Illingworth, *AIDS and the Good Society* (London: Routledge, 1990), 15; J. Lauritsen, *The AIDS War: Propaganda, Profiteering and Genocide from the Medical-Industrial Complex* (New York: Asklepios, 1993), 188–90.

24. S. Kane, *AIDS Alibis: Sex, Drugs and Crime in the Americas* (Philadelphia: Temple University Press, 1998), 33; N. Krieger, introduction to *AIDS: The Politics of Survival*, ed. N. Krieger and G. Margo (Amityville, NY: Baywood, 1994), ix.

25. J. Cavailhes et al., *Rapport gai: Enquête sur les modes de vie homosexuels en France* (Paris: Personna, 1984), 92–95; Martet, *Les combattants du sida*, 46; J. Girard, *Le mouvement homosexuel en France 1945–1980* (Paris: Syros, 1981), 187–88.

26. S. Strickland, *Politics, Science, and Dread Disease: A Short History of United States Research Policy* (Cambridge, MA: Harvard University Press, 1972), 213.

27. D. Kirp, "The Politics of Blood: Hemophilia Activism in the AIDS Crisis," in *Blood Feuds: AIDS, Blood, and the Politics of Medical Disaster*, ed. E. Feldman and R. Bayer (New York: Oxford University Press, 1999), 312.

28. M. Hayry and H. Hayry, "AIDS and a Small North European Country: A Study in Applied Ethics," *International Journal of Applied Philosophy* 3 (1987): 59.

29. P. Baldwin, "The Return of the Coercive State? Behavioral Control in Multicultural Society," in *The Nation-State Under Challenge: Autonomy and Capacity in a Changing World*, ed. J. Hall et al. (Princeton, NJ: Princeton University Press, 2003); E. Fee, "Public Health and the State: The United States," in *The History of Public Health and the Modern State*, ed. D. Porter (Amsterdam: Rodopi, 1994), 260; A. Yankauer, "Sexually Transmitted Diseases: A Neglected Public Health Priority," *American Journal of Public Health* 84 (1994): 1896.

30. S. A. Månsson, "Psycho-Social Aspects of HIV Testing: The Swedish Case," *AIDS Care* 2 (1990): 8; B. Henriksson and H. Ytterberg, "Sweden: The Power of the Moral(istic) Left," in *AIDS in the Industrialized Democracies*, ed. D. Kirp and R. Bayer (New Brunswick, NJ: Rutgers University Press, 1992), 325; B. Henriksson, *Social Democracy or Societal Control? A Critical Analysis of Swedish AIDS Policy* (Stockholm: Glacio, 1988), 28; Swiss Institute of Comparative Law, *Comparative Study on Discrimination against Persons with HIV or AIDS* (Strasbourg: Council of Europe, 1993), 21.

31. "Stellungnahme der Deutschen Gesellschaft für Innere Medizin zu AIDS," *AIDS-Forschung* 7 (1989): 379.

32. J. Lott, *More Guns, Less Crime: Understanding Crime and Gun-Control Laws* (Chicago: University of Chicago Press, 1998).

33. *Medical Times and Gazette* 11 (1855): 31–35, 84–88.

34. N. Fowler, *Ministers Decide: A Personal Memoir of the Thatcher Years* (London: Chapmans, 1991), 253.

35. Bundestag, Drucksache 11/7200, 31 May 1990, 340.

36. M. Isbell, "AIDS and Public Health: The Enduring Relevance of a Communitarian Approach to Disease Prevention," *AIDS and Public Policy Journal* 8 (1993): 160, 168.

37. R. Bayer, "AIDS Prevention and Cultural Sensitivity: Are They Compatible?" *American Journal of Public Health* 84 (1994): 895–97.

38. J. Rechy, *The Sexual Outlaw* (New York: Grove Press, 1977), 31.

39. J. de Savigny, *Le Sida et les fragilités françaises: Nos réactions face à l'épidémie* (Paris: Albin Michel, 1995), 315.

Chapter Two

The Social Contract of Health in the Twentieth and Twenty-First Centuries

Individuals, Corporations, and the State

DOROTHY PORTER

Health as a Social Right

When the French National Assembly declared health, along with work, a right of man in 1792, it laid the political foundations that would form the basis of a social contract of responsibility for population health between the democratic state and its citizens.[1] By the middle of the nineteenth century, the British state translated the idea of health citizenship into a universal equal right under the law to protect the population from epidemic disease.[2] In 1848, a French and a German revolutionary—Jules Guérin in the *Gazzette médicale de Paris* and Rudolf Virchow in his reports on typhus in Upper Silesia—interpreted health citizenship as constituted through democratic freedom, universal education, and amelioration of social and economic inequality.[3]

Throughout the nineteenth century, central European states adopted increasingly interventionist legislation to protect populations against the threat of infectious disease. In the United States and Canada, "sanitary revolutions" took place at local and regional levels, but federal interventions were less comprehensive. By the last quarter of the century, the effects of local, regional, and central state actions began to be effective in reducing mortality from infectious diseases in industrial societies. The most significant changes were registered in lower infant mortality, as the result of the increasingly comprehensive supply of clean, noncontaminated water in urban environments.

As infectious diseases declined in industrialized urban societies at the turn of the twentieth century, the attention of public health authorities and medical academics turned toward the control of chronic diseases. This chapter explains how, following World War II, prescriptions for the prevention of chronic diseases removed responsibility for population health from the state to the individual through lifestyle management, thus shifting the focus of disease etiology from social-structural and environmental causes to the behavior of individuals. It also argues, however, that during the early twenty-first century, a new covenant of health is being advocated by reformers in the United States that not only returns responsibility to political states but also insists on a primary role for large-scale economic corporations in addressing the environmental causes of chronic epidemics, such as obesity. This chapter also argues that although U.S. health reformers have influenced international dialogues on the environmental causes of chronic disease, the social contract of health within the United States itself continues to prioritize individual responsibility for population health.

Chronic Illness, Lifestyle Medicine, and Social Behavior

A limitless labor supply was the fuel necessary to drive the economic engines of eighteenth- and nineteenth-century industrializing societies. Thus, preventing premature mortality from infectious diseases was a major political priority.[4] Reducing the costs of caring for ever larger numbers of chronically sick, aging populations replaced this policy in the largely infectious-disease-free, technologically advanced, wealthiest societies from the middle of the twentieth century on.[5]

The impact of epidemiological transition and demographic transformation became compelling to medical and public health intellectuals from the interwar years on, as new statistical models of population structures stimulated panic over falling birth rates, declining mortality, and possible disastrous imbalances between productive and nonproductive populations.[6] During the 1920s, statisticians working within the life insurance industry had begun to examine the relationships between lifestyle, overweight, morbidity, and mortality. Louis Israel Dublin produced surveys on overweight and mortality for the Metropolitan Life Insurance Company in 1924 and 1929 and completed surveys on lifestyle and chronic disabling diseases, including asthma and heart disease, with Herbert H. Marks in the 1940s.[7] At the end of World War II, the U.S. Public Health Service initiated new studies of the impact of the epidemiological transition to chronic diseases when Joseph Mountain hired Gilcin Meadors in 1946 to found what eventually became the Framingham study of heart disease in 1947.[8] Meadors set up the initial study with the express purpose of producing "recommendations for the modification of personal habits and environment" that could prevent the development of chronic heart disease (CHD).[9] In the 1950s the Framingham study highlighted the role played by diet and cholesterol in the disease. At the same time, in Britain, Jerry Morris and his colleagues at the Medical Research Council's Social Medicine Unit were highlighting another lifestyle determinant of CHD, exercise.[10] In the meantime, in 1948 Iwao Milton Moryama and Theodore Woolsey produced a large analysis of cardiovascular disease in relation to age changes in the population, using the U.S. Population Survey Data. This also included discussions of lifestyle issues such as obesity.[11] In October 1952, the National Vitamin Foundation funded a symposium at Harvard University on "Overeating, Overweight, and Obesity" which included papers on lipogenesis, the psychology of overeating, and the physiology of overweight, as well as a paper by P. C. Fry on "Obesity: Red Light of Health."[12] The public and individual health implications of overweight and obesity attracted increasing attention throughout the 1950s. Numerous public health authors took up the issue of *Your Weight and Your Life*,[13] offering advice on *The Low-Fat Way to Health and Longer Life: The Complete Guide to Better Health through Automatic Weight Control, Modern Nutritional Supplements, and Low-Fat Diet.*[14] Psychology research students, such as Barbara Levy at Berkeley, undertook studies such as the "Dimensions of Personality as Related to Obesity in Women."[15]

Lifestyle began to replace traditional structural explanations of core public health concerns such as infant mortality. Since the nineteenth century, studies of infant mortality had identified economic inequality as the major cause of steep differential gradients according to class. However, new sociological investigations began to explore other factors in the early 1950s. Because at that time it was extremely difficult to determine the intrauterine events that might have led to the death of babies within the first four weeks of life, often the cause of death on certificates was simply listed as "prematurity." Stewart, Webb, and Hewitt from the Oxford Institute of Social Medicine suggested that this term really described a way of dying rather than an actual cause. In 1955, they attempted to correlate 1,078 stillbirths and neonatal deaths with a variety of factors, including the mother's physique during the antenatal period.[16] However, the investigation of what appeared to be the biological conditions pertaining to death again identified social behavior as a major factor. In their 1955 study Stewart, Webb, and Hewitt discovered that "medium" and "thin" women did not differ in their ability to produce live infants, but among the 212 women described as "obese," the risk of stillbirth or neonatal death was 60 percent, above the standard. This risk appeared to be still greater among women who were described as both "obese" and "short."[17]

The established structural explanation of the relationship between poverty and infant mortality was thus challenged by a new argument that the mother's physique, in particular obesity, was the major determinant of stillbirth and neonatal death. This argument implied that *lifestyles* involving unhealthy behaviors, such as excessive food consumption and lack of exercise, created major risks, rather than *life conditions,* such as economic inequality.

One of the most dramatic demonstrations of the relationship between lifestyle habits and chronic illness was established by the Doll and Hill correlation of cigarette consumption with rising levels of lung cancer published in the *British Medical Journal* in 1950. Later they confirmed their original tentative conclusions with an analysis of the causes of death of doctors between 1951 and 1956 in relation to nonsmoking, present smoking and exsmoking groups at those dates.[18]

Although smoking was considered a habit rather than a dependency in the strict psychological definition of addiction, it was portrayed as an individual responsibility.[19] The antismoking campaigns in Britain and the United States that followed the Doll and Hill results exemplified the new message of a clinical model of chronic-disease prevention. The key to the social management of chronic illnesses—such as lung cancer—was emphasizing individual prevention, raising health consciousness, and promoting self-health care.

Following the antismoking campaign, the prevention of chronic disease through the education of the individual gathered momentum. Subsequent postwar campaigns offered lifestyle methods for preventing heart disease, various forms of cancer, liver disease, digestive disorders, venereal disease, and obesity. This model of prevention was grounded in epidemiology's new, legitimate authority. The analysis of the relationship between smoking and lung cancer gave epidemiology new credibility as the authoritative source on a bio-, psycho-, socio-, medical model of chronic disease. It became a critical heuristic device and legitimated a new approach to disease prevention through controlling individuals' lifestyles.

The Healthy Lifestyle and Health Citizenship in the Twenty-first Century

The shift in public health to controlling individual behavior to prevent and manage chronic illness through the institution of the healthy lifestyle expanded exponentially during the postwar period. This shift created new, international economic empires among the sports and leisure industries. But the politics of the healthy lifestyle also became fraught with conflict in which the interests of political states, professional groups, and corporate markets competed for power.

In the last quarter of the twentieth century, an international dialogue produced congruous messages in health propaganda campaigns that focused on preventing cardiovascular diseases, digestive disorders, cancer and, most recently, sexually transmitted diseases and HIV/AIDS, in states with high levels of chronic illnesses among aging populations. The healthy lifestyle was increasingly presented as the best chance that affluent nations had for reducing the morbidity consequences and exponentially increasing health costs of having 25 percent of their populations over eighty years old. The Combined Health Information Database, which was produced by a range of federal health agencies and provided comprehensive coverage of health promotion and education materials and program descriptions, listed over nineteen hundred items that it published in the last quarter of 2004 alone on healthy lifestyle promotion.[20]

The political implications of the prevention of chronic illness through the promotion of healthy lifestyles for health citizenship was vividly demonstrated in the most recent developments in what could be described as a "health war" over obesity. Since the late 1970s, postmodern fat lands have been feeling the weight of their fast-food economies and sedentary, high-tech, nonlabor-intensive modes of production. According to the National Center for Disease Prevention and Health Promotion, "In the United States, obesity rose at an epidemic rate during the last two decades of the twentieth century. One of the national health objectives for the year 2010 became a reduction in the prevalence of obesity among adults to less than 15 percent. The most recent research, however, continued to indicate that the situation was worsening rather than improving." According to the *Surgeon General's Call to Action to Prevent and Decrease Overweight and Obesity* (2001), in the United States in 1999, 61 percent of adults, 13 percent of children 6 to 11 years old, and 14 percent of adolescents aged 12 to 19 were overweight or obese. The prevalence of obesity tripled for adolescents over the previous two decades. The increases in overweight and obesity occurred in "all ages, racial and ethnic groups, and both genders" producing "300,000 deaths each year" in diseases associated with obesity such as "heart disease, certain types of cancer, type 2 diabetes, stroke, arthritis, breathing problems, and psychological disorders, such as depression." The Surgeon General's Office (SGO) estimated that "The economic cost of obesity in the United States was about $117 billion in 2000." Health disparities figured prominently in the structure of the epidemic, with women in poverty having a 50 percent higher risk of obesity than either men or women with higher socioeconomic status. Although the SGO acknowledged that genetics could be a cause of obesity, it identified behavioral causes as primary and offered behavioral and cultural change as the route to achieving a fat-free future for individuals and the nation.[21]

The Surgeon General's Office emphasized the need to communicate the significance of obesity and its causes in insufficient activity, unhealthy food, and overconsumption to individuals, social groups, and health-care providers. Health-care providers needed to become health advisors "across the life-span" and strong health promotion campaigns needed to be established in schools. The SGO also highlighted communication about breastfeeding and the health education of prospective parents about child obesity as another priority. Breastfeeding, the SGO assumed, would reduce the likelihood of infant obesity and help mothers to "return to pre-pregnancy weight more quickly."[22]

In 2001 SGO demanded, "The Nation must take action to assist Americans in balancing healthful eating with regular physical activity" and that individuals and groups "across all settings must work in concert" to ensure that

- high-quality physical education in schools establishes attitudes and skills for a physically healthy life, and nutritional instruction is given to promote healthy eating choices and patterns

- healthy activity levels is promoted among adults—a minimum of thirty minutes of moderate physical activity on most days of the week—by creating more opportunities for physical activities at worksites and encouraging employers to make facilities available

- reduction in television watching is promoted, along with the replacement of sedentary with active leisure pastimes

- a broad cultural promotion of healthy food choices is undertaken, including five servings of fruits and vegetables per day along with "reasonable portion sizes at home, in schools, at worksites, and in communities."[23]

Beyond using health promotion and persuasion to bring about cultural and behavioral change, the SGO highlighted potentially more coercive interventions such as the restriction of the availability of high-calorie, high-fat foods and beverages on school campuses by

- enforcing existing U.S. Department of Agriculture regulations that prohibit serving foods of minimal nutritional value during mealtimes in school food-service areas, including in vending machines

- adopting policies specifying that all foods and beverages available at school contribute to eating patterns that are consistent with the Dietary Guidelines for Americans

- providing more food options that are low in fat, calories, and added sugars, such as fruits, vegetables, whole grains, and low-fat or nonfat dairy foods

- reducing access to foods high in fat, calories, and added sugars and to excessive portion sizes.[24]

The SGO addressed the vexed question of payment for care by urging that mechanisms be created "for appropriate reimbursement for the prevention and treatment of overweight and obesity."[25] And finally, the SGO demanded that the nation make a major investment into further research and intervention planning. The latter was subsequently established through Centers for Disease Control (CDC) state-based programs that produced a wide variety of strategic plans by individual state health departments. These plans focused on different types of intervention, from targeting social groups through different agencies for health promotion to evaluating the impact of breastfeeding on infant and maternal obesity.[26]

From the beginning of the twenty-first century, federal and state health and disease agencies have pursued strategies that set a high priority on education and persuasion to encourage behavioral change. Coercive intervention was only recommended within the context of the prevention of childhood and adolescent obesity.[27] But the politics of the healthy lifestyle and obesity had already become highly charged in the 1990s, with self-styled nutrition activists accusing government health agencies of being "gutless" in failing to tackle the ultimate cause of obesity, which they claim is a toxic environment created by corporate capitalist greed.[28]

According to health reform campaigners from the Center for Science in the Public Interest (CSPI), Michael Jacobson, its director, and Kelly D. Brownell, Yale professor of health psychology and director of the Yale Center for Eating Disorders, Tommy Thompson, the U.S. health and human services secretary (2001–4), was "brandishing popguns" when his department needed to be getting out "howitzers and announcing a war to overhaul the nation's diet."[29] Jacobson ridiculed Thompson's 3:00 A.M. public-service announcements telling people to use the stairs rather than elevators and to work around the house, along with Thompson's proposal to make food labels display calorie numbers in slightly larger print. Instead Jacobson, Brownell, and the CSPI argued that the health department needed to require restaurants to publish calories on menus, to take steps to force junk food out of schools, and to make large food corporations pay for pushing obesity by taxing high-fat, high-calorie foods.[30] Jacobson argued that the FDA and the Department of Agriculture also needed to take decisive action to reduce the sale of unsafe, unhealthy food substances such as quorn and olestra, and to prevent the sale of phony products falsely labeled as "whole-grain," "all-fruit," and "natural." The food-supplement market was, according to Jacobson, a con artist's paradise, and he accused the FDA of doing nothing to police it effectively.[31] The CSPI advocated that the war against Big Food and corporate capitalism should be fought through political activism, pressuring government for change at the national and local state levels.

Like CSPI, other radical organizations such as "Adbusters" (created by Kalle Lasn, the author of *Culture Jam*[32]), identified corporate capitalism and its powerful ideological tool, advertising, as creating a cultural, social, and material toxic environment. Lasn argued through his web-based *Adbusters* magazine that the route to "beating Big Food" along with the rest of corporate capitalism should be a campaign of noncooperation such as a "Buy Nothing Day."[33] Multinational corporatism, according to *Adbusters,* created societies in which everyone became a "terrorist consumer."[34] *Adbusters'* rhetoric matched that of other anti-capitalist campaigners who joined to protest against the production of "consumer terrorism" in riots and vandalism attacks on McDonald's during G7, World Trade Summits from the 1990s.

Anti–Big Food campaigners provoked an equally radical backlash among defenders of consumer freedom and corporate capitalist production. The Center for Consumer Freedom (CCF) accused CSPI of trying to create a "nanny state"[35] and Kalle Lasn and Adbusters of being anti–corporate capitalism hypocrites.[36] CCF and Republican policy theorists such as Peter Ferrar, director of the Institute for Innovative Policy and the International Center for Law and Economics;[37] Bruce Bartlett, Fellow of the National Center for Policy Analysis;[38] and campaigners for feminist individualism such as Wendy McElroy[39] identified food reform as "food fascism."[40] A ideological war of attrition developed among food-reform advocates, the food industry, and conservative organizations such as the CCF. The war intensified starting in 1994 when, in an Op-Ed piece in the *New York Times,* Kelly Brownell presented a four-part plan aimed at fighting diet-related illness in the United States that included levying a tax on high-fat, high-calorie foods, such as fast-food burgers and snacks such as Twinkies—the infamous "Twinkie tax."[41]

Despite, or perhaps because of, being a psychology professor, Brownell argued that focusing on individual behavior would not solve the obesity epidemic. Government intervention must address what he called an "American crisis" and control a toxic food environment by subsidizing healthy foods, taxing unhealthy foods and regulating advertising. Like Kalle Lasn, Brownell believed that corporate power and advertising were poisonous forces creating a toxic food environment. "What's the difference between the effect of Joe Camel and Ronald McDonald? . . . It's McDonald's stated corporate goal to have no American more than four minutes from one of their restaurants. If a tobacco company put up a 'Billions and Billions Sold' sign, we'd be outraged."[42] (Lasn's Adbusters' posters represented Joe Camel as Joe Chemo, sitting sad, sick, and bald in a hospital bed.) Brownell, together with CSPI, argued that the tax collected on junk food could be used to support education campaigns to change what Jacobson believed was the essential inclination of human nature toward "sloth and gluttony."[43] Yet both Jacobson and Brownell believed that this approach stopped blaming individuals and instead attacked the environment they live in.[44]

A predictable response from conservatives raging against the "sin tax" and what they depicted as Nazi-style authoritarianism was not the only concern voiced about differential food taxes.[45] Medical-journal editorials, such as those in the *British Medical Journal*, highlighted the implication for civil liberties in interfering with what individuals chose to eat.[46] Jacobson, Brownell, and others responded by comparing their proposals with the antismoking campaign, which equally undermined individual liberty and attacked the corporate environment for the benefit of community health. They cited as a model to be reproduced the successes of the antismoking campaign and the benefits gained from reducing morbidity and mortality due to smoking-related diseases.[47]

The comparison between the marketing strategies of Big Food and Big Tobacco hold out the hope to the food radicals of legally indicting and publicly regulating the corporate food industry's culpability for its contribution to the burden of morbidity and premature mortality, not only in postindustrial societies but beyond them in the globalized capitalist economic system. In 1999, the U.S. Department of Justice brought legal suit against the owners of the former British-American Tobacco Co, Philip Morris Inc, the producers of, among others, Marlborough cigarettes, for "a pattern of racketeering activity" to "conceal the health risks of cigarette smoking and the addictiveness of nicotine."[48] This case was seen as the most powerful achievement yet of the antismoking lobby, and it pivoted around the concept of nicotine addiction. Food reformers subsequently drew parallels between the addictiveness of nicotine and that of junk food, hoping to use the parallels as a lever through which food reformers could gain influence on the production and marketing strategies of the large food corporations. Morgan Spurlock, an independent documentary filmmaker, reached blockbuster audience levels with his film *Supersize Me*, in which he experimented with eating only foods and soda beverages from McDonald's for thirty days. Apart from documenting the significant physiological damage to his liver and cardiovascular system and his unprecedented, massive weight gain, Spurlock's film powerfully expressed an argument about the addictive nature of McDonald's fast food and drinks. Toward the end of the thirty-day experiment, Spurlock claimed that he had literally become a McDonald's junkie, craving his next fix, living only a half life of depressed debility between meals and snacks.[49] In the film, Spurlock spoke about his addiction over images of Ronald McDonald selling burgers to small children, emphasizing how both the tobacco and food industries use pediatric addiction as a marketing tool.

Despite concerns over civil liberties, in 2003 the World Health Organization (WHO) supported the introduction of taxes on high-fat, calorie-dense, low-nutrition foods and the use of tax revenue for subsidizing healthy foods in affluent nations to reduce morbidity from obesity and its related diseases.[50] The WHO also recommended that governments work with private industry and voluntary organizations to promote healthy lifestyles, including using market incentives to encourage entrepreneurial enterprise and cooperation in bringing about social change in population diets, physical activity, and consumption patterns. Without directly attacking large-scale corporate capitalism, the WHO 2003 Draft Strategy reproduced a number of the recommendations that had been forwarded by groups such as CSPI for over a decade, including the regulation of marketing, advertising, and food labeling, especially to protect the most vulnerable members of a population—children. The Draft Strategy received the full support of CSPI's director of legal affairs, Bruce Silverglade.[51] CCF responded by repeating its criticism of taxing food. CCF's Mike Burita argued, "You're going down a pretty dangerous path on a number of fronts," because "who is going to be the food czar who decides what gets taxed?" He added that most people believed that obesity is a matter of personal responsibility and that such taxation would be unfair, "especially to the people who do enjoy those foods in moderation and practice a healthy lifestyle."[52]

By firmly linking tax to subsidy, the WHO recommendations explicitly addressed an issue that neither the CSPI nor the CCF had highlighted but was raised by Tom Marshall of the University of Birmingham in the UK. Marshall declared, "Low-income groups, who tend to eat higher-fat diets, would disproportionately bear the greatest tax burden."[53] The only other party to highlight this issue was the food industry itself. Its business depends on knowing the structure of its markets and the socioeconomic stratification of its consumers. Jim McCarthy of the Snack Food Association responded to the WHO Draft Strategy by pointing out that any food tax would create the most financial hardship for the poor.[54] The food industry offered a collective perception of the cultural environment in which it operated. John Peters, the head of Procter & Gamble's Nutrition Science Institute, suggested, "Here's the problem as I see it: Our American view of value right now is stuck in the 'more for less' domain" and that "servings are big because that's what people want."[55]

Where one industry nervously contemplated market restriction and instability, however, another spied an opportunity. "Fast-casuals" such as Panera Bread, Au Bon Pain, and Briazz began expanding rapidly, starting in the late 1990s. City Blends cafés and juice bars have earned huge profits out of making "the country healthier . . . one city at a time."[56] However, Bonnie Liebman and Jayne Hurley of CSPI remained skeptical about the extent to which health retailers, such as the healthy supplement producers, live up to their name.[57] The sportswear, sports equipment, fitness-center, and commercial-diet industries continued to grow exponentially into the twenty-first century to serve insatiable consumers. When Dr. Robert C. Atkins's death was announced on news reports throughout the world, other inventors of diet systems became international figures.

Although national governments continued to navigate a treacherous path through the political food wars while seeking the most effective means of addressing the obesity epidemic, perhaps the most significant signs of change appeared within corporate capitalism itself. As Liebman and Hurley pointed out, in December 2002 McDonald's announced its first quarterly loss since 1965.[58] Jacobson attributed the slump to angry parents and outraged consumers who finally turned off from 540-calorie supersize soda drinks and heart attacks inside sesame buns.[59] During the early 2000s, fear of profit loss and new competitors in a changing food-cultural environment began to motivate the traditional fast-food industry to get on board the healthy-eating profit-share train before it left the station. Ronald McDonald disappeared from McDonald's advertising, which began to promote "loving" their new salad menus instead. The low-carbohydrate craze begun by Dr. Atkins and his imitators created the fastest food-marketing transformation ever witnessed. Starting in 2000, the corporate food world began offering alternatives from Round Table low-carb pizzas to burgers without buns to Subway's sandwiches. Beer brewers and soda companies from Budweiser to Coca Cola and Pepsi Cola equally celebrated a reduced-carb love feast, only to be outdone by the "0 carbs, 0 calories, 0 caffeine, 0 sodium, 0 compromise" of Dr Pepper/Seven Up's Diet Rite. Low-carb corporate strategic adjustment appeared to follow Jacobson's assertion that the politics of food will ultimately be won by consumers turned into activists by political agitators.

Conclusion

The alliance of medicine, social science, and public policy in trying to modify social behavior has altered the social contract of health between the modern state and its citizens. The relative weight of the obligations of the state vis-à-vis those of the individual in democratic societies changed over the course of the late twentieth century as postindustrial, affluent societies modified their aims. The promotion of the healthy lifestyle became a rearguard action to reduce the exponentially increasing costs of redeeming chronically broken bodies in an ever aging population.

Making lifestyle transformation the basic strategy for achieving population health transformed the concept of health as a right of citizenship that had been created by the French and American revolutionaries in the eighteenth century. From the time French revolutionaries declared health to be a right of man in 1792 it also became a responsibility. As Ludmilla Jordan-ova has pointed out, the *idéologue* Constantine Volney reminded the citizen of the new republic that his body was an economic unit belonging to the community, and he had a sociopolitical duty to lead a healthful, temperate existence in order to ensure his value for the commonwealth.[60] In the late twentieth century democratic states reasserted this feature of the social contract of health by making it an individual responsibility. Using public information to persuade individuals to take up prescribed healthy lifestyles, postmodern states employed a vast array of expertise to prevent chronic disease, following a model that had been created in the campaign against lung cancer and other smoking-related diseases. The most recent developments in lifestyle disease prevention in the face of rising obesity rates have, however, yet further reconfigured the relationship not only between states and citizens, but also between citizens, states, and large-scale corporate economic organizations in the social contract of health.

Despite state and popular focus on preventing obesity through the reform of individual behavior, this epidemic has engaged the responsibility of government for intervening in the broader political, economic, and social environment, as well as in individual liberties, on behalf of the health of the community. The obesity epidemic has illustrated that although lifestyle-disease prevention ostensibly shifts responsibility for community health toward individual citizens, government responsibility for controlling environments remain undiminished in the social contract of health in late- or postindustrial democratic societies. Although national governments have undertaken activities and degrees of intervention to promote cultural and behavioral change, the step toward intervention in large-scale economic organization is a political quagmire that no government has yet been prepared to confront. In the United States, where the largest multinational food corporations originate, the rhetoric and constrained activism of radical health reformers have had little or no impact on bringing about a change in government health policy toward the food industry. Citizens themselves have made more of an impact, in this case not through political activism but by changing patterns of consumption. The extent to which governments like the United States will be co-opted by citizens into making political interventions (such as taxation or legal prohibition) in the environments in which obesity epidemics develop may, however, depend on another location of power in what the historian Alan Brandt identifies as a "heterogeneous state."[61] Historians such as Alan Brandt, David Rosner, and Gerald Marcowitz have highlighted how the battle between the citizenry and large-scale economic corporate organizations has shifted to the juridical theater.[62]

American health-reform campaigning, however, has been quite influential in the international dialogue on the role of state intervention in the prevention of chronic diseases such as obesity. The environmental etiology has been reemphasized over individualized behavioral explanations, and taxation and regulation of corporate production and marketing has been proposed by the WHO.

But some contemporary critics have identified potentially negative implications of the rise of lifestyle-disease prevention for health citizenship and population health: the creation of a worried well society and the transformation of health-care providers into a behavioral police force. Michael Fitzpatrick, a Stoke Newington–based doctor, believes that government promotion of the healthy lifestyle and the media promotion of health-scare panics have created a culture of hypochondria. This culture has in turn exponentially stimulated the market for alternative healing—or complementary medicine—and turned the British G.P., at least, into a medical policeman of deviant behavior trying to impose medical regulation on everyday life.[63] The conservative medical journalist James Le Fanu indicts the preoccupation with the social relations of health for producing unnecessary anxiety over health and illness.[64] And the historian Edward Shorter has identified the rise of a hypochondriacal society at the end of the twentieth and beginning of the twenty-first century as the result of an excessive psychologization of illness.[65] The question of the rise of a hypochondriacal society as the outcome of these developments or of what, in 1975, Ivan Illich identified as the medicalization of everyday life[66] or what Michel Foucault identified as the rise of a surveillance society[67] would, however, require another paper to consider.

Notes

1. D. Weiner, "Le droit de l'homme à la santé: Une belle idée devant l'Assemblee constituante 1790–1791," *Clio Medica* 5 (1970): 208–23; D. Weiner, "Public Health Under Napoleon: The Conseil de salubrité de Paris 1802–1815," *Clio Medica* 9 (1974): 271–84.

2. D. Porter, "Public Health and Centralisation: The Victorian State," in *Third Oxford Text Book of Public Health*, ed. Roger Detels et al., 1:19–34 (Oxford: Oxford University Press, 1997).

3. See D. Porter, *Health, Civilization and the State* (London: Routledge, 1999), 46–78.

4. J. Duffy, *The Sanitarians: A History of American Public Health* (Chicago: University of Illinois Press, 1990); A. Hardy, *The Epidemic Streets: Infectious Disease and the Rise of Preventive Medicine, 1856–1900* (Oxford: Clarendon, 1994); A. Wohl, *Endangered Lives: Public Health in Victorian Britain* (London: Dent, 1983).

5. D. Porter, "The Healthy Body in the Twentieth Century," in *Medicine in the Twentieth Century*, ed. R. Cooter and J. Pickstone, 201–16 (Amsterdam: Harwood Academic Publications, 2000).

6. D. Porter, "Eugenics and the Sterilization Debate in Sweden and Britain before World War II," *Scandinavian History* 24 (2000): 145–62.

7. L. I. Dublin, "Mortality of Overweights According to Spine Length" (presented for the Committee at the Annual Meeting of the Association of Life Insurance Medical Directors at Newark, New Jersey, October 23, 1924; New York: Committee on

Dryer Measurements in Relation to Life Insurance Underwriting Practice, Report No. 2, 1924); L. I. Dublin, "The Relation between Overweight and Cancer: A Preliminary Examination of Evidence from Insurance Statistics" (Proceedings of the Association of Life Insurance Medical Directors of America, vol. 15; New York: Association of Life Insurance Medical Directors of America, 1929); L. I. Dublin and H. H. Marks, "Mortality Risks with Asthma" (read at the Forty-fourth Annual Meeting of the Association of Life Insurance Medical Directors of America, October 1933; New York: Press of Recording and Statistical Corporation, 1934); L. I. Dublin, ed., "The American People: Studies in Population," *Annals of the American Academy of Political and Social Science* 188 (1936); L. I. Dublin and H. H. Marks, "Mortality among Insured Overweights in Recent Years" (read at the Sixtieth Annual Meeting of the Association of Life Insurance Medical Directors of America, October 11–12, 1951; New York: Association of Life Insurance Medical Directors of America, 1952).

8. G. Oppenheimer, "Becoming the Framingham Study 1947–1950," *American Journal of Public Health* 95 (2005): 602–10.

9. Oppenheimer, "Becoming the Framingham Study," 603.

10. J. N. Morris et al., "Coronary Heart-Disease and Physical Activity of Work," *Lancet* 257 (1953): 1053–57.

11. I. M. Moriyama et al., *Statistical Studies of Heart Disease*, 1–9 (Washington, DC: Public Health Reports, 1948).

12. National Vitamin Foundation, "Overeating, Overweight, and Obesity" (proceedings of the nutrition symposium held at the Harvard School of Public Health, Boston, Massachusetts, October 29, 1952, Nutrition Symposium Series; New York: National Vitamin Foundation, 1953).

13. G. A. Lewis, *Your Weight and Your Life: A Scientific Guide to Weight Reduction and Control* (New York: Norton, 1951).

14. L. M. Morrison, *The Low-Fat Way to Health and Longer Life: The Complete Guide to Better Health Through Automatic Weight Control, Modern Nutritional Supplements, and Low-Fat Diet* (Englewood Cliffs, NJ: Prentice-Hall, 1958).

15. B. K. Levy, "Dimensions of Personality as Related to Obesity in Women" (PhD diss., University of California at Berkeley, 1955).

16. A. M. Stewart, J. W. Webb, and D. Hewitt, "Observations on 1,078 Perinatal Deaths," *British Journal of Social Medicine* 9 (1955): 57–61.

17. Stewart et al., 61.

18. R. Doll and A. B. Hill, "Smoking and Carcinoma of the Lung," *British Medical Journal* 2 (1950): 739–48; R. Doll and A. B. Hill, "Lung Cancer and Other Causes of Death in Relation to Smoking," *British Medical Journal* 2 (1956): 1071–81.

19. V. Berridge, "Science and Policy: The Case of Post-War British Smoking Policy," in *Ashes to Ashes: The History of Smoking and Health*, ed. S. Lock, L. Reynolds, and E. M. Tansey, 143–70 (Amsterdam and Atlanta: Rodopi, 1998); V. Berridge, "Morality and Medical Science: Concepts of Narcotic Addiction in Britain," *Annals of Science* 36 (1979): 67–85.

20. "The Combined Health Information Database, 2004," discontinued as of September 1, 2006. Available at http://198.232.250.114/ (accessed September 14, 2006).

21. United States Department of Health and Human Services, *The Surgeon General's Call to Action to Prevent and Decrease Overweight and Obesity* (Washington, DC:

United States Department of Health and Human Services, Office of the Surgeon General, 2001).

22. *The Surgeon General's Call to Action*, 1.

23. *The Surgeon General's Call to Action*, 1.

24. *The Surgeon General's Call to Action*, 2–3.

25. *The Surgeon General's Call to Action*, 2.

26. See "Overweight and Obesity: State-Based Programs," Centers for Disease Control and Prevention, Department of Health and Human Services, Chronic Disease Prevention and Health Promotion. Available at http://www.cdc.gov/nccdphp/dnpa/obesity/state_programs/index.htm (accessed August 31, 2007).

27. *The Surgeon General's Call to Action*, 6–10.

28. M. Jacobson, "FDA: Gutless Tiger," *Nutrition Action Healthletter*, July–August 2003, 2.

29. M. Jacobson, "Big Problem, Small Solution," *Nutrition Action Healthletter*, May 2004, 2.

30. Jacobson, "Big Problem," 2.

31. Jacobson, "FDA: Gutless Tiger," 2.

32. K. Lasn, *Culture Jam: The Uncooling of America* (New York: Morrow, 1999).

33. D. Meadows, "The Global Citizen: Kalle Lasn is as Mad as Heck," *AlterNet*, May 15, 2000. Available at http://www.alternet.org/story/9147/ (accessed August 31, 2007).

34. "I Terrorist,"*Adbusters* 54 (July–August 2004).

35. Center for Consumer Freedom, "Attacking Food Using the Tobacco Model," May 30, 2000. Available at http://www.consumerfreedom.com/news_detail.cfm?headline=283 (accessed August 31, 2007).

36. Center for Consumer Freedom, "Anti-Corporate-Hypocrites [*sic*]: Walk a Mile in Our Shoes," February 27, 2004. Available at http://www.consumerfreedom.com/news_detail.cfm?headline=2385 (accessed August 31, 2007).

37. P. Farrera, "The Rise of Food Fascism," *Washington Times*, June 1, 2003, B03.

38. B. Bartlett, "Targeting Big Food," National Center for Policy Analysis, April 3, 2006. Available at http://www.ncpa.org/edo/bb/2002/bb040302.html (accessed August 31, 2007).

39. W. McElroy, "The Food Fascists," July 13, 2000. Available at http://www.wendymcelroy.com/rockwell/mcelroy000713.html (accessed August 31, 2007).

40. Farrera, "The Rise of Food Fascism."

41. M. Ball, "Brownell Calls for Food Tax to Fight Epidemic," *Yale Herald*, February 13, 1998.

42. Ball, "Brownell."

43. M. Jacobson, "Obesity in America: Inevitable?" *Nutrition Action Healthletter*, March 2000, 2; N. Hellmich, "Obesity is the Target," *USA TODAY*, May 8, 2003, D.01.

44. Jacobson, "Obesity in America: Inevitable?"

45. D. Dowd Muska, "Sin Tax Error," *Nevada Journal*, June 2003.

46. T. Marshall, "Exploring a Fiscal Food Policy: The Case of Diet and Ischaemic Heart Disease," *British Medical Journal* 320 (2000): 301–5.

47. Ball, "Brownell."

48. *U.S. v. Philip Morris, Inc.*, September 22, 1999. Available at http://www. usdoj.gov/civil/cases/tobacco2/complain.pdf#search='united percent2ostates percent2ovs percent2ophilip percent2omorris' (accessed August 31, 2007).

49. *Supersize Me: A Film of Epic Proportions*, directed by Morgan Spurlock (New York: Roadside Attractions/The Con and Samuel Goldwyn Films, 2004).

50. World Health Organization, *Integrated Prevention of Noncommunicable Diseases: Draft Global Strategy on Diet, Physical Activity and Health* (Geneva: World Health Organization, 2003).

51. A. Srikameswaran, "WHO Wants 'Twinkie Tax' to Discourage Junk Foods," *Pittsburgh Post-Gazette*, December 6, 2003.

52. Srikameswaran, "WHO Wants 'Twinkie Tax.'"

53. Marshall, "Exploring a Fiscal Food Policy."

54. Hellmich, "Obesity."

55. Hellmich, "Obesity."

56. City Blends Smoothie Cafe, "Making the country healthier . . . one city at a time." Available at http://www.cityblends.com/ (accessed August 31, 2007).

57. B. Liebman and J. Hurley, "Beyond Fast Food: 'Fast Casuals' Come of Age," *Nutrition Action*, April 2003, 10–16.

58. Liebman and Hurley, "Beyond Fast Food."

59. Jacobson, "Obesity in America: Inevitable?"

60. L. Jordanova, "Guarding the Body Politic: Volney's Catechism of 1793," in *1789: Reading Writing Revolution, Proceedings of the Essex Conference on the Sociology of Literature, July* 1981, ed. F. Barker et al., 12–21 (Colchester: University of Essex Press, 1982).

61. A. Brandt, "Public Health and the Heterogeneous State" (paper presented at the symposium on Public Health and the State: Yesterday, Today and Tomorrow, Columbia University, New York, October 17 and 18, 2005).

62. G. Markowitz and D. Rosner, *Deceit and Denial: The Deadly Politics of Industrial Pollution* (Berkeley and Los Angeles: University of California Press, 2002).

63. M. Fitzpatrick, *The Tyranny of Health: Doctors and the Regulation of Lifestyle* (London: Routledge, 2000).

64. J. Le Fanu, *The Rise and Fall of Modern Medicine* (London: Little Brown, 1999).

65. E. Shorter, *From Paralysis to Fatigue: A History of Psychosomatic Illness in the Modern Era* (New York: Free Press, 1993).

66. I. Illich, *Limits to Medicine: Medical Nemesis, the Expropriation of Health* (London: Marion Boyars, 1976).

67. M. Foucault, *The Order of Things: An Archeology of the Human Sciences* (London: Tavistock, 1972).

Part Two

Carving Out the International

Chapter Three

American Foundations and the Internationalizing of Public Health

PAUL WEINDLING

Foundations as International Organizations

American foundations have been powerhouses of international health reform. They supported a broad spectrum of policies, encompassing laboratory research, public health training, and sanitary fieldwork. Infectious and parasitic diseases, mental health, and drug therapy have at various times appeared on foundation agendas. These programs have involved strategic evaluation of some fundamental problems: how to measure health and disease and their economic costs, how most efficiently to turn discoveries in the laboratory into preventive policies, and how to calculate the prospects for wholesale eradication of infectious diseases. Foundations have had greater freedom than state agencies to support experimental projects and to disseminate standards based on best practice derived through international training programs.

The foundations' varied activities have given rise to conflicting interpretations of their role as social agencies. Some scholars have taken the medical programs at face value as promoting disinterested advancement of medicine for human benefit. According to these accounts, in their visionary support for cultural and medical projects, donors such as John D. Rockefeller, Jr. assume an almost saintly quality.[1] Since the mid-1970s, a wave of critical studies examined foundations as agencies of imperialism, including cultural imperialism, disseminating American cultural and political values in expert-led public health programs.[2] These studies claimed that the foundations expressed the class interests of trustees, who were generally recruited from elites in industry and banking, leavened by professional leaders in law and medicine.[3] They were active in areas of American commercial and strategic interest, for example, Latin America, China, and, during the 1920s, the newly independent states of eastern Europe, which were seen as buffers against the spread of communism.

Acccording to a third interpretive approach, in establishing systems for the professional management of health and welfare, foundations were building expert and professional elites. The highly prestigious Rockefeller Foundation Fellowships boosted the careers of men, whom it was hoped would take positions of social leadership in their countries. The foundation periodically noted that public health elites in countries of substantial intervention such as Poland or in international agencies such as the United Nations Relief and Rehabilitation Administration (UNRRA) had been Rockefeller trainees and former fellows.[4]

This chapter is predicated on two caveats. First, we cannot assume a dynamic flow of expert knowledge from elite agencies in the United States to peripheral locations. Foundations and their advisers learned from model schemes elsewhere. In short, the approach to the formation and implementation of policy was an interactive one. The second caveat concerns the dominance of studies of the Rockefeller Foundation for the first half of the twentieth century. The operations of the Rockefeller became an interpretive testing ground. But other foundations were also involved in international health—both as talking partners of the Rockefeller and as independent sources of innovation. The public health element in other foundations merits analysis.

An Emerging Force

Before World War I, international health was limited to conventions and treaties among countries to halt the spread of contagious diseases. State policy was essentially negative, aimed at safeguarding the given nation's health by halting the spread of infectious, epidemic diseases from overseas.

The period 1900–1914 was the crucible for the new type of corporate foundation with an immensely wealthy single donor, trustees, and executive staff, in contrast to a medical research institute sustained by mass donations (such as the Pasteur Institute) or state agencies (such as Koch's institute). The trinity of John D. Rockefeller Senior and Junior and their visionary mentor, Frederick Gates, was mesmerized by the French and German development of diphtheria antitoxin at the Pasteur and Koch institutes, as this showed the immense potential of financing an institute for pure medical research. They established the Rockefeller Institute for Medical Research in 1901, thereby establishing the model of a research institution with outstanding facilities in the United States.[5]

Confronted by the imperialist agendas of Great Britain, France, and Germany, the powerful new organizations sought to emulate if not to outdo their rivals in terms of science. The Rockefeller Sanitary Commission (1909–14) and International Health Board (1916–27) intervened on behalf of mass education and populist participation. It extended the evangelizing antihookworm campaigns to Latin America and the Pacific. It then tackled malaria, yellow fever, yaws, and schistosomiasis.[6] Foundation officers regarded with some satisfaction the displacement of British, French, and German medical influence, which they condemned as scientifically narrow. If the foundation could maintain distance between itself and the U.S. State Department on the one side, and recipient states on the other, then surely its aims would be taken as purely altruistic.

When it was established in 1913, the Rockefeller Foundation (RF) linked its public health initiatives to an elitist agenda formulated by the Carnegie Foundation for the Advancement of Teaching to improve standards of medical education in the United States. Abraham Flexner reported that standards of medical education in the United States were lamentably uneven, when compared with those of Germany, with its full-time professors.[7] This set a pattern of remedying deficiencies in the United States by emulating best practice elsewhere. The Rockefeller strategy came to rely on major international centers at Johns Hopkins and Harvard and at the expanded London School of Hygiene and Tropical Medicine as world training centers in public health. The Rockefeller Foundation sponsored the Johns Hopkins School of Public Health as a flagship scheme that trained numerous Rockefeller staff members as well as public health personnel from around the world.[8] The RF's China Medical Board (established in 1914) opened the Peking Union Medical College in 1919, which they regarded as "the Johns Hopkins of China." Its international staff was to raise standards of medicine and public health.[9]

During World War I and its cataclysmic aftermath of epidemics and mass starvation, the RF and other foundations rallied with philanthropic relief to ravaged areas of France and Belgium, and then to Poland and Russia. When U.S. sanitary reformers supported reconstruction in liberated Serbia from 1919, they carried with them Ralph Waldo Emerson's *Conduct of Life* as a tract promoting health as part of an optimistic philosophy of self-reliance in the struggle against disease, ignorance, and selfishness.[10] By avoiding short-term emergency measures and developing schemes for long-term and fundamental reconstruction, the reformers hoped to avert major subsistence crises and epidemics.[11] The goal was not just to prevent disease, but also, by tackling the social roots of distress, to prevent another war.

One way of achieving this goal was to develop preventive, primary health care. Although assisted by U.S. finance and expertise, the new public health clinics were far from just "an American show." In war-ravaged Serbia, socialized primary health care developed as part of a community-building program of providing public health in the form of a network of civic health centers run by citizens' councils, or *zadrugas,* on a democratic basis. Education, self-help, and a healthy lifestyle were fundamental, and in this respect the *zadrugas* and the U.S. health demonstration units merit comparison. As the delegate of Elizabeth Milbank Anderson, who endowed the Memorial Fund in 1905 (renamed the Milbank Memorial Fund in 1921), John A. Kingsbury, named the fund's first full-time chief executive in 1921, supported such democratic initiatives, while stressing the need for statistical analysis of their efficacy. Kingsbury's internationalism is less well known than his radicalism and support for health insurance.[12] He expected that the United States and eastern Europe could provide reciprocal models of innovation.[13] He believed that philanthropic support for Serbia would measurably improve the health of the current and next generations, not only in the localities assisted but also in many other parts of the world.[14]

By 1921 the Rockefeller Foundation had turned away from relief projects as ephemeral and as treating symptoms of deprivation rather than providing any fundamental cure. The RF set about making surveys of health conditions and services on a country-by-country basis throughout the world.[15] The surveys ushered in the most creative period, during the 1920s and thirties, of U.S. foundation support for international health. Alan Gregg compiled several of the surveys, and when the foundation switched to the funding of programs he became director for the medical sciences. During the isolationist period of U.S. foreign policy in the 1920s, foundations were perversely at their most interventionist in working within state administrations and exerting pressure for the development of public health policies and institutions. Rockefeller Foundation support for the American Commission for the Prevention of Tuberculosis in France galvanized with new energy a sluggish and bureaucratized French public health system.[16] Another option was to reconstruct international health as based on voluntarist, community-based initiatives. The RF supported multiple strategies—research in a central laboratory, training public health personnel, and sanitary operations in peripheral locations. This was part of a wider effort to transform assistance in self-sustaining, democratic communities. In this process, the RF and other innovators faced suspicions that preventive medicine was socialized medicine.[17] But the foundations were not content with simply internationalizing research and public health training programs. A fourth strategy crystallized. The foundations embarked on a series of experimental schemes designed as models of international health reform. René Sand, the Belgian advocate of sociological medicine, remarked that the U.S. foundations, "by introducing a rational reformatory policy, have stimulated health organisation throughout the world."[18]

The Rockefeller Foundation systematically observed conditions of public health on a global basis, but it was highly selective in its funding. In Europe, its officials worked closely with government departments of public health in France, and in the new central European states of Czechoslovakia and Poland.[19] The case of Germany illustrates how different branches of the RF adopted divergent policies. The RF started a special German program after World War I to assist the medical sciences, but its International Health Division kept out of Germany, considering its public health system to be excessively geared toward laboratory sciences. The Rockefeller Foundation also sought to supplant German medical influence in such countries as Bulgaria and Greece. It preferred major interventions in the successor states of central Europe, notably Poland, Hungary, and Czechoslovakia, hoping that these would act as a democratic buffer. The International Health Board helped establish schools of public health in no less than sixteen countries, ranging from Brazil to Yugoslavia.[20] The foundations guided and supported the League of Nations Health Organisation at a time when nation-states were suspicious of a genuinely international approach.[21]

To date, most historical analyses have focused on the Rockefeller Foundation without considering how it acted in concert with other foundations, notably the Milbank Memorial Fund (MMF, founded in 1905), the Commonwealth Fund (founded in 1918), and the conglomerate of Carnegie endowments.[22] One branch of the Carnegie trusts was drawn into a decade of support for the Eugenics Record Office at Cold Spring Harbor, and another into education to secure global peace, when it published assessments of health in World War I. Frederick Keppel, president of the Carnegie Corporation of New York, was international minded, although he had to resort to convoluted tactics to get around strictures on funding outside the United States when he wished to pay for projects in East and South Africa. The Commonwealth Fund limited its international funding to mental hygiene and child guidance and to assistance for hospitals.[23] Only the Rockefeller Foundation and the Milbank[24] considered international health problems in the round and had diversified programs for international medical assistance. When state investment in medical research was low and central state administrations equivocated about their obligations to health care, expectations of foundation support ran high.

Program officers and a new community of international health experts considered governments restrictive and rigid, resisting innovation in international health. States were also somewhat ambivalent about, and often resentful of, the League of Nations' efforts to promote measurement of health conditions in the community. Governmental representatives were concerned that international measures of disease and malnutrition would expose social deprivation—as happened in Britain during the depression, when scientists worked through the combined International Labour Organization and League of Nations Technical Commission on Nutrition. Rockefeller Foundation support for the League of Nations Health Organisation gave this body freedom to innovate international health standards and the measurement of the medical consequences of inadequate diet, housing, and occupational hazards. Select American cities, towns, and rural communities became laboratories of international health reform. The American approach to public health, as established in the new schools of public health at Johns Hopkins, Harvard, and Yale universities, combined organizational questions, health education, and the practicalities of sanitary technologies with high-powered laboratory research on vaccines and pathogens.[25]

American public health experts were interested in both sides of a quite fundamental divide between primary health care and grassroots sanitary provision for whole communities and regions and single-issue, scientifically based preventive campaigns. The U.S. foundations had faith that their approach, combining scientific innovations with prescriptions for a hygienically reformed lifestyle, was superior to the rival, laboratory-based approaches of the Pasteur Institute or of German bacteriology. The RF officers had no love for imperialism, which they associated with European efforts to maintain the preeminence of the Pasteur Institute and the London School of Hygiene and Tropical Medicine. But the program officers were resigned on pragmatic grounds to investing in these central institutions as the best way to influence standards in the respective colonial spheres. On the other hand, the foundation officers were convinced that a synthetic approach to public health had genuine advantages. The International Health Board's single-disease campaigns, under the direction of Wickliffe Rose, came to be regarded as too narrow.[26] The more synthetic approach paid attention to statistical monitoring and methods and to organizational questions. The aim was systematically to measure, control, and reduce the incidence of death and disease by combining science with a supreme effort of economic investment in health and enlightening the people.[27]

This doublethink suggests that the foundation often pursued multiple objectives: for example, yellow fever exemplified the dichotomy between prevention through sanitation and laboratory-based innovations.[28] The officers of the foundation drew up ambitious and visionary plans for disease elimination. The foundation's support for biological research on the physical basis of life and molecular biology accelerated a laboratory-based approach to the study of all aspects of the human condition, from psychology to physical sickness. The laboratories of the Rockefeller Institute for Medical Research were crucibles for solving global problems of disease control. Yet "making the peaks higher" (Wickliffe Rose's maxim, expressing the foundation's drive to promote academic excellence) involved community-based schemes.[29] These too were of a broader international significance. The efforts to establish community-based standards adds not only a significant dimension to international health studies, but also allows general points to be drawn about U.S. foundations' role in the wider world of international health.

Both within the United States and internationally, the foundations' contributions to primary health initiatives have been largely overlooked. The assumption has been that because the United States lacked a federal department of health (as had been established in most European states immediately after World War I), health insurance and socialized medicine did not materialize in the United States during the 1930s, and that public health and primary heath care were therefore in the doldrums. It is necessary to appreciate that innovative work on new international health standards involved not just the technical agenda of providing biological standards for vaccines, pharmaceuticals (as Salvarsan for syphilis), and vitamins, but had the more general purpose of evaluating and comparing community health. In terms of social policy, American program officers and certain public health experts viewed socialization of health services and compulsory medical insurance as too costly and disruptive. These considerations shaped initiatives to transfer and refine experimental projects in community health.

Trustees and Experts

In many ways, the foundations were only as good as their human capital of program officers and field workers. Here, we can identify two rich tiers of interaction: creative, but haphazard, relations, first, between donors and their advisers; and second, between program officers and recipients of grants, whether individual academics or institutions. The second tier, which developed once the foundations were securely established, was more routinized and bureaucratic, and yet in many ways was able to advance whole fields of activity, when a foundation officer identified the most innovative academics and professional leaders. Wickliffe Rose took a top-down view: getting it right at the center was sure to have an impact at the peripheries. Others were more interactionist, placing first priority on the community, and the interaction of its components, as a health-producing organism. Here the role of the dynamic and innovative Alan Gregg, acting on behalf of the Rockefeller Foundation, and a succession of creative figures within the Milbank—notably John Kingsbury, the medical statistician Edgar Sydenstricker, and the nutrition and housing expert Frank Boudreau—merit attention. Academic advisers and program officers did much to sustain the internationalism of policy formation and program implementation.

Although the Rockefeller Foundation had far greater resources (its assets in petroleum and mining being vastly more lucrative than the dairy products of the Borden Milk Company, which supported the Milbank), it was frequently the MMF's technical board that steered Rockefeller largesse. Examples include the setting up of the U.S. county health demonstrations, the founding of the League of Nations medical statistics service, and the tackling of population questions.[30] By the 1930s, the Rockefeller officers looked to the Milbank's mercurial advisory council for tuberculosis demonstrations and to its technical board for new thinking. John D. Rockefeller, Jr. and Albert G. ("Bert") Milbank kept in touch on topics of common interest. They were on friendly terms, had attended the same high school, and had cochaired the United War Work Campaign.[31] Astute program officers knew that they could gain support for an adventurous program if a trusted adviser of J. D. Rockefeller, Jr. (say, W. H. Welch) could prompt him to write to Albert Milbank to gain support for a particular project. They knew that their board members would be swayed by the knowledge that a notable figure supported a venture. Relations were close between the Rockefeller Foundation's Medical Sciences Program Officer Alan Gregg, and the Milbank employees Sydenstricker, Kingsbury, and later Boudreau. Milbank and Rockefeller undertook linked ventures when they agreed on the shift of priorities from funding medical relief in France to health demonstration units. The Milbank and Rockefeller Foundations supported the Ting Hsieng experiment in mass health movements in China, regarding this as the logical extension of the international motives underpinning health demonstration unit projects in New York.[32] The foundations viewed the demonstrations as "laboratories" in which principles for "application to the country at large" could be formulated.[33]

In the cohort of internationally minded foundations officers, not all were trained physicians. An excellent case in point was Charles-Edward Winslow, a biologist and professor of public health at Yale University. Winslow took a strategic lead in both America and internationally. His evocative accounts of community health demonstrations were couched in evangelistic rhetoric, with titles such as *The Road to Health, Health on the Farm and in the Village,* or *A City Set on a Hill.* Winslow's descriptions had a deliberately homespun, local quality, designed to elicit support and participation arising from commitment to public health as rooted in organized community efforts. Yet Winslow and his fellow reformers derived much of their medical expertise and organizational skills from an unspoken but committed internationalism in public health reform. Winslow visited Russia during the turbulence of 1917, where he was impressed with *zemstvo* community-based health care. Although the *zemstvos* were a relic of liberal tsarist reforms that were too limited to stem the tide of revolution, there was a moment in 1917 when a radical liberal agenda seemed a real possibility before the Bolshevik seizure of power.[34] These local projects reinforced Winslow's views on the community-building role of public health and the preventive value of health education, already taking shape under the tutelage of Hermann Biggs of the New York City Board of Health.[35] The health demonstration units of the city of Syracuse, New York (beginning in 1923); the Bellevue-Yorkville district of New York City (1924–33); Cattaraugus County, New York (1922–29); and Winslow's home base of New Haven (beginning in 1919) became medical and demographic laboratories for the resolution of fundamental problems in the provision and measurement of health care. The idea of a healthy life as a theme of sanitary evangelism was transformed into preventive primary health care and improved efficiency of public health systems. Health reformers launched these local units as experiments in social medicine, aiming to transform international public health in the global arena.[36]

Winslow was also the medical director of the League of Red Cross Societies (LRCS), which was an offshoot of the American Red Cross. The LRCS mobilized mass public philanthropy between 1919 and 1923, although it was not itself a corporate foundation with a single donor. Henry P. Davison, head of the War Council of the American Red Cross and founder of the League, formulated controversial plans for Red Cross–sponsored community health clinics, moving the organization away from war and disaster relief and into working for "positive health."[37]

Winslow publicized the community program with eloquence, enthusiasm, and critical acumen. His activities ranged from health promotion in New Haven to international plans for health indicators. *Health on the Farm and in the Village,* published in 1931, was influenced by the rural health initiative of the LNHO: Winslow served on the League of Nations Health Committee in 1921 and from 1927 to 1930. He argued that the United States was a cultural debtor nation, borrowing international models of clinic organization, health education, and community involvement. Controversies surrounding sickness insurance acted as a brake on extending physician-based services in the United States. But seeking an alternative way forward, public health experts and the foundations still made progress by developing the role of public health nurses, social workers, and teachers, as well as attention to housing and nutrition. When Winslow evaluated European health insurance schemes in 1929, he recognized that these compulsory state- and employer-financed devices could not readily be transposed to the United States. Yet the presence of sickness insurance in Europe provided possibilities for morbidity studies, such as those sponsored by the League of Nations Health Organisation. Rather than seeing the interwar period as characterized by an isolationist United States turning its back on socialized forms of European health care, a foundation-based approach reveals a dynamic international movement for public health.[38] Here were constant interactions. Winslow insisted on the value of the health demonstrations "to the whole world."[39]

Many of the donors had been influenced by the relief efforts of World War I. The Serbian example is illuminating. The war had seen massive Allied intervention in Serbia with international public health teams to control typhus epidemics. The sweeping influenza epidemics left a sense that more was necessary in terms of primary prevention.[40] With postwar reconstruction came a new movement for establishing a public health infrastructure and mass education. The convergence of populism with sanitary expertise in measuring and analyzing disease linked community medicine to health promotion and socialized primary care. "Sound statistical methods" were held to be essential to evaluate district health. As an American representative of the Serbian Relief scheme remarked to the Croatian medical reformer Andrija Štampar in December 1920, "Then we will know where we are 'shooting' when we undertake a public health campaign there."[41]

The American reformers' international partners included Štampar, recognized by the MMF and Rockefeller Foundation as "the ablest health officer in Europe"; Ludwik Rajchman, director of the new hygiene institute in Warsaw, and from 1921 until 1938 secretary of the League of Nations Health Organisation;[42] and Sir Arthur Newsholme, who as former medical officer to the Local Government Board for England and Wales advocated a liberal health policy, based on a local health service providing preventive and therapeutic care.[43] This international network of medical reformers recognized that the United States was a key player in interwar public health reform; it saw how American ideas and resources could ensure that medicine would underpin democracy in eastern Europe. At the same time, the Europeans felt that they had something to offer in terms of organizing health care for the community. Their reciprocal projects were to reshape the international agenda of public health.

John Kingsbury played a crucial role as secretary of the Milbank between 1921 and 1935. When he moved from the Serbian Child Welfare Association of America (generously financed by Elizabeth Milbank Anderson as a private initiative) to the Milbank Memorial Fund, he set out to reconstruct ideas on primary health care.[44] Diverse elements were blended into the new concept of the health center. On the one hand, René Sand regarded the health center as a U.S. innovation, comparable with a department store as a grouping of specialized clinics or health shops (a model used in the East Harlem Health Center experiment).[45] On the other hand, European variants incorporated a multiplicity of specialized services for which the costs of treatment came from sickness insurance or from state funds. Sand considered the Yugoslav clinics as pioneers in the idea of the health center as a social center with recreational facilities.[46]

The extension of public health from disease prevention to health promotion involved appraisal of some fundamental issues, which motivated the launching of the New York health demonstrations:

1. How are health and disease measured, especially improvements in health?

2. How is health delivery in the community best organized?

3. How can health be most effectively improved and sickness prevented in terms of improving the conditions of life, for example, nutrition and housing?

4. What are the costs of sickness, and how much will the community invest in health?

5. How can knowledge of maintaining health be disseminated to the public, so that a healthy lifestyle will be achieved?

The above questions came onto the agenda of the advisory council of the Milbank Memorial Fund in 1922.[47] Social scientists, social work experts, and medical scientists focused on how economic and nutritional factors determined health. Bacteriologists realized the necessity of collaborating with social scientists, statisticians, and social workers. W. H. Welch recognized how control of bacterial pathogens and facilitation of a healthier lifestyle went together. Winslow hailed this agenda as "the new public health" in that it brought hygienic knowledge to the individual in his or her home or shop.[48] The public health approach shifted from philanthropic to social scientific, coinciding with the post–World War I sense of the need to determine "the conditions for a better life."[49]

Statistical Solutions

The Milbank's role in strategic health planning on an international basis was a significant one. It viewed metropolitan and rural health demonstrations as scientific experiments, requiring causality and proof. In May 1922, W. H. Welch recommended Raymond Pearl, an expert in population genetics, to the Milbank because of his insistence on sound statistical methods in public health research. Its advisory council demanded a new demographic and economic rigor, so that the outcome of service provision could be evaluated.[50] The call for proof was answered by the progressive-minded statistician Edgar Sydenstricker of the U.S. Public Health Service. Between 1916 and the mid-1920s, he pioneered measures of morbidity statistics for selected population groups. Sydenstricker argued for the need to shift away from mortality statistics to the burdens of chronic diseases, initially hookworm and pellegra, and then cancers and heart disease. Kingsbury realized that by drafting the talented Sydenstricker, he could target the energies of the antituberculosis campaigners at a broader spectrum of pathogenic causes, as well as applying those energies on a cost-effective, efficient basis.[51]

Sydenstricker's mission was to realize the "dream" of a view of health rather than death by evaluating the balance among biological, economic, and environmental pathogens in community and family studies. He masterminded the U.S. Public Health Service study of Hagerstown, Maryland from 1921 to 1924, when he used the family as the unit of observation. His aim was to gain insight into the typical, by measuring the weekly incidence of illness in a general population group over a three-year period. He demonstrated the higher importance of respiratory diseases in morbidity rather than mortality.[52] The originality of Sydenstricker's contributions to measuring community health was considerable. He analyzed the causation of diseases in the community and identified the major mortality and morbidity among age groups and social sectors. He pioneered the study of sample populations, using the resources of health centers. With his appointment in 1926, the Milbank gained a figure of substance who could put analysis of the prevalence of sickness at the forefront of international thinking and strategy. Although Sydenstricker was convinced that some form of sickness insurance on the European model was desirable, the community initiatives were deliberately kept separate from the insurance issue with public and voluntary provision.

As with the citizen-controlled Serbian health *zadrugas,* the result was an organized community program. This citizen-based model contrasted with the typical municipal health department headed by a full-time physician who functioned as (to borrow the phrase of the British medical statistician Major Greenwood) a virtual "medical dictator" also in charge of a school health department and specialized services with public health nurses. The division between community-accountable and expert-led dispensary clinics had caused much fractious discussion (the classic case was in Berlin in 1848–51) and highlighted a fundamental dichotomy in terms of political control. But again, the U.S. projects synthesized both elements. Once the general principles of health service organization were clarified, the model of the health demonstration could be disseminated both nationally and internationally.[53]

In 1925 the Milbank commissioned Sydenstricker to analyze the effects of health promotion.[54] The fund contributed massively to the health demonstrations at Syracuse as an "average city" and Cattaraugus as an average rural area. Three New York counties were selected as "control communities," raising issues of the comparability of racial and social status and whether controls were possible in a strictly scientific sense. Sydenstricker established a system of vital statistics as a "model for national standards in the field."[55] By now the director of the Division of Research of the Milbank, he overhauled the health-demonstration design. The Bellevue-Yorkville health demonstration in midtown New York typified the new approach, having been converted into a health center from a model public bathhouse donated by Elizabeth Milbank Anderson. Starting in 1929, the Bellevue-Yorkville program provided a new statistical basis for measuring the efficacy of public health interventions, reinforced by collaboration with the New York City Board of Health. This demonstration posed major questions concerning the costs and conditions for securing medical improvements. The population of one hundred fifty thousand was a pool for evaluating a range of services and was intensively screened for tuberculosis.[56] Winslow (then a member of the Technical Board of the

Milbank) looked at the costs of sickness in context. For example, he asked, How much might a family have to pay for medical care as a result of a whole series of illnesses that could well coincide with a birth?[57]

However, Sydenstricker was not without his critics. Newsholme, the British advisor of the Milbank, was irritated by Sydenstricker's wish to shift from tuberculosis to cancer and heart-disease control.[58] Their conflict showed that Sydenstricker had grasped a fundamental shift in twentieth-century mortality and the necessity to modify public health strategies accordingly. Sydenstricker encouraged a survey of morbidity in twelve hundred families in Syracuse, which was completed in 1931. U.S. health-service organization has generally been regarded as a failure for not providing a system of funding for universal health care. This may be seen in the negative response to the president's research committee on social trends of 1929, or in Kingsbury's departure from the Milbank in 1935.[59] Yet the demonstration units suggest positive and durable results, which were of international significance. Sydenstricker's 1933 tract on health and environment was the culmination of an analysis of disease as a multifactorial process. His statistical insights did much to reshape international public health agendas.[60]

International Activism

The convergence between the aspirations of the "health demonstrators" and international health can be seen in Sydenstricker's temporary transfer to the League of Nations Health Organisation to establish its statistical service in 1923–24. The Geneva interlude confirmed the technical excellence of Sydenstricker's use of medical statistics. When the Milbank asked Sydenstricker to review its programs, he was succeeded by Frank Boudreau as the statistician-epidemiologist in Geneva in 1925. This succession was significant because when he later followed Sydenstricker at the Milbank, Boudreau imported the League of Nations' radical new thinking on the relation between nutrition and the social causes of disease. Predictably, Sydenstricker pushed forward into analysis and comparison of morbidity in localities, for which he had the backing of the Rockefeller Foundation. In the mid-1920s, the RF contributed well over one-third of the finances of the League of Nations. Yet often it was the Milbank's Technical Board that set the pace in formulating the agenda for action.

Sydenstricker's sojourn in Geneva paved the way for a new wave of morbidity studies, such as Siegfried Rosenfeld's investigation of tuberculosis morbidity in Vienna and that of Emil Eugen Roesle of the German Reich Health Office. The program was given a holistic rationale by René Sand's concept of positive health, which dated from the mid-1920s. As general secretary of the League of Red Cross Societies from 1921 and as its technical adviser from 1927, Sand supported the shift from prevention of infections to promotion of a healthy lifestyle for the family, underpinned by a public health infrastructure. In 1927 Sand transplanted the idea of the health demonstration to the Belgian town of Jumet. He was impressed by Sydenstricker's analysis of the impact of economic factors on disease and mortality.[61]

The global spillover can be seen in the Ting Hsien experiment of 1930. The Mass Education Movement in China health program offered the chance to use a demonstration model in a rural area, where health improvements were linked to providing basic literacy. Sydenstricker (who was born in China of missionary parents) travelled there in 1930—for "setting up among a sample population a survey which will reveal certain facts about the health conditions of the Chinese people." This was a joint Rockefeller-Milbank initiative, with Welch persuading John D. Rockefeller, Jr. to gain the support of Albert Milbank.[62] Soon the LNHO's director, Ludwik Rajchman, became deeply involved in China. Sydenstricker evaluated the plan to survey the health of one thousand Chinese families, approving the attempt to link health to education and rural work.[63] The project was a follow-up to the Rockefeller Foundation's investment in elite medical education in China and had potential implications for global implementation.

By the late 1920s, European welfare experiments prompted U.S. medical analysts to probe more deeply into the costs and structures of health. James T. Shotwell, president of the Carnegie Endowment for International Peace, commended the Milbank for supporting research in other countries than the United States "in order to be able to apply, by the use of the comparative method, those things most worthwhile which come to light in other quarters of the world."[64] In 1928, Welch reported on programs in Scandinavia and Yugoslavia as potential models for financing heath care. Boudreau, the deputy director of the League of Nations Health Organisation and in many ways its mainstay, reviewed European insurance schemes.[65] In 1934, Sand proposed to Kingsbury parallel American and European surveys on medical care: "Sir Arthur's [Newsholme] International Studies as well as Medicine and the State, the publications of the Committee on the Costs of Medical Care, the demonstrations of Cattaraugus County, Syracuse and Bellevue-Yorkville, all organized or sponsored by the Milbank Memorial Fund, have gathered a considerable wealth of materials. The fundamental revelation is that in the USA no class of the population receives at present adequate medical service. . . ."[66] Although foundations could launch model programs, their acceptance on a universal basis required political will and state measures that went beyond foundations' scope of action.

The sources of inspiration were diverse. Between 1929 and 1931, Newsholme had analyzed the relations between private and official medicine in thirteen continental countries and Great Britain. With Milbank support, he produced three volumes of comparative international studies.[67] The enterprise was completed when Kingsbury joined Newsholme on a visit to the Soviet Union in 1932. Their adventurous book, *Red Medicine*, evaluated the Soviet experiment in social medicine. Albert Milbank remarked to Sydenstricker that he would have gladly paid a retainer for the book not to have been written. In contrast, John D. Rockefeller, Jr. was more complimentary.[68]

In 1936, as a League of Nations Representative, Charles-Edward Winslow surveyed Soviet experiments in public health and was more critical than Kingsbury or Henry Sigerist. Foundation men such as Alan Gregg became convinced that doctors were the obstacle to progress in public health, particularly to its rational reorganization within the community.[69] The fascination with the Soviet Union exposed the limitations of the U.S. health demonstration units in terms of providing fully comprehensive medical care. On the other hand, the more conservatively inclined questioned whether the Soviet health system had a democratic basis. The difference of opinions on Soviet medicine between the critical Newsholme and the admiring Kingsbury and Sigerist should not obscure a common focus on the health demonstrations.[70] Internationally the rise of the Nazi and fascist movements polarized thinking on the organization of health. Winslow avoided the political contention of the mid-1930s, retaining a more pragmatic perspective on what was feasible within the United States, and counseled caution in regard to the socialization of health. At the same time, the shift in emphasis to mental health and nutrition meant that the public health initiatives moved into politically less fractious areas.

Evolving Health Indicators

In 1935, the Milbank joined with the League of Nations Health Organisation in commissioning Isidore Falk to study the operation of European health insurance programs. This move can be counted among Kingsbury's legacies after he left the Milbank because of the insurance issue.[71] Falk had been working with Sydenstricker on plans for health insurance in the United States for the Presidential Committee on Economic Security.[72] Although Sydenstricker's premature death in 1936 was a blow, he left a generation of able disciples. As Kingsbury predicted, their future was secure provided they did not push health insurance, birth control, or "a real V.D. program."[73]

Other foundations applied limited resources to achieving global impact. The Commonwealth Fund targeted mental health, which during the 1930s was regarded as ripe for medical scrutiny. A positive mental outlook was fundamental for preventive medicine; the international movement for mental hygiene spanned World War II. The diverse initiatives by many agencies can be seen as part of a movement to develop holistic studies of the human physiology and psyche.[74] In 1936, Raymond Fosdick, the president of the Rockefeller Foundation, pronounced body and mind indivisible.[75] This theme was taken up by Winslow and Gregg, who came to view psychological aspects of health and disease as a major area for intervention, whether at the level of neurobiology or in terms of community mental-health provision and education.

The economic crisis of the early 1930s accelerated concerns with measuring the effect of social deprivation on health in both urban and rural contexts. The Spanish demand for rural health studies, made to the League of Nations in 1931, spurred interest in local health topographies. The Rockefeller Foundation continued substantial grants to the League's Health Organisation, allowing it to develop an ambitious program on the social bases of disease. The Milbank defrayed the costs of American delegates who attended the League's conference on the effects of the depression on health, held in Berlin in a last democratic gasp in December 1932.[76]

The culmination of the internationalizing of the health demonstrations came in 1935–36 with the program of "health indices" (a term coined by Ludwik Rajchman of the League of Nations Health Organisation). The indices were a simplified form of the "health appraisal" system used in the U.S. health demonstrations, and in City and Rural Health Conservation Contests, first held in 1929. In 1936, the Milbank imported the League of Nations officer, Knud Stouman, to work with Falk and Winslow in New Haven in formulating an experimental system of health measurements. New Haven was selected as an American town of average size, and, conveniently, it was Winslow's home base for community health experiments.[77] In 1937, Frank Boudreau was appointed to succeed Sydenstricker as scientific director at the Milbank. Boudreau imported the economic perspectives of the League of Nations into the American context. He remained active on housing and nutrition committees of the LNHO while deploying his skills to secure reform in America. Once the United States joined the war in 1941, Boudreau was in demand as an adviser on national policy because of his nutritional expertise, and in planning the nascent Food and Agricultural Organization (FAO) and World Health Organization (WHO).

The purpose of the health indices was to measure the health of population groups within a specific community, as well as associated environmental and administrative factors. Stouman and Falk blended the League's measures with the criteria of the City and Rural Health Conservation Contests in the United States.[78] The eleven headings ran from population to examinations of physical fitness. After the initial New Haven trial, the indices were applied in a rural district of eastern Hungary in 1937. In 1938 several member countries agreed to experimental application of the indices. The culmination came in a 1938 study of Brussels, made by Stouman with the support of René Sand, by now the secretary general of the Belgian Ministry of Health. Brussels was chosen because of its complexity and the difficulties in obtaining morbidity and mortality data: unlike in American cities there were no annual "health contests" or appraisals.[79] Parallel rural studies were made in Belgium and Poland, using a set of simplified indices selected in April 1938 by eastern European public health experts. In October 1938, the LNHO sponsored an experts' meeting, which endorsed the value of indices as an international standard. The new system was designed as to correct aggregate national health statistics, which masked regional, social, age-specific differentials.

As in World War I, during World War II U.S. foundations again became involved in emergency relief and also in operationalizing scientific innovations for public health. The Rockefeller Foundation assisted in transferring penicillin development to the United States and in devising methods for the production and application of DDT. These were momentous innovations. The Rockefeller's International Health Division officer, Fred L. Soper, looked forward to the wholesale eradication by DDT of insect vectors of diseases.[80] Penicillin initiated a raft of saturation programs with pharmaceuticals. The RF thus saw the birth of a new era in international health. But it rapidly withdrew, leaving the terrain to a new set of agencies, such as the World Health Organization and UNICEF, the burgeoning nongovernmental organizations, and finally bilateral programs of medical assistance between states, not least to counteract Soviet influence in international public health and medical education. The Rockefeller Foundation phased out its International Health Division in 1951, merging it with the medical sciences program. The foundation felt that the IHD's very success in international work meant the time was ripe to seek new challenges in other related fields, notably agriculture and population studies.[81] Reacting to the first salvos of the cold war, during the McCarthy era the Milbank's Technical Board decided that "it was impossible to initiate a large scale program of international medical research." Further, governmental agencies of the National Institutes of Health were more likely to be involved in any new international initiative. Although public health had escaped being a major casualty of cold war politics, the foundations felt that prudence was advisable in any new initiative supporting foreign public health services. It was considered necessary to secure State Department approval for specific programs such as cholera suppression in Calcutta and Bangkok.[82] Thus, during the second half of the twentieth century, U.S. foundations exerted only an indirect influence on international health by tackling the linked issues of population size and nutritional resources. At the point when medicine could fulfil the vision of effective pharmaceuticals and disease eradication—virtually the vision with which Gates inspired the Rockefellers—the Rockefeller Foundation withdrew from sanitary fieldwork and public health research.

Conclusion

From a modern perspective, the belief in the international transferability of public health organizational models might appear naïve. American medical philanthropists saw a Serbia without ethnic tensions and consistently overlooked the vulnerability of minorities.[83] It seemed to matter little that Andrija Štampar was a Croat among Serb counterparts. No questions were asked about whether Albanians were part of the health *zadrugas* in the Kosovo region. The philanthropists were similarly naive about the "Red medicine" of the Soviet Union as a model. The Rockefeller Foundation officers were interested in the new Soviet Union partly because of its potential for research, and partly because of its collectivized medical organization. Some fellowships in library assistance were granted, but the trustees drew the line at major involvement in Russia.[84] In like fashion, the foundation officers did not grasp the lethal dangers of fascism to world peace. The RF funded an ambitious malaria program in fascist Italy until America entered the war.[85] After the Nazi takeover in Germany, the RF program to assist refugee scholars did not include the dismissed German experts in social medicine and public health. Overall the RF's program for displaced German scholars amounted to less than the funding for a major institute of scientific and medical research, to which it remained committed. At the start of World War II, the Rockefeller Foundation flirted with the idea of a European program in Vichy and occupied France, Hungary, and greater Germany—until the foundation president, Raymond Fosdick, reined in his renegade program officers and field workers.[86] But after World War II, when Fosdick and John D. Rockefeller III wanted a German program, foundation officers did everything they could to prevaricate and delay.

Yet set against such political naïveté was the faith that, with careful measurement of epidemiological and demographic conditions and with an understanding of human psychology, health reform of humanity was achievable. The techniques steadily became more sophisticated, thanks to the blend of Sydenstricker's analyses and the endeavors of health educators in disseminating understanding of good health to the public. The experimental demonstration units were crucibles not only in the United States, but also for international endeavors stretching from Serbia to China. Education and improved sanitation in domestic and working arrangements would lead to better health and fuller, more satisfied lives within more stable, democratic, and equitable societies. It was a noble vision. Sanitary reformers courageously drew attention to the cost issue, linking it to communal democracy. As Winslow recognized, this did not mean American health insurance on a European model, but once a grassroots will to promote community health could be attained, other solutions were appropriate for the United States.

Notes

1. R. Fosdick, *The Story of the Rockefeller Foundation* (New York: Harper & Bros., 1952); J. Ettling, *The Germ of Laziness: Rockefeller Philanthropy and Public Health in the New South* (Cambridge, MA: Harvard University Press, 1981); E. R. Brown, *Rockefeller Medicine Men: Medicine and Capitalism in America* (Berkeley: University of California Press, 1975).

2. E. R. Brown, "Public Health and American Imperialism: Early Rockefeller Programs at Home and Abroad," *American Journal of Public Health* 66 (1976): 897–903; D. Fisher, "Rockefeller Philanthropy and the British Empire: The Creation of the London School of Hygiene and Tropical Medicine," *History of Education* 7 (1978): 129–43; A.-E. Birn, *Marriage of Convenience: Rockefeller International Health and Revolutionary Mexico* (Rochester, NY: University of Rochester Press, 2006); A.-E. Birn, "A Revolution in Rural Health? The Struggle over Local Health Units in Mexico, 1928–1940," *Journal of the History of Medicine* 53 (1998): 43–76.

3. C. Kiser, *The Milbank Memorial Fund: Its Leaders and its Work* (New York: Milbank, 1975), 154–57.

4. See the various essays in P. Weindling, ed., *International Health Organizations and Movements, 1918–1939* (Cambridge: Cambridge University Press, 1995).

5. G. Corner, *A History of the Rockefeller Institute, 1901–1953: Origins and Growth* (New York: Rockefeller Institute Press, 1965); R. Fosdick, *John D. Rockefeller Jr.: A Portrait* (New York: Harper & Bros., 1956), 110–15.

6. A.-E. Birn, "Eradication, Control or Neither? Hookworm vs. Malaria Strategies and Rockefeller Public Health in Mexico," *Parassitologia* 40 (1998): 137–48; M. Cueto, "Science Under Adversity: Latin American Medical Research and American Private Philanthropy, 1920–1960," *Minerva* 35 (1997): 233–45; M. Cueto, "The Cycles of Eradication and Latin American Public Health, 1918–1940," in Weindling, *International Health*, 222–43 (Cambridge: Cambridge University Press, 1995).

7. A. Flexner, *Medical Education in the United States and Canada: A Report to the Carnegie Foundation for the Advancement of Teaching* (New York: Carnegie Foundation for the Advancement of Teaching, 1910); A. Flexner, *Medical Education in Europe: A Report to the Carnegie Foundation for the Advancement of Teaching* (New York: Carnegie Foundation for the Advancement of Teaching, 1912); cf. E. Condliffe Lagemann, *The Politics of Knowledge: The Carnegie Corporation, Philanthropy, and Public Policy* (Middletown, CT: Wesleyan University Press, 1989); S. Wheatley, *The Politics of Philanthropy: Abraham Flexner and Medical Education* (Madison: University of Wisconsin Press, 1989).

8. E. Fee, *Disease and Discovery: A History of the Johns Hopkins School of Hygiene and Public Health, 1916–1939* (Baltimore: Johns Hopkins University Press, 1987).

9. M. Ferguson, *China Medical Board and Peking Union Medical College* (New York: China Medical Board of New York, 1970); M. Bullock, *An American Transplant: The Rockefeller Foundation and the Peking Union Medical College* (Berkeley: University of California Press, 1980); Q. Ma, "The Rockefeller Foundation and Modern Medical Education in China" (PhD diss., Case Western Reserve University, 1995); Q. Ma, "The Peking Union College and the Rockefeller Foundation's Medical Programs in China," in *Rockefeller Philanthropy and Modern Biomedicine: International Initiatives from World War I to the Cold War*, ed. W. Schneider, 159–83 (Bloomington: Indiana University Press, 2002).

10. Kojic to Doharty, Board of Managers, Serbian Child Welfare Association, May 2, 1924, 2, Kingsbury Papers (hereafter JAK), Part II, Box 65 (hereafter II/65), Manuscript Division, Library of Congress (hereafter LC), Washington, DC; *Co-operative Reconstruction: A Report of the Work Accomplished in Serbia by the Serbian Child Welfare Association* (New York: Serbian Child Welfare Association, 1924).

11. Kingsbury to Hoover, December 23, 1920, JAK, II/28, LC.

12. Elizabeth Milbank Anderson, letter of recommendation for Kingsbury, January 6, 1918, JAK, II/5, LC; Kingsbury on Elizabeth M. Anderson's contribution to the health *zadrugas*, address delivered at Slovac, September 2, 1934, Milbank Memorial Fund papers (hereafter Yale MMF), Box 11, Folder 14 (hereafter 11/14), Sterling Library, Yale University. On the MMF and sickness insurance, see R. Shryock, *The Development of Modern Medicine* (Madison: University of Wisconsin Press, 1977), 409.

13. Yugoslav trip, Belgrade, August 27, 1924, JAK, II/65, LC.

14. Kingsbury to Reeder, October 27, 1924, JAK, II/30, LC.

15. S. G. Solomon, "Local Knowledge or Knowledge of the Local: Rockefeller Foundation Officers' Site Visits to Russia in the 1920s," *Slavic Review* 62 (2003): 710–33.

16. L. Murard and P. Zylberman, "La Mission Rockefeller en France et la création du comité international de défense contre la tuberculose, 1917–1923," *Revue d'histoire moderne et contemporaine* 34 (1987): 257–81.

17. Fee, *Disease and Discovery*, 228.

18. R. Sand, *The Advance to Social Medicine* (London: Staples, 1952), 223.

19. P. Weindling, "Public Health and Political Stabilization: Rockefeller Funding in Interwar Central/Eastern Europe," *Minerva* 31 (1993): 253–67.

20. Fee, *Disease and Discovery*, 220; Z. Dugac, "New Public Health for a New State: Interwar Public Health in the Kingdom of Serbs, Croats, and Slovenes (Kingdom of Yugoslavia) and the Rockefeller Foundation," in *Facing Illness in Troubled Times: Health in Europe in the Interwar Years, 1918–1939*, ed. I. Borowy and W. Gruner, 277–304 (Frankfurt am Main: Peter Lang, 2005).

21. P. Weindling, "Philanthropy and World Health: The Rockefeller Foundation and the League of Nations Health Organisation," *Minerva* 35 (1997): 269–81.

22. But see J. Seelander, *Private Health and Public Life: Foundation Philanthropy and the Reshaping of American Social Policy from the Progressive Era to the New Deal* (Baltimore: Johns Hopkins University Press, 1997).

23. A. McGee Harvey and S. Abrams, *"For the Welfare of Mankind": The Commonwealth Fund and American Medicine* (Baltimore: Johns Hopkins University Press, 1986).

24. The original name from 1905 to 1921 was the Memorial Fund Association.

25. E. Fee and R. M. Acheson, eds., *A History of Education in Public Health* (Oxford; New York: Oxford University Press, 1991); J.-P. Gaudillière, "Rockefeller Strategies for Scientific Medicine: Molecular Machines, Virus and Vaccines," in "The Rockefeller Foundation and the Biomedical Sciences," ed. I. Löwy and P. Zylberman, special issue, *Studies in History and Philosophy of Biology and Biomedical Sciences* 31C (2000), 491–509. For analysis of the curricula of schools of hygiene in Germany, Poland, Hungary, Yugoslavia, and Greece, to all of which the RF contributed, see C. Prausnitz, *The Teaching of Preventive Medicine in Europe* (Oxford: Oxford University Press, 1933).

26. R. Acheson, *Wickliffe Rose of the Rockefeller Foundation, 1862–1942* (Cambridge: Cambridge University Press, 1992).

27. On economic dimensions, see Sydenstricker, Future Policy of the Milbank Memorial Fund, Yale MMF, 10/981; see also Winslow on the economic value of public health, letter to Boudreau, January 8, 1951, Yale MMF, 27/55.

28. J. Farley, "The International Health Division of the Rockefeller Foundation: The Russell Years, 1920–1934," in Weindling, *International Health*, 203–21 (Cambridge: Cambridge University Press, 1995); J. Farley, *To Cast Out Disease: A History of the International Health Division of the Rockefeller Foundation, 1913–1951* (New York: Oxford University Press, 2004).

29. For the broader significance of local health interventions, see RG 1.1, Series 235 (hereafter 1.1/235), Rockefeller Archive Center (hereafter RAC), Tarrytown, New York. The phrase "making the peaks higher" is alternatively attributed to Émile Picard, secretary of the French Academy of Sciences, in 1925.

30. Sydenstricker, memorandum to Kingsbury (notes on trip to Geneva and England, June 5, 1934), JAK, II/19, 3, LC; D. M. Fox, "The Significance of the Milbank Memorial Fund for Policy: An Assessment at Its Centennial," *Milbank Quarterly* 84, no. 1 (2006): 5–36.

31. For an example of Milbank-Rockefeller contact, see William Welch to John D. Rockefeller Jr., November 16, 1932; Albert Milbank to John D. Rockefeller Jr., November 21, 1932, RG III.2E/11/114, RAC. Milbank and Rockefeller both attended Cutler School from 1886 to 1889. See the letters in JAK, II/15, 1949, LC.

32. Kingsbury to Welch, requesting that he intercede with John D. Rockefeller, Jr., November 16, 1932, JAK, II/22, LC.

33. Resolution to fund the Chinese Mass Education Movement, July 1, 1935, RG 1.1, 1/601/7/69, RAC.

34. J. Hutchinson, *Politics and Public Health in Revolutionary Russia* (Baltimore: Johns Hopkins University Press, 1990); J. Hutchinson, "'Who Killed Cock Robin?': An Enquiry into the Death of Zemstvo Medicine," in *Health and Society in Revolutionary Russia*, ed. S. G. Solomon and J. Hutchinson, 3–26 (Bloomington: Indiana University Press, 1990); W. Rosenberg, "The Zemstvo in 1917," in *The Zemstvo in Russia: An Experiment in Local Self-Government*, ed. in T. Emmons and W. Vuchinich, 383–422 (Cambridge: Cambridge University Press, 1982).

35. A. Viseltear, "C.-E. A. Winslow: His Era and His Contribution to Medical Care," in *Healing and History*, ed. C. Rosenberg (New York: Dawson, 1979), 207; C.-E. A. Winslow, "Public Health Administration in Russia in 1917," *Public Health Reports* 445 (December 28, 1917): 2191–2219.

36. Sand, *The Advance to Social Medicine*, 217–18.

37. J. Hutchinson, "'Custodians of the Sacred Fire': The ICRC and the Post-War Reorganisation of the International Red Cross," in Weindling, *International Health*, 17–35; B. Towers, "Red Cross Organisational Politics, 1918–1922: Relations of Dominance and the Influence of the United States," in Weindling, *International Health*, 36–55; J. Hutchinson, *Champions of Charity* (Boulder and London: Westview Press, 1996).

38. For context, see D. Porter, *Health, Civilisation and the State* (London: Routledge, 1999), 220–30.

39. Technical Board minutes f. 981, program of November 20, 1931, 11/78, Yale MMF.

40. A. W. Crosby, *America's Forgotten Pandemic: The Influenza of 1918* (Cambridge: Cambridge University Press, 1990); P. Weindling, *Epidemics and Genocide in Eastern Europe* (Oxford: Oxford University Press, 2000), 87–89.

41. Reeder to Štampar, December 22, 1920, JAK, II/28, LC.

42. Kingsbury to Armstrong, March 6, 1925, JAK, II/30, LC; M. Balinska, *Une vie pour l'humanitaire: Ludwik Rajchman 1881–1965* (Paris: La Découverte, 1995).

43. J. Eyler, *Sir Arthur Newsholme and State Medicine, 1885–1935* (Cambridge: Cambridge University Press, 1997), 393.

44. Kiser, *The Milbank Memorial Fund,* 23–25.

45. "The New York Tuberculosis Association: Five Formative Years, 1919–1924," cited as offprint. Photo of the Health Shop in the East Harlem Health Center, which evolved from the Health Corner at First Avenue and 15 Street.

46. Sand, *Advance to Social Medicine,* 217.

47. Advisory Council minutes, November 16, 1922, Yale MMF, 1/1. On the establishment of the Advisory Council, see W. H. Welch to Kingsbury, May 1, 1922, JAK, II/22, LC.

48. C.-E. A. Winslow, *The Evolution and Significance of the Modern Public Health Campaign* (New Haven: Yale University Press, 1923), 52.

49. W. H. Park, "The Social Implications of a Longer Life," in Yale MMF, box 1, file 5 f. 22, Advisory Council Minutes, dinner meeting, 1924.

50. Advisory Council minutes, discussions of Framingham and new demonstration plans, March 22, 1922, Yale MMF, 1/1, f. 23; W. H. Welch to Kingsbury, May 1, 1922, JAK, II/22, LC.

51. Announcement by Kingsbury, November 19, 1925, Yale MMF, 10/73, f. 293; Technical Board minutes, October 7, 1929, Yale MMF, 11/78, f. 707.

52. E. Sydenstricker, "The Incidence of Illness in a General Population Group: General Results of a Morbidity Study from December 1 1921 through March 31 1924, in Hagerstown, Maryland," *Public Health Reports* 49 (1925): 271–91.

53. L. Farrand, "The Philosophy of Health Demonstrations," *American Journal of Public Health* 17 (1927): 1–22.

54. In 1925, Sydenstricker was seconded by the U.S. Public Health Service. On April 15, 1926, he joined the MMF payroll as statistical consultant.

55. C.-E. A. Winslow, *A City Set on a Hill: The Significance of the Health Demonstration of Syracuse, New York* (Garden City: Doubleday, Doran and Company, 1934), 74.

56. Bellevue-Yorkville Health Demonstration, Yale MMF, 3/30–31/1–6; C.-E. A. Winslow and S. Zimand, *Health under the "El": The Story of the Bellevue-Yorkville Health Demonstration in Midtown New York* (New York: Harper & Bros., 1937).

57. C.-E. A. Winslow, *The Road to Health: The Jayne Foundation Lectures for 1929* (New York: Macmillan, 1929), 107.

58. Technical Board minutes, May 12–13, 1928, Yale MMF, 11/77, 570; Eyler, *Sir Arthur Newsholme and State Medicine,* 357–58.

59. Kiser, *The Milbank Memorial Fund,* 55–62.

60. E. Sydenstricker, *Health and Environment* (New York: McGraw-Hill, 1933).

61. R. Sand, "The Jumet Health Demonstration," *The World's Health* 8 (1927): 110–15; J. A. Kingsbury, "The Effect of the Anti-Tuberculosis Campaign," *The World's Health* 6 (1925): 63–70; also in Yale MMF, 11/10, on Framingham. See also P. Zylberman, "Hereditary Disease and Environmental Factors in the 'Mixed Economy' of Public Health: René Sand and French Social Medicine, 1920–1934," in *Heredity and Infection: The History of Disease Transmission,* ed. J.-P. Gaudillière and I. Löwy (London: Routledge, 2001), 261–81.

62. Welch to John D. Rockefeller, Jr., December 19, 1932, RG III.2E/11/114, RAC; J. D. Rockefeller Jr. to Albert Milbank, November 30, 1932, RG III.2E/11/114, RAC.

63. A. G. Milbank to J. D. Rockefeller Jr. on continuing MMF funds for Ting Hsien, December 8, 1932, JAK, II/18, LC; John D. Rockefeller Jr. to Kingsbury on "Dr. Welch and Mr. Rockefeller—Ting Hsien project," JAK, II/18, LC; Welch to Kingsbury, November 21, 1932, JAK, II/23, LC; Technical Board minutes, January 16, 1930, Yale MMF, 11/78, f. 741–42; Technical Board minutes, May 22, 1930, Yale MMF, 11/78, f. 779; Balinska, *Une vie pour l'humanitaire*, 75.

64. Shotwell to Kingsbury, October 13, 1932, JAK, II/38, LC.

65. Technical Board minutes, October 26, 1928, Yale MMF, 11/ 77, f. 603.

66. Sand to Kingsbury, August 28, 1934, JAK, II/19, LC.

67. Kingsbury to Newsholme, March 24, 1931, JAK, II/16, LC; Cf. Eyler, *Sir Arthur Newsholme and State Medicine*, 341–76.

68. Kingsbury to Boudreau, June 29, 1932, JAK, II/65, LC; Kingsbury to Newsholme, November 9, 1935, JAK, II/65, LC; John D. Rockefeller Jr. to Kingsbury, December 30, 1933, RG III.2E/11/114, RAC.

69. Technical Board minutes, October 20, 1932, Yale MMF, 11/78, f. 956; J. Hutchinson, "'Dances with Commissars': Sigerist and Soviet Medicine," in *Making Medical History: The Life and Times of Henry E. Sigerist*, ed. E. Fee and T. Brown, 229–58 (Baltimore: Johns Hopkins University Press, 1997).

70. Sigerist to Newsholme, December 5, 1937, JAK, II/19, LC.

71. Technical Board minutes, April 18, 1935, Yale MMF, 11/80; Newsholme to Kingsbury, April 28, 1935, JAK, II/16, LC. For background, see J. Kingsbury, *Health in Handcuffs: The National Health Crisis—and What Can Be Done* (New York: Modern Age Books, 1939).

72. Kingsbury to Newsholme, April 30, September 4, 1935, JAK, II/16, LC; Newsholme to Kingsbury, July 3, 1935, JAK, II/16, LC.

73. Kingsbury to Boudreau, May 23, 1935, JAK, II/39, LC.

74. McGee Harvey and Abrams, *For the Welfare of Mankind*, 175, 185.

75. J. Pressman, "Human Understanding: Psychosomatic Medicine and the Mission of the Rockefeller Foundation," in *Greater than the Parts: Holism in Biomedicine, 1920–1950*, ed. G. Weisz and C. Lawrence (New York: Oxford University Press, 1998), 190.

76. Welch to Kingsbury, November 21, 1932, JAK, II/23, LC.

77. C.-E. A. Winslow, *Health Survey of New Haven: Conducted Under the Auspices of the Community Chest* (New Haven: Yale School of Medicine, 1928).

78. K. Stouman and I. S. Falk, "Health Indices: A Study of Objective Indices of Health in Relation to Environment and Sanitation," *Quarterly Bulletin of the Health Organisation* 5 (1936): 901–66; L. Murard, "Atlantic Crossings in the Measurement of Health: From the U.S. Appraisal Forms to the League of Nations's Health Indices," in *Medicine, the Market and the Mass Media*, ed. V. Berridge and K. Loughlin, 19–54 (London: Routledge, 2005).

79. K. Stouman, "Health Indices Established in an Experimental Study of the City of Brussels," *Quarterly Bulletin of the Health Organisation* 7 (1938): 122–67; Anon., "Health Indices: Their Place in Public Health Reports," *Bulletin of the Health Organisation* 8 (1939): 60–86.

80. F. Soper, *Building the Health Bridge: Selections from the Works of Fred L. Soper*, ed. J. A. Kerr (Bloomington: Indiana University Press, 1970).

81. A. J. Warren, "The Program in Medicine and Public Health," Trustees' Confidential Report, December 1951, RG 1.1, 3/920/1/3, RAC.

82. Technical Board minutes, December 16, 1958, Yale MMF, 12/98; W. E. van Heyningen and J. Seal, *Cholera: The American Scientific Experience, 1947–1980* (Boulder: Westview Press, 1983); J. L. Brand, "The United States Public Health Service and International Health, 1945–1950," *Bulletin of the History of Medicine* 63 (1989): 579–98.

83. Mitchell Report on the Public Health in Southern Yugoslavia (circa 1925), RG 1.1, 710/2, RAC.

84. S. G. Solomon and N. Krementsov, "Giving and Taking Across Borders: The Rockefeller Foundation and Russia, 1919–1928," *Minerva* 39 (2001): 265–98.

85. D. Stapleton, "Internationalism and Nationalism: The Rockefeller Foundation, Public Health, and Malaria in Italy, 1923–1951," *Parasitologia* 42 (2000): 127–34.

86. W. H. Schneider, "War, Philanthropy, and the Creation of the French National Institute of Hygiene," *Minerva* 41 (2003): 1–23.

Chapter Four

Maneuvering for Space

International Health Work of the
League of Nations during World War II

Iris Borowy

The "space" within which an organization acts is shaped by its mandate, its
financial and material resources, and its prestige, as well as the qualifica-
tion, imagination and dedication of its staff. An organization's "space" may
become contentious because of conflicting interpretations of the organization's function or because of alterations in the landscape in which that
organization is embedded. For the League of Nations Health Organization
(LNHO), which had been instrumental in establishing international public
health during the interwar period, all of the above factors operated simultaneously during World War II. This chapter explores how the LNHO coped
with and navigated the challenges of reduced and altered space.

The LNHO was particularly vulnerable for several reasons. To begin
with, its functions were only vaguely defined. An early resolution listed the
tasks of the LNHO as advising the League of Nations and voluntary organizations in matters affecting health, organizing a rapid interchange of
information on epidemics and health missions, cooperating with the International Labour Organization (ILO) and the League of Red Cross Societies (LRCS) and providing a framework for international agreements.[1]
However, these points were put forth at the very early and provisional
stages of the LNHO. They were not restated for the formation of the Permanent Health Organization in 1923, nor were new objectives ever negotiated. Indeed, the practice during eighteen years of LNHO policy clearly
went beyond these narrow early limits. For all practical purposes, the
LNHO could deal with anything anywhere as long as it could be construed

to mean health. It consisted of a Health Committee that met once or twice a year to decide on the work program, and a Health Section, a part of the League Secretariat, that implemented those decisions. The ill-defined mandate of the LNHO could—and did—give rise to overlap with other organizations. Sometimes that overlap was put to good use, as in the creation during the 1930s of mixed committees for such large topics in social medicine as nutrition and rural health. At other times, it created counterproductive tension and rivalry, as other bodies considered LNHO activities an infringement on their space. The political environment in which the agency existed further complicated its room for action. The 1930s saw intense nationalism, almost constant economic crisis, and an erosion of the prestige attached to international cooperation. In 1920, when it was first established, the League had given the LNHO space to exist, but as the League's own standing, confidence, and means diminished, its framework came to restrict rather than protect its technical organizations.

To be sure, even before the war, the working space of the LNHO was threatened. Until the end of the 1930s, these difficulties were obscured by its many activities, including some impressive successes. Inspired by enthusiastic members, particularly its dynamic Medical Director, Ludwik Rajchman, the LNHO assumed a very broad, though somewhat unsystematic, field of work, which stretched across continents and medical disciplines, ranging from infectious diseases through biological standardization, from assistance in building national health systems to nutrition, rural hygiene, housing, and other large areas of social medicine. In geographic terms, the LNHO had a virtually global reach: its epidemiological service covered some 72 percent of the world population.[2] Over the course of its existence, people from some eighty countries or dependent regions cooperated in one form or another with the LNHO.[3]

But as international tensions heightened, cooperation among different countries and their representatives became increasingly delicate: conflicting national interests in colonial, foreign, and economic affairs; border disagreements; claims of ethnic minorities; and diverse ideas about international administration gave rise to multiple points of friction among practically all member states. Of course, the League of Nations and all its organizations had traditionally been committed to strict neutrality, but this concept had been fragile at all times. As the conflicts of the 1930s, ranging from Manchuria, Danzig, and Ethiopia to Spain, showed, the League trod a thin line between neutrality and passive support for the strong. Indeed, it was relatively easier for a health organization to remain "apolitical" than for many other administrative bodies within the League, but that does not mean that it was ever easy or even possible. In January 1939, Secretary General Joseph Avenol dismissed Medical Director Rajchman, ostensibly for financial reasons but actually because Rajchman's socialist leanings, his outspoken opposition to the Munich accord, and his activities in China made him unpalatable to various governments as well as to the conservative Avenol himself.[4] Rajchman had been unloved in many quarters, but there is no doubt that the loss of his energy and determination profoundly weakened the LNHO.[5] His successor, the Swiss expert for public health Raymond Gautier, could not hope to fill the void.

With war looming, neutrality became the gospel in Geneva. As early as April 1939, Swiss authorities expressed concern that the German government might seize on the presence of the League in Geneva as a pretext for an invasion. Anxious to avoid expulsion, Secretary General Avenol made arrangements that would allow the transfer of the entire Secretariat to Vichy, France, on short notice (before Vichy became a politically charged locale).[6] Neutrality was tested in LNHO circles outside of Geneva as well. In May 1939, the president of the Health Committee, the Frenchman Jacques Parisot, developed a plan that would effectively have tied the LNHO to the Allied powers in coordinated sanitary services during the upcoming war. His ideas, circulated in French government circles, were eventually rejected by France's Foreign Ministry, which was unwilling to open itself to the charge of preparing the collusion of a technical agency of the League with one group of belligerent countries.[7] The League recognized neutrality as the ticket to surviving a war that posed threats to its "space" from many directions.

Defending Neutrality—Claiming Space in Time of War

The mobilization in European countries called several Health Section members to arms, increasing the workload for those that remained.[8] There was no information about the whereabouts of the Polish scientists who had collaborated with the LNHO, including two former or current Health Committee members, Witold Chodzko and Gustaw Szulc. Requests to the International Red Cross produced some information about and postcards from some of the scientists and allowed the tracing of their fates during the winter of 1939–40.[9] Meanwhile, Acting Medical Director Gautier acted according to the principle of "carry[ing] on with every possible activity which [could] be pursued in present circumstances."[10] But exactly what these activities were still had to be defined. A whole range of scheduled meetings was postponed indefinitely, including the large European Conference on Rural Life, which had been in preparation for years.[11] But new tasks presented themselves almost immediately. On September 14, 1939 the Romanian minister of health called attention to the Polish refugees streaming into his country and asked whether any coordination of antiepidemic activities had been planned for countries involved.[12] This demand, with its eerie sense of déjà-vu, seemed an invitation to relive the past. To a large extent, the LNHO owed its creation to a massive typhus epidemic that had raged in eastern Europe after

World War I nineteen years earlier.[13] However, this time around, the task was limited—and partly spoken for. After his return from a fact-finding mission to Bucharest, Budapest, and Belgrade, Gautier reported that the number of Polish refugees was limited and that no more were to be expected, since the Red Army had invaded Poland. Health problems were few and under control, though epidemics could not be precluded for the upcoming winter. In any case the American Red Cross was preparing to send drugs, disinfectants, and warm clothing.[14]

Nevertheless, relief for refugees became an important topic when Health Section members developed guidelines for the changed conditions. The LNHO, they claimed, must deal with new problems arising out of the war because at "a time when the movements of population and evacuations are creating important problems of nutrition and health protection, it [was] obvious that . . . no body [was] better fitted than the Health Organisation to give technical advice. . . ." In addition, some of the permanent services, for example, the Epidemiological Intelligence Service, the Singapore bureau, and the Commission on Biological Standardization, should be kept because, once interrupted, they would be difficult to restore.[15] Commissions should continue their work whenever "this could be done without placing too heavy a strain on the resources and staff of the Health Organisation."[16]

This plan appeared reasonable, but it presupposed the continuation of amiable relations among the international members. The Health Committee meeting of November 1939 made clear that such harmony could not be taken for granted. With the outbreak of war, even long-time committee members could not help regarding one another as allies or enemies. The majority openly sided with the Western allies. Parisot opened with words of sympathy and appreciation for the Polish colleagues whose whereabouts were unknown and hailed the presence of Dr. Jerzy Babecki, as a sign that Poland was "alive and true to its traditions." In a similar vein, the U.S. surgeon general, Hugh Cumming, greeted Parisot with "Vive la France." In contrast, the former long-time committee president, the serologist Thorvald Madsen of Denmark, was isolated in his pro-German sympathies. He had been instrumental in drawing Germany into the LNHO many years earlier. Now a French source reported him as blaming France and Great Britain for wanting to destroy Germany and flaunting maps of central Europe with much-reduced territory for Poland.[17] Even if logistically possible, further committee meetings might have proved politically difficult.

The Health Section recommendations were adopted with very minor changes.[18] The Health Committee never met again.

Efforts to reconceptualize the working "space" proved only partly successful. For some weeks, the issue of refugees and evacuations dominated LNHO attention. In January 1940, the Health Section began work on elaborate guidelines for health work before, during, and after large population transfers.[19] In retrospect, these activities appear naïve, since the upcoming reality of mass displacement would have little to do with these theoretical ideas for an orderly evacuation. Besides, they could seem like anticipatory subservience to the displacing powers. In fact, they were probably neither of these things but rather a frantic attempt to find and claim areas of recognized expertise. An exchange of views with national health agencies revealed broad interest in the issue but increasing security concerns, which made governments unwilling to disclose their plans.[20] Further discussions held on March 4–7, 1940 resulted in a lengthy paper that detailed a long list of measures to accompany population transfers.[21] In retrospect, the text reads more like guidelines for travel agencies serving groups with special health needs than rules for wartime activities.

The German occupation of Denmark and Norway in April–May 1940 brought the full reality of war to Geneva. Because an invasion of Switzerland seemed imminent, plans were made to relocate LNHO working space. In what appears to have been virtual panic and chaos, League archives were sent to Vichy, only to be returned a few days later.[22] Gautier would later recall "the incredible turmoil we experienced in May 1940, when half of our files were sent to Vichy in expectation of an exodus which never materialised."[23] But the League effectively disintegrated. During the summer, the Economic, Financial and Transit Department moved to Princeton, New Jersey. A little later the treasury and Refugee Department moved to London, the Drug Traffic Department to Washington, and the ILO to Montreal.[24] The Health Section remained in a corner of the now grotesquely oversized Palais des Nations, with plenty of space but few people and none of the sections with which they had cooperated in the past. League finances consisted almost entirely of payments by Great Britain and Commonwealth countries and of reserve funds from prewar times, forcing ever more drastic cuts in personnel.[25]

As of June 1940, the Health Section consisted of only a handful of people: Raymond Gautier as acting medical director; Yves Biraud, a French expert on epidemiology; and a small clerical staff.[26] The continuation of the LNHO for the following four years would rest on their shoulders. Thorvald Madsen, who had been the Health Committee president for nineteen years, wrote two postcards in German from occupied Copenhagen saying that his institute was continuing to produce sera, but that it was impossible for him to come to Geneva.[27] There was no more news from him until the end of the war. Meanwhile, his Belgian colleague on the Health Committee, René Sand, was deported to Germany.[28] Jacques Parisot, the current Health Committee president, was captured but released in October 1940 and returned to France. He did not contact the Health Section until April 1941 and then supplied supportive words but no tangible help.[29]

Evidently, the work of commissions on specific topics was no longer possible and the bulk of LNHO activities virtually collapsed. Biraud and Gautier had to find ways to act in what little space was left, with little money, unreliable mail service, expanding war zones, and difficult travel conditions, and with those few remaining colleagues who were neither mobilized nor deported nor dismissed for financial reasons. The permanent services dealing with biological standardization and epidemiological intelligence fared best. The Copenhagen Sera Institute was still operational and produced and distributed standards, but it had become part of the Axis world and could no longer supply all of Europe. As an emergency countermeasure, the British Medical Research Council decided to supply the standard sera to countries under Allied control, while emphasizing that the "real" standards were those in Copenhagen. Over the course of the war, both laboratories supplied thirty-five standard agents, reproduced these standards, and even adopted two new standards (for vitamin E and heparin).[30]

Under these circumstances, serving as a clearinghouse of information on all health-related matters became a relatively more important part of the Health Section work. Routine correspondence had been a necessary but unloved duty for many years. Now it became a central task because it ensured visibility. Yves Biraud answered requests, drawing on a collection of five thousand technical reports, now referred to as "documentation centre" and carefully documented them.[31] In return, various humanitarian organizations, such as the American Friends Service Committee, sent their reports to Geneva.[32] This exchange of information, mostly on infectious diseases or on hygienic conditions in refugee camps was helpful, but processing a little over one request per week could hardly be considered proof of indispensability.

The Epidemiological Intelligence Service became another cornerstone of wartime activity. But difficulties increased as military security concerns reduced the amount of data governments were willing to communicate, and the expansion of warfare progressively restricted the service's sphere of action.[33] The Far Eastern Bureau ceased receiving data from Indochina in early 1940, followed by India and the other British colonies, and it closed hastily just days before the occupation of Singapore in February 1942.[34] This was a grave setback, since the epidemiological data of virtually all of Asia, Australia, and the Indian Ocean region had traveled through this bureau. Its employees had been able to escape to Australia but were unable to establish a substitute base there.[35] The loss of the Far Eastern Bureau was grievous not only for practical reasons. Whoever had access to and control over data and transfer lines in that area could justifiably claim competence for international health issues in a large part of the world.

Other disruptions were more unexpected. Yves Biraud was surprised to find that after September 1940, U.S. Public Health Reports no longer arrived at the LNHO. Since they continued to reach other European health institutions, this failure was obviously not accidental. Biraud commented drily, "It does seem hard luck that there should be more interference with the communications from our friends than with communications from our 'enemies'!"[36] His comment reveals the awkwardness of the LNHO's situation. Although it was officially neutral, its sympathies were certainly on the Allied side. But abandoning the principle of neutrality would go against the law of the League and would mean the loss of Axis epidemiological data, on which the service increasingly relied. In 1940, the price of neutrality was U.S. data.

It was also potential embarrassment. In 1942, a member of Parliament, apparently aware of League information material naming Germany as a recipient of LNHO data, asked the British government which countries had received advice on health matters from the League in recent months. The Foreign Office staff feared that this information might strengthen opponents of the League. But as Neville Goodman, a former member of the LNHO Committee and a senior official in the British ministry of health, made clear, His Majesty's Government was not concerned about possible advantages Germany might gain from LNHO information. On the contrary, "the British health authorities would very much regret any action being taken which led to any fettering of the League's discretion to answer such enquiries, since the League was able to obtain in return valuable information from enemy countries which became immediately available to British authorities."[37] Goodman was unconcerned about Allied information reaching Germany, because, assuming that everything he sent to Geneva would eventually find its way to Germany, he only sent nonsensitive data. He was convinced that Great Britain was gaining more valuable insight into Germany than vice versa.[38] This episode reveals the intensity of the wartime trade in information in Geneva: representatives of governments and humanitarian and international relief organizations traded information, goods, and favors.[39] For a while, the former German Health Section member, Otto Olsen, regularly informed the German Health Bureau about LNHO activities. He received documents from Yves Biraud, who sometimes added good wishes to the bureau president, Hans Reiter. Olsen then sent reports on recent LNHO work to Germany.[40] Thus, at this point neutrality may have worked in the sense that it preserved a flow of information. The German attitude to this flow is unknown. If Germany was as confident as Britain, the LNHO may merely have preserved some working space for itself by distributing useless information.

For Biraud, isolated in Geneva, the increasing unpopularity of the League made it tempting to abandon neutrality. In September 1940, Biraud sought the views of the Rockefeller Foundation about potential options for the LNHO: separating completely from the League but staying in Geneva, or staying with the League but transferring to the United States, either to Washington, DC or to Princeton.[41] Either way, he believed the Health Section and particularly his beloved Epidemiological Intelligence Service would be more viable than they were under current conditions. Neither option materialized. Acting Secretary General Seán Lester was unwilling to transfer the Health Section for fear that the departure of this last body might result in Swiss pressure to close down the Secretariat completely, which would deal a fatal blow to the League of Nations.[42] And the Rockefeller Foundation showed no interest in adopting the Health Section.

Roughly eighteen months later, a different option presented itself. In January 1942, Britain's War Office foresaw an urgent need for nutrition in large parts of Europe, which would have to be met at the end of the war. In view of the predictable pressure on limited shipping space, the War Office considered it "prudent to accumulate stock not only of the essential bulk foods such as cereals but also proportionately large stock of the various concentrates which are now available to counteract specific dietetic deficiencies." In this context, they were interested in nutritional data in presently occupied countries: food rations consumed before and during the war, foodstuffs most suitable for distribution in concentrated form, vitamin-deficiency diseases, and similar information. Mindful of the interwar League work on nutrition, they asked Geneva for help.[43] Apparently, the information they received was so satisfactory that shortly afterward British authorities invited a member of the LNHO Health Section to London to cooperate with Allied bodies.[44] This choice between risking virtual dissolution by cutting the already minimal leftover staff in Geneva or risking irrelevance by missing out on essential developments in the international health scene cannot have been easy, particularly because the decision involved retaining or jettisoning the principle of neutrality.

In October 1942, Raymond Gautier moved to the League bureau in London. Together with inter-Allied services, he prepared contingency plans for the distribution of available resources in medical staff, sera, vaccines, drugs, and medical equipment to meet the most urgent needs of the countries presently occupied.[45] He remained in London until early 1943, by which time his work was essentially done. He was reluctant to return to Geneva, where both food and contacts were clearly more scarce than in London, and began sounding out opportunities in the United States.[46] In March 1943, a call from the State Department enabled him to cooperate with several Allied institutions in Washington. For three months he worked as a consultant for the Office of Foreign Relief and Rehabilitation Operations and then for another six months for the Office of Lend-Lease Administration.[47] These occupations would keep him in Washington until late 1944.

For his part, Yves Biraud remained as the only medical member of the Health Section in Geneva. Increasingly, he had to fight isolation, lack of resources, and intellectual theft as obscure, self-styled officials purported to represent new institutions seeking to encroach on the LNHO's domain.[48] Biraud's priority was to keep the Epidemiological Intelligence Service alive. He was still receiving regular reports from most European countries and limited data from overseas.[49] Although he had to suspend the monthly and yearly epidemiological reports, he did succeed in retaining the *Weekly Epidemiological Record* in Europe throughout the war.[50] Increasingly, epidemiological service became an argument for LNHO existence and legitimacy. The second central LNHO publication, the *Health Bulletin*, whose continuation had been much in doubt in May 1940, endured, although it appeared less frequently.[51] For these publications, Biraud had to draw on prewar papers and on the standardization projects based in the laboratories in Copenhagen and Hampstead.

Defining International Health—Claiming Space for the Postwar Period

During the winter of 1942–43, as the defeat of Germany was coming into sight, planning for the future began to dominate international health discourse. In October 1942, before Raymond Gautier's departure, Yves Biraud was already sketching preliminary ideas.[52] From London, abandoning all pretence of neutrality, Gautier discredited the Office International d'Hygiène Publique (OIHP), whose director, Robert Pierret, he claimed, was "more Nazi than the Nazis."[53] In an elaborate draft plan, he imagined pooling the best of interwar public and private organizations and associations. In phrases later transposed to the World Health Organization charters, he laid down the principle of health as "more than the absence of illness . . . namely, physical, mental and moral fitness."[54] Prewar LNHO studies had already made strides in this direction, and, he stressed, they should form the basis of postwar efforts.

Two weeks later, he repeated his ideas in comments on a project under discussion in Washington circles that linked a future health organization to relief and to plans for a United Nations organization. A permanent health organization, he insisted, should be separate from relief and should benefit from interwar experience. In particular, such experience should inform consideration of a decision-making committee of the organization, which could be in the hands of leading independent scientists (the LNHO policy), or of government representatives (the OIHP policy). The former approach would ensure innovative ideas and scientific excellence, whereas the latter would ensure that ideas carried weight in the real world. Gautier opted for a "mixture of both—officials and non-officials" as "the only workable proposition." He sketched an organization whose advisory council would consist of representatives of national health administrations but was otherwise practically identical to the structure of the present LNHO. The main decision-making body, the health committee, would continue to consist of "experts selected for their technical knowledge."[55]

This design would form the basis of all succeeding plans. Half a year later, in October 1943, Biraud called for an "amalgamation of international health institutions" that would eliminate the competition and mistrust that existed between the LNHO and the OIHP. His proposed Health Assembly, consisting of heads of national health administrations, would have a mainly consultative function. A Managing Health Committee would represent the assembly and would be responsible for most administrative activities. Daily work would rest with the Secretariat and its director. Various regional offices would ensure its global scope and extra-European work.[56] To create a unified health organization, the OIHP would have to be dissolved. This measure had been tried after World War I but had failed due to the political clout that the OIHP wielded in several countries. Now, to ensure success, Biraud was willing to entertain the idea of an OIHP-type of Health Assembly. As he admitted in a letter to Secretary General Seán Lester:

> [T]he amalgamation I proposed is really an absorption of the Office by the League's Health Organisation. . . . This was inspired by the study of the opposition aroused to the absorption of the Office in a more comprehensive League Organisation in 1920–21.[57]

Meanwhile, events were unfolding at different places and in uncontrollable ways. In May 1943, an Allied meeting in Hot Springs, Virginia laid the foundation for an international agency in charge of food and agriculture, the future Food and Agriculture Organization (FAO). In November 1943, early Allied relief initiatives received a larger international framework when forty-three countries signed the United States–sponsored institution of a United Nations Relief and Rehabilitation Administration (UNRRA), which counted international health work as part of its task.[58] Due to unprecedented funding, UNRRA developed into the largest-ever body for international health work. In 1946 alone, it spent $82 million, as compared with $414,000 for the LNHO in 1931.[59]

These new agencies affected Biraud's assessment of LNHO options in late 1943. He identified three priorities—feeding and nutrition, reconstruction and housing, and the fight against epidemics—all of which had been major fields of work for the LNHO before the war. Responsibility for nutrition had now gone to the FAO, whereas practical work on epidemics became the province of UNRRA, which left housing as the only issue of importance where the LNHO faced no competition. Biraud urged Parisot, Secretary General Lester, and Neville Goodman of the British Ministry of Health to support a new initiative in the field, but remained unsuccessful.[60] Instead, UNRRA began expanding its activities in the field of health and became interested in utilizing LNHO expertise. After some exchange of views in the spring of 1944 with Secretary General Lester about cooperation, Herbert

H. Lehman, the director general of UNRRA, suggested the institution of an LNHO "research unit" to interpret data from Geneva and other sources and to assist UNRRA in gaining a realistic assessment of health conditions in Europe and Asia. On May 15, 1944, the new unit—consisting of Gautier, the LNHO statisticians Knud Stouman and Zygmunt Deutschman, and several clerks—began work.[61] In the following months, it issued a weekly digest of recent developments on one or two infectious diseases, but to Gautier's disappointment, the flow of information was quite one sided from the LNHO to UNRRA. Worse, direct communication between the LNHO and Allied government authorities was not welcome, and Gautier felt excluded from crucial UNRRA meetings. In addition, he faced an uphill struggle with his efforts to resurrect the Far Eastern Bureau in India or Australia. But his ideas clashed with stiff competition: Allied plans favored an UNRRA institution in Chungking, China.[62] And the OIHP director, Pierret, tried to rebuild a bureau in Saigon.[63]

In 1943, Biraud attempted to mark out new spheres of competence. He began focusing on *Health Bulletin* publications. Fulfilling a request of the International Red Cross, he put together a multilingual glossary of over five thousand terms dealing with infectious diseases in twenty-four languages. Several hundred reprints were distributed to the Red Cross and other pertinent institutions.[64] Later volumes included a report on "hunger disease and its treatment in detention camps," written by Joseph Weill of the Oeuvre de Secours aux Enfants (OSE) and describing the activities of humanitarian organizations in detention camps in southern France.[65] A subsequent assessment of public health in Europe painted a surprisingly positive picture: there had been neither an extraordinary rise in the mortality rate nor an outbreak of a large epidemic, although some infectious diseases, such as diphtheria, scarlet fever, meningitis, and typhus had increased regionally. Malnutrition had probably increased the tuberculosis rate and the mortality rate among elderly people, but serious famine existed only in Greece and in prisons, detention camps, underprivileged urban quarters, and ghettos.[66] Biraud was quite aware of the relatively positive note of his study and sought to distance himself from other, more somber reports that he considered counterproductive. In a letter to Gautier, he criticized "the kind of alarmist propaganda based on selective material, such as has been issued by the I.L.O. on 'Health of Youth in Occupied Europe,' produced in 1943," which, he felt, had misled Allied journalists and, when found wrong, actually impeded relief work.[67] Gautier sought to distribute Biraud's study of health in wartime Europe in special reprints in the Anglo-Saxon countries as "proof [of] our vitality."[68]

For the same reason, Biraud insisted on a revival of the *Chronicle of the Health Organisation,* an information brochure created in 1939 but suspended in 1940. But this step only highlighted the main problems. By 1944, mail service had so deteriorated that a regular exchange of information even between Biraud and Gautier was all but impossible, leaving Biraud to reconstruct developments in Washington from short, cryptic cables.

At this time, with the perceived need to update the 1926 Sanitary Convention to regulate air and sea travel, international sanitary cooperation became topical. The Health Research Unit estimated that after the war, 50 million people would be on the move.[69] This prospect, coupled with medical advances, particularly against yellow fever, made regulations and control urgent. In May 1943, a committee of quarantine experts set up by UNRRA drafted the revisions of the 1933 and 1926 conventions that secured provisional agreement at the second UNRRA conference in Montréal in September.[70] As UNRRA assumed direct responsibility for administering epidemiological data, a supplementary "research unit" became superfluous. However, since the unit's members and their LNHO contacts were the leading experts around Washington UNRRA, it was suggested that the unit's statistical staff get leave to remain in Washington on UNRRA's payroll. The LNHO statistician Knud Stouman recommended this strategy because anything else would have meant "sawing off the branch on which" the LNHO was sitting.[71]

After the dissolution of the "research unit," Gautier's presence in Washington became pointless. He remained in London, where he had helped organize a penicillin conference, and eventually rejoined Biraud in Geneva in the early summer of 1945. Meanwhile, Stouman and his LNHO statistician-colleague Zygmunt Deutschman transferred to UNRRA in London and Washington, respectively.[72]

Meanwhile, Biraud was losing ground in his attempts to keep hegemony over epidemiological services. Toward the end of 1944, UNRRA opened its own service to handle the data of the signatory countries of the Sanitary Convention, while the OIHP would act on behalf of the neutrals and others not wishing to sign.[73] Including a service run by the Allied military, this brought to four the number of existing epidemiological services.[74] None of the Allied parties (neither Soviet nor English nor American) sent data to Geneva.[75] Biraud's control over information evaporated as the Allied front advanced.[76] In November 1944, he considered moving to Britain to join the London UNRRA office. Gautier disagreed. He feared that in joining forces with UNRRA, the LNHO Epidemiological Intelligence Service would end its neutral stand and thereby lose its distinctive nature. Besides, by tying its fate to a temporary institution such as UNRRA, it might forfeit its chance to join a new international organization.[77] Biraud reluctantly conceded: contravening the principle of neutrality, he even offered to suspend sending the epidemiological weekly to Germany and German-controlled territories if the Americans would provide their data.[78] By that time, neutrality seemed increasingly like a luxury of the past.

Toward a New Organization

The new focus was staking claims for the postwar world. The arrangements made at Hot Springs, Virginia in 1943 had already set a precedent in the field of nutrition. When conditions began to improve in Paris after its liberation in late August 1944, the OIHP made an unexpected comeback with its claim to be a caretaker of the Sanitary Conventions. Having sought refuge in the French provincial town of Royat, the OIHP had for years retained only minimal mailing contact with the outside world via its Swiss member.[79] In Gautier's and Biraud's views, it was profoundly discredited by its pro-Axis leanings. But in late 1944, as in 1920, the French government, which disliked the prospect of the future health body located outside France with a predominantly non-French staff, urged the maintenance of the OIHP.[80] However, French insistence weakened when it became clear that UNESCO would be placed in the French capital.[81] Robert Pierret was supported by Britain. British views were certainly influenced by Pierret's links to M. T. Morgan, a senior official in the British Ministry of Health.[82] But more important, the British government hoped to gain French agreement to a temporary administration of a draft sanitary convention by UNRRA in exchange for support for OIHP. The government also saw the OIHP as a counterbalance to the social approach of the LNHO, whose focus on state responsibilities for the well-being of populations and on international intervention threatened deeply ingrained British traditions of liberalism, limited public welfare, and national sovereignty. The activist approach of the LNHO may also have raised the specter of the equality of League members, a prospect against which Melville Mackenzie, an official of the British Ministry of Health who had worked for the Health Section for fifteen years, railed in 1942. He proposed

> to frame the Constitution of the Committee that, in voting, each country carries a weight in proportion to its responsibilities and the amount its resources allow it to play in the development of its own health services as well as in international collaboration.

As a solution, he recommended the OIHP principle that member countries were entitled to different numbers of votes according to the amount of their annual contribution.[83]

Voting in categories was no longer publicly discussed in 1945, but the basic concerns were played out in controversies over who should sit in the decision-making body of the new health organization. Spokesmen for the British Ministry of Health criticized the inclusion of experts, who were not government representatives and who could therefore not commit their governments.[84] This line of argument reversed course from the British prewar insistence that LNHO decisions should *not* commit governments. Presumably, the idea was not so much that representatives would commit their governments but that these governments would commit their representatives and the body they sat in. Thus, the new institution would be much less likely to voice demands or proclaim governmental duties. In this vein, existing OIHP structures were eminently compatible with British desires for governmental freedom of action.

This view was diametrically opposed to LNHO traditions and to Gautier's schemes for the future, and consequently no friendly thoughts about the LNHO could be expected from London. In fact, for a while, the LNHO tended to be overlooked altogether. A member of the British Foreign Office referred to the LNHO as "a sort of rival office of the Paris office" which "was not looked very friendly on by our health authorities" and whose activities should not be revived.[85] In late 1944, London thinking envisioned a

> single international organisation connected with the Social and Economic Council of the United Nations and situated in the U.S.A. which would maintain a Bureau of central information and have the general direction of research. It would be linked with the Paris Office which would be concerned with quarantine regulations and possibly with another Bureau for the Standardisation of Drugs but these Offices would not be directly subordinate to it.[86]

British plans explicitly foresaw the "discontinuance, as such, of the Health Section of the League, its records, equipment and staff being transferred to the new organisation. . . ."[87]

For their part, during the interwar years American agencies had increasingly seen merit in a strong international health structure and were now determined to play a central role in it. Some of the new interest derived from visionary humanitarian concerns. Charles-Edward Winslow appealed to global responsibilities in the face of mass misery and to the capability of international health policies to "raise the world society to a level it has never known before."[88] The Senate Committee on Education and Labor found a more down-to-earth phrasing: "Improved world health will increase our markets."[89] Unlike their British colleagues, the Americans had no special preference for the OIHP or its model. Nor did they support the LNHO, which they perceived as no longer functioning. U.S. opinion favored a fresh start with a totally new organization, preferably with a seat in Washington, DC.[90] At the same time, plans included the survival of the Pan-American Sanitary Bureau and possibly the establishment of other regional offices.[91]

Gautier's and Biraud's earlier plans had been little more than "a concealed pro-League plea."[92] As it became increasingly clear that the days of both the LNHO and the League were numbered, Gautier and Biraud turned their efforts to saving several central elements: a single, unified health institution; a holistic idea about health as more than the mere absence of disease;

a strong focus on social medicine; a tripartite structure with an assembly, a secretariat, and a committee that would be a scientific "brain trust"; and preferably a seat in Europe.[93]

There was a real struggle over the location. International health was felt to be primarily organized by Europeans, and—probably more important—Biraud feared that a seat in the United States would place the new institution in the hands of the Pan-American Sanitary Organization.[94] Geneva proved acceptable to most countries, except the U.S.S.R., which remained bitterly opposed to everything that smacked of the League, from which it had been expelled in 1940.[95]

There was substantial consensus on some other points. Almost everybody wanted an institution with a tripartite structure, an epidemiological intelligence service, some sort of standardization agency, a clearinghouse for health-related information, assistance to national health services, and technical commissions on individual topics. Other controversies concerned the degree of autonomy of the future health organization from the emerging United Nations Organization (UNO), whether the future members of the decision-making body of the health organization should necessarily represent governments, and the extent to which prewar institutions would survive or be carried over into new institutions.

In 1945 these discussions on the future international health organization were dominated by the establishment of the United Nations. In San Francisco in April 1945, the votes of the Brazilian and Chinese delegates ensured that the United Nations would take charge of international health.[96] To influence subsequent lively discussions, Gautier tried to publicize in Washington his and Biraud's plan to amalgamate the LNHO and the OIHP but initially met with little interest. Indeed, the situation was very confusing because people met and discussed plans in various circles, and it was difficult even for insiders to detect any coherent development. Biraud and Gautier hoped that some of their friends from earlier LNHO times might inform them if and when something tangible evolved.[97]

Although the LNHO had maintained a continuous, albeit minimal, existence, many of its prewar members were scattered in different parts of Europe with little knowledge of each other or the state of affairs. Thorvald Madsen wrote a bewildered note to Gautier asking, "Have you had any contact with the other members and who are they now? What about Parisot?"[98] Jacques Parisot had been arrested by the Gestapo in June 1944 and taken to a concentration camp in Czechoslovakia as a hostage. At the time, Biraud had undertaken an intense campaign for his release, using all official and inofficial contacts available. These efforts did not free Parisot, but Biraud did succeed in supplying him with urgently needed medicine via the YMCA.[99] In May 1945, Parisot was freed from captivity, but in July, there was still no contact with him. Andrija Štampar had survived four years in a concentration camp and resumed teaching social medicine in Zagreb, and Witold Chodzko was also alive. Biraud and Gautier considered the need for a Health Committee meeting but doubted its usefulness before the development of the United Nations became clearer.[100] Nevertheless, Gautier tried to fill the ranks of the Committee, finding substitutes for those members, such as the Turkish member Husamettin Kural, who had not survived the war. To avoid completely new faces, he persuaded the secretary general to appoint former associates such as René Sand and Alfred Gigon as substitute members.[101] Toward the end of 1945, Gautier discussed the idea of calling a meeting with influential committee members of prewar times, such as Thorvald Madsen, Hugh Cumming, and René Sand, but met with little enthusiasm.[102] Parisot, who would naturally have been in charge of convening such a meeting, remained strangely vague and inactive on this issue.[103]

Gautier's efforts to revive commissions on particular subjects, such as the standardization commission, the malaria commission or the expert group on pharmacopeia were similarly unsuccessful. The reconstitution of any LNHO commission was hampered by the lack of expert personnel and funds and a decline in international interest in LNHO activities. The liberation of Singapore in 1945 temporarily improved chances for the reopening of the Far Eastern Bureau. Gautier received authorization from the League Supervisory Commission for six months of funding. But UNRRA had founded two independent offices in Chungking and Sydney, and the British were urging them to reopen the Singapore office as well. Consequently, the idea of an LNHO-organized Far Eastern Bureau provoked resistance in London.[104]

In the fall of 1945, Biraud and Gautier once again revised their draft constitution into an even more elaborate and detailed paper, using the FAO constitution as a model. To give the draft a more conservative touch, they highlighted the role of government officials in the Health Assembly; to compensate, Gautier added a preamble that contained the more social, progressive elements.[105] The chances for Biraud's and Gautier's ideas were improved somewhat by the change in government in Great Britain.[106] However, Gautier still felt that, "[i]n the minds of our British colleagues it means a representative of the Ministry of Health. Enough said!"[107]

Gautier and Biraud sent their draft and further explanations to numerous key people, especially in the Anglo-Saxon world, notably Hugh Cumming, Melville Mackenzie, Jacques Parisot, René Sand, Charles-Edward Winslow, Thorvald Madsen, Knud Stouman, and Frank Boudreau. Clearly, the draft it made its way into many places, including the U.S. State Department.[108] In addition, they presented a detailed plan for the next steps necessary in establishing the organization they proposed.[109] Listing these activities was an act of some *chutzpah*, considering that so far nobody had asked their advice or even their opinion. An interdepartmental body under the chairmanship of Surgeon General Thomas Parran began working on plans. In October 1945, forty U.S. health experts, invited by the State Department, met to consider ideas for a totally new organization. The chief issue was the extent to which this body should be allowed to interfere with national policies.[110] Only few of those present, such as the former surgeon general Hugh Cumming or Frank Boudreau of the Milbank Memorial Fund had prewar experience in the field, an indication of the extent to which these preparations broke with the past.[111] The principal architects of international health in the United States and Great Britain, James Doull (of the State Department) and Melville Mackenzie, hoped to restrict the planning activity to a small group of people. Although this strategy proved impractical, it was clear that the important questions would be decided in Washington and London.[112]

In December, Biraud traveled to the United States, ostensibly for a meeting on multiple causes of death, but he used his stay in Washington and a stopover in London to propagate LNHO views regarding the future health organization and the Far Eastern Bureau. In London, he found a willingness to cooperate with a reopened bureau among those powers with a vested interest in the area—the French, Dutch, and Chinese—but still stiff resistance from the British, who appeared to rely on a perceived direct agreement between the South Eastern Asia Command and UNRRA.[113] Biraud's stopover in London on his way back from Washington coincided with the crucial meeting of the UN Economic and Social Council in February. Health was not a priority issue in that context. Only one representative of health concerns was present: Andrija Štampar , who was, however, vice president of the meeting. Štampar had frequently cooperated with the LNHO during recent years, and had even briefly been a member of the Health Section. His close ties to the LNHO, particularly his former friendship with Ludwik Rajchman, ensured his attention to ideas emanating from Geneva. In fact, on his way to London, Štampar had passed through Geneva, where he received a briefing from Gautier and another draft constitution by Biraud. Having Štampar, a man of no apparent direct LNHO connections, present these ideas was useful "*pour éviter certaines susceptibilités.*"[114]

The preparation of the founding conference for the new health organization was entrusted to the Technical Preparatory Committee.[115] Its chairmanship was first offered to Biraud, but "strong opposition" (interestingly, from other quarters than the OIHP) to him and his identification with LNHO ideas was an obstacle.[116] Retroactive changes in the resolution of the meeting upgraded the standing of the OIHP as institution and Paris as locale, leading Biraud to suspect behind-the-scenes meddling by Pierret.[117] Indeed, by that time, Pierret's activities went hand in hand with last-minute French attempts to influence the postwar health scene. At the invitation of the French government, two OIHP meetings in April and October 1946 enjoyed a somewhat larger format than called for in regular committee work, bringing together some ninety to 110 participants who received special rations of wine, spirits, Champagne, and cigarettes—material "arguments" that were beyond LNHO means.[118]

Yet gradually, Biraud's and Gautier's strategy appeared to pay off. Whether by chance or due to their tireless efforts, the steps taken toward a new health organization followed Biraud's suggestions. Conceptual thinking in Washington also came very close to LNHO concepts.[119] From March 18 to April 5, 1946, the Technical Preparatory Committee met under the chairmanship of René Sand, a member of the last emergency subcommittee of the LNHO, who had been released from German detention. Biraud and Parisot represented the LNHO. Other participants with prewar ties to the LNHO—although they now took part in different capacities—included Andrija Štampar , Hugh Cumming, and Neville Goodman (long-time members both of the Committee and of the OIHP); Wilson Jameson (a member of the commissions on health effects of the depression and on housing); Martin Kacprzak (a member of committees on rural life and on the revision of the international list of causes of death); and Melville Mackenzie (a long-time member of the LNHO Health Section).[120] The Technical Preparatory Committee worked out a draft constitution of the future international health organization.[121] Special subcommittees discussed several related issues, among them the relation between the future organization and existing institutions. Here, Biraud fought—unsuccessfully—to gain support for the reopening of the Far Eastern Bureau in Singapore. Pierret fought—also unsuccessfully—to gain support for the continued independence of the OIHP.[122]

In the end, conceptual planning proved more influential than political clout. In the summer of 1946, a month-long conference of representatives of sixty-one countries worked out a constitution for a new World Health Organization, whose LNHO roots were undeniable. In the end, Gautier and Biraud's hope for a single, united institution was realized. The introductory sentence in its constitution—"Health is a state of complete physical, mental and social well-being and not merely the absence of disease or infirmity"— was derived directly from Gautier's wartime writing and reflected the strong social approach to health issues that the WHO inherited from the LNHO.[123] Similarly, the organizational structure, though vastly more elaborate, was based on the plan Biraud had drafted in October 1943.[124]

The later fate of the WHO further confirmed its LNHO legacy. Its seat has been in Geneva, and for several years it was in the premises of the former League. The breadth of its work program surpassed the objectives of all previous organizations, but it bears closest resemblance to the LNHO with its seemingly unlimited scope.[125] Practically all of the agenda items were derived in some way from work of the LNHO, particularly its work on standardization of biological agents; on lists of pharmacopeia, diseases, and causes of death; on epidemiological intelligence; on vital statistics; and on a large number of specific diseases. Naturally, over the course of the last decades, more diseases have been added than the LNHO could have approached during its short life.[126] Serial publications include the *Bulletin,* the *Weekly Epidemiological Record,* and the annual *World Health Report,* all of which were begun by the LNHO.

By comparison, the OIHP, despite the support it enjoyed in government circles, fared much worse. None of its key elements—a focus on sanitary conventions, a uninational staff, voting power of countries according to categories of financial contribution, and a function as strictly a service institution to governments—survived. It is in the membership of the WHO Assembly and the Executive Committee, comprising both officials of health administrations and independent experts, that some of its legacy has remained.

An interim commission was formed in the summer of 1946 to bridge the time interval until the WHO became operational.[127] Biraud became deputy executive secretary under Brock Chisholm. In that position, he offered new WHO contracts to LNHO staff members in Geneva. In August 1946, he transmitted his satisfaction with developments to Seán Lester:

> To you I may add that the survival of the traditions of the Health Organization of the League in the W.H.O. is assured not only by the transfer of its functions but also by the transfer of its staff which, on my suggestion, the Interim Commission and the Executive Secretary have readily agreed to.[128]

In October 1946, all LNHO functions were transferred to the WHO.[129]

Conclusion

In retrospect, it is fascinating to observe how an institution dealt with the steady and inexorable disappearance of its working space. After a frustrating struggle to defend the LNHO's remaining but shrinking territory, the last members switched strategies, turning their attention to the enormous space opened up by the creation of new postwar organizations. Echoing unrelated processes going on elsewhere, the LNHO was an institution without space in search of space without an institution. This adaptability made possible the successful transfer of key LNHO characteristics—such as epidemiological research, metastudies, and inquiries into the social determinants of health—into WHO space. We can read the narrative of the LNHO during World War II as a case study in translocation as a strategy for intellectual survival in the face of institutional erosion.

Notes

I would like to thank the *Deutsche Forschungsgemeinschaft* for its generous support of the research project on the League of Nations Health Organization, GR 880, which has made work on this paper possible.

1. Recommendation of the International Health Conference Relating to the Establishment of an International Health Organisation under the League, April 16, 1920, Assembly Document 14 (12/3943/126), League of Nations Archive, Geneva (hereafter LNA); Rules of Procedure of the Health Committee, undated, C.H. 197, LNA.

2. "Report of the Health Organisation for the Period October 1932 to September 1933," *Bulletin of the Health Organisation* 2 (1933): 543.

3. Database established by Rainer Karczewski and Iris Borowy as part of an ongoing research project on the League of Nations Health Organization.

4. See J. Barros, *Betrayal from Within* (New Haven and London: Yale University Press, 1969), 186–88; "Composition du Comité d´Hygiène," author unknown, Note pour le Ministre, January 11, 1939, série SDN. IL—Hygiène, Nr. 1562, Archive of the Ministère des Affaires étrangères, Paris (hereafter MAE).

5. See J. A. Gillespie, "Social Medicine, Social Security and International Health 1940–60," in *The Politics of the Healthy Life*, ed. E. Rodríguez-Ocaña (Sheffield: EAHMH, 2002), 222.

6. F. P. Walters, *A History of the League of Nations* (London: Oxford University Press, 1952; reprint: 1969), 802.

7. Ministre de la Santé Publique to Président du Conseil, Ministre de la Défense Nationale et de la Guerre, Composition du Comité d´Hygiène, June 13, 1939, and attached scheme outline, untitled, unsigned, and undated, série SDN. IL—Hygiène, Nr. 1562, MAE; Président du Conseil to Ministre des Affaires étrangères, Composition du Comité d´Hygiène, July 4, 1939, série SDN. IL—Hygiène, Nr. 1562, MAE; Ministre des Affaires étrangères to Président du Conseil, Ministère de la Défense nationale et de la Guerre, Composition du Comité d´Hygiène, stamped July 27, 1939, série SDN. IL—Hygiène, Nr. 1562, MAE.

8. Biraud to Dunn, November 20, 1939, R 6202, 8D/38544/1993, LNA.

9. Czeslaw Wroczynski was found in a Soviet prisoner of war camp. Ludwik Anigstein moved to New York. Rudolf Weigl, director of the Biology Institute of the University of Lwow and father of the typhus vaccine, stayed at an institute in Lwow. Marcin Kacprzak, Josef Celarek, Gustaw Szulc, Zygmunt Rudolf, Alexander Szniolis, and Witold Chodzko all were in Warsaw. See correspondence, Health Section and ICRC, winter 1939–40, R 6062, 8A/39646/985, LNA.

10. Gautier to Selskar Gunn, November 15, 1939, RG 1.1, Series 100, Box 22, Folder 181 (hereafter 1.1/100/22/181), Rockefeller Archive Center, Tarrytown, New York (hereafter RAC).

11. Note on the Continuation of the Health Organisation's Studies in the Fields of Nutrition, Housing, Physical Fitness and Clothing, August 21, 1939, 2, C.H. 1429, LNA; League of Nations, *Chronicle of the Health Organisation*, vol. I, no. 11 (November 1, 1939) in SDN Chronique de l'Organisation d'Hygiène 1939–1945, Collection No. 934–5 (hereafter Chronique) 70, LNA; League of Nations, *Chronicle of the Health Organisation*, Special Number, December 1945, Chronique, 3–4, LNA.

12. Médecin Général N. Marinesco, Ministre de la Santé Publique de Roumanie to LNHO, September 14, 1939, R 6149, 8A/39052/39052, LNA.

13. M. A. Balinska, "Assistance and Not Mere Relief: The Epidemic Commission of the League of Nations, 1920–1923," in *International Health Organizations and Movements, 1918–1939*, ed. P. Weindling, 81–108 (Cambridge: Cambridge University Press, 1995).

14. Gautier estimated that there were ten thousand refugees in Romania and six thousand in Hungary. Report by Dr. R. Gautier on His Mission to Romania, Hungary, and Yugoslavia, October 3, 1939, R 6149, 8A/39052/39052, C.H. 1430, LNA; Gautier to Cumming, October 9, 1939, R 6149, 8A/39052/39052, LNA.

15. This regulation applied to work on cancer of the cervix uteri, heroic drugs, rabies, certain malaria studies, and nutrition in Asia.

16. Thirty-First Session of the Health Committee, Current Work of the Health Organisation and Adaptation of its Activities to Present Circumstances, November 15, 1939, 14–16, C.H. 1443, LNA.

17. Memorandum, untitled and unsigned, November 26, 1939, 193–96, SDN, IL-Hygiène 1561, MAE.

18. League of Nations, *Chronicle of the Health Organisation*, vol. I, no. 12 (December 1, 1939), Chronique, 75, LNA.

19. Medical Aspects of Evacuation, November 1, 1940, R 6149, 8A/39701/39545, LNA.

20. Gautier, Problèmes d´ordre Médical et Sanitaire soulevés par les Evacuations, January 27, 1940, R 6149, 8A/39823/39545, LNA. Bela Johan, in the Hungarian Ministry of Interior, feared excessive secrecy. B. Johan, Ministère Royal Hongrois de l'Intérieur, to Gautier, February 9, 1940, R 6149, 8A/39701/39545, LNA.

21. They included the constant presence of doctors and nurses; preparations at the place of arrival (including the presence of doctors, dentists, public health officers, sanitary inspectors, midwives, health visitors, social workers, and personnel of the Red Cross and first-aid organizations); systematic vaccinations; special care for the elderly, pregnant women, and children; and in particular, the comprehensive coordination of all activities by all relevant authorities. Medico-Social Questions Arising out of the Movements of Civil Populations, March 12, 1940, C.H. 1448 (1), LNA.

22. Walters, *A History of the League of Nations*, 809.

23. Gautier to Aykroyd, October 24, 1941, R 6076, 8A/38171/2133, LNA.

24. Walters, *A History of the League of Nations*, 809.

25. Walters, *A History of the League of Nations*, 810. But in 1941, the budget was only a third of what it had been during the past three years, and it was shrinking further. Record of an Inter-Allied Meeting to discuss the work of the Supervisory Commission of the League of Nations, undated, FO 371/26662, Public Record Office, London (hereafter PRO).

26. League of Nations, *Chronicle of the Health Organisation*, Special Number, December 1945, Chronique, 5–6, LNA.

27. Madsen to Gautier, July 5 and 24, 1940, R 6061, 8A/3931/985, LNA.

28. N. Goodman, *International Health Organizations and Their Work*, 2nd ed. (Edinburgh and London: Churchill Livingstone, 1971), 132.

29. Cramer, ICRC, to Gautier, October 11, 1940, R 6062, 8A/13441/985, LNA; Parisot to Secretary General, April 19, 1941, R 6062, 8A/13441/985, LNA.

30. League of Nations, *Chronicle of the Health Organisation*, Special Number, April 1945, Chronique, 3–10, LNA.

31. The *Chronicle of the Health Organisation*, a brochure in which the Health Section presented its work, gave detailed lists: in 1941, the LNHO received sixty-five requests from seventeen countries, among them seven from international institutions and twenty-seven from national or regional health bureaus. League of Nations, *Chronicle of the Health Organisation*, Special Number, October 1943, Chronique, 8–9, LNA; League of Nations, *Chronicle of the Health Organisation*, Special Number, December 1945, Chronique, 6, LNA.

32. See various correspondence in R 6149, 8A/39701/39545 and LNA, R 6113, 8A/41753/11327, LNA.

33. League of Nations, *Chronicle of the Health Organisation*, Special Number, December 1945, Chronique, 6, LNA.

34. Biraud to Gautier (London), November 15, 1944, R 6159, 8A/42474/42474, LNA. L. Manderson, "Wireless Wars in the Eastern Arena: Epidemiological Surveillance, Disease Prevention and the Work of the Eastern Bureau of the League of Nations Health Organisation 1924–1942," in *International Health Organization and Movements, 1918–1939*, ed. P. Weindling (Cambridge: Cambridge University Press, 1995), 127–28.

35. League of Nations, *Chronicle of the Health Organisation*, Special Number, October 1943, Chronique, 6–7, LNA.

36. Biraud to Cumming, January 27, 1941, R 60601, 8A/4922/985, LNA. Biraud to V. Akin, U.S. Public Health Service, January 27, 1941, R 60601, 8A/4922/985, LNA.

37. Such information included data on typhus incidence in German-occupied countries. M. A. Williams, Parliamentary Questions, September 7 and 8, 1942, FO 371/30991, PRO.

38. M. A. Williams, Parliamentary Questions, September 7 and 8, 1942, FO 371/30991, PRO.

39. See J.-C. Favez, *The Red Cross and the Holocaust* (Cambridge: Cambridge University Press, 1999), 24.

40. See correspondence Olsen/Biraud/Reiter, 1941, R 6069, 8A/41083/1263, LNA.

41. Biraud to Sawyer, September 1, 1940, 1.1/100/22/181, RAC.

42. Deutschman to Strode, December 27, 1941, 1.1/100/22/181, RAC.

43. George Crystal to Acting Secretary General, February 6, 1942, 371/30991, PRO; A. Baster, Offices of the War Cabinet, to R. M. Makins, Foreign Office, January 13, 1942, 371/30991, PRO.

44. Neville Goodman, Ministry of Health, Whitehall, to Biraud, March 23, 1942, R 6151, 8A/42219/41674, LNA.

45. League of Nations, *Chronicle of the Health Organisation*, Special Number, December 1945, Chronique, 7, LNA; League of Nations, *Chronicle of the Health Organisation*, Special Number, October 1943, Chronique, 4–5, LNA.

46. Gautier, International Health of the Future, March 5, 1943, 1.1/100/22/182, RAC; Gautier to Cumming, January 27, 1943, R 6061, 8A/4922/985, LNA.

47. Gautier to Madsen, July 24, 1945, R 6061, 8A/3931/985, LNA; League of Nations, *Chronicle of the Health Organisation*, Special Number, October 1943, 4–5, LNA.

48. See correspondence in R 6151, 8A/41674/41674, LNA, and R 6062, 8A/13441/985, LNA.

49. Biraud to Aykroyd, March 21, 1943, R 6076, 8A/38171/2133, LNA.

50. Biraud to Urrutia, Santiago de Chile, May 21, 1941, R 6204, 8D/38544/1993, LNA.

51. Gautier to Aykroyd, May 31, 1940, R 6076, 8A/38171/2133, LNA; Biraud to Gautier, July 7, 1943, R 6083, 8A/8862/2353, LNA.

52. Biraud to Cumming, October 16, 1945, R 6150, 8A/41755/41755, LNA.

53. J. K. Roberts, General Department, memo of conversation, November 23, 1942, FO 371/30991, PRO. See also Gautier to Cumming, January 27, 1943, R 60601, 8A/4922/985, LNA; Gautier, International Health of the Future, March 15, 1943, 1.1/100/22/182, RAC.

54. Gautier, International Health of the Future, March 15, 1943, 1.1/100/22/182, RAC.

55. Gautier, Future Health Organisation, May 31, 1943, R 6150, 8A/42169/41755, LNA.

56. Biraud, Suggestions for the Post-War Amalgamation of International Health Institutions, October 25, 1944, R 6151, 8A/42231/41674, LNA.

57. Biraud to Lester, November 6, 1943, R 6150, 8A/42169/41755, LNA.

58. Goodman, *International Health Organizations*, 139–40.

59. Goodman, *International Health Organizations*, 138.

60. Biraud to Parisot, November 10, 1943, R 6062, 8A/13441/985, LNA; Biraud to Goodman, November 13, 1943, R 6062, 8A/35566/985, LNA.

61. "Dr. Gautier's material for P.G.'s report 1944," received December 18, 1944, R 6151, 8A/42231/41674, LNA; V. St., *Collaboration with UNRRA*, R 6151, 8A/42231/41674, LNA; Biraud, Staff for Washington League Health Unit, April 13, 1944, R 6151, 8A/42231/41674, LNA; League of Nations, *Chronicle of the Health Organisation*, Special Number, December 1945, 7–10, LNA; Deutschman to Strode, December 27, 1941, 1.1/100/22/181, RAC; Lester to Jacklin, March 23, 1944, 1.1/100/22/181–82, RAC.

62. Gautier, Research Unit Washington, to Jacklin, LON Treasury, London, summer 1944, received in Geneva December 1944, R 6150, 8A/4247/4247, LNA; Gautier, "The Reasons for Reopening a Health Bureau in the Far East with a Branch Office in Australia," attached to Gautier to Strode, May 24, 1944, 1.1/100/22/182, RAC; Stouman to Gautier, November 29, 1944, R 6150, 8A/42474/42474, LNA; Biraud to Parisot, March 8, 1946, R 6062, 8A/13441/985, LNA.

63. Biraud to Gautier, November 1944, R 6159, 8A/42472/42472, LNA.

64. Biraud to Gautier, March 22, 1943, R 6083, 8A/8862/2353, LNA; Biraud to Gautier, July 7, 1943, R 6083, 8A/8862/2353, LNA; Biraud to Professor Tomcsik, University of Basel, January 26, 1944, R 6185, 8D/42284/1992, LNA; League of Nations, *Chronicle of the Health Organisation*, Special Number, October 1943, LNA, 9; Y. Biraud, "Lexique polyglotte des maladies contagieuses: Contibution à la Nomen-clature nosologique internationale," *Bulletin de L'Organisation d'Hygiène* (Geneva), 10 (1942–44): 201–556; Biraud to Gautier, March 25, 1944, R 6185, 8D/35950/1992, LNA.

65. J. Weill, "La maladie de la faim et son traitement dans des camps d'internes," *Bulletin de L'Organisation d' Hygiène* (Geneva), 10 (1942–44): 730–80.

66. Y. Biraud, "L'état sanitaire de l'Europe. Etude de la situation au point de vue des épidémies et de la nutrition," *Bulletin de L'Organisation d'Hygiène* (Geneva), 10 (1942–44): 557–706.

67. Biraud to Gautier, London, November 15, 1944, R 6159, 8A/42474/42474, LNA.

68. Gautier to Lester, Washington, July 1, 1944, R 6151, 8A/42503/41674, LNA. Apparently, these reprints only materialized a year later but met with substantial interest on the part of U.S. health authorities then, including the State Department and the Social Security Board. Knud Stouman, UNRRA, to Biraud, November 14, 1945, R 6151, 8A/42231/41674, LNA.

69. Health Research Unit, Digest of Current Information, No. 16, September 1944, R 6150, 8A/43321/ 42474, LNA.

70. Goodman, *International Health Organizations*, 75–76 and 146–47.

71. Stouman to Gautier, December 11, 1944, R 6159, 8A/42474/42474, LNA.

72. However, Deutschman apparently remained "very loyal to the League." Gautier to Madsen, November 12, 1945, R 6061, 8A/3931/985, LNA; Stouman to Gautier, November 14, 1944, R 6159, 8A/42474/42474, LNA.

73. Stouman to Gautier, December 11, 1944, R 6159, 8A/42474/42474, LNA; Lehman to Pierret, March 24, 1945, OIHP papers, microfilm, T 19, WHO Archive, Geneva.

74. Biraud to Gautier, London, November 15, 1944, R 6159, 8A/42474/42474, LNA; Biraud to Lester, August 15, 1944, R 6151, 8A/42231/41674, LNA.

75. See Foreign Office to H. M. Embassy, Washington, DC, December 5, 1944, FO 371/40864, PRO.

76. Biraud did profit from the French data sent by his former colleague, Veillet-Lavallé, who worked in the French National Health Institute. Biraud to Parisot, March 8, 1944, R 6062, 8A/13441/985, LNA.

77. Gautier to Lester, November 23, 1944, R 6150, 8A/42474/42474, LNA; Gautier to Stouman, November 24, 1944, R 6150, 8A/42474/42474, LNA. Gautier did not know that the main source of German figures, the *Reichsgesundheitsblatt*, had ceased to exist in October. Biraud to Gautier, December 22, 1944, R 6150, 8A/42474/42474, LNA.

78. Biraud to Gautier, December 22, 1944, R 6150, 8A/42474/42474, LNA.

79. Note sur les relations techniques entre l'Office International d'Hygiène publique et les États-Unis d'Amérique du 10 juin au octobre 1944, OIHP papers, microfilm, A 62, WHO Archive. Biraud claimed that the OIHP data were mere copies of his data. Biraud to Gautier, London, November 15, 1944, R 6159, 8A/42474/42474, LNA.

80. Note pour M. Schneiter, Secrétaire d'Etat aux Affaires Etrangères à propos de l'Office International d'Hygiène publique, de l'U.N.N.R.A. et de la future Organisation mondiale internationale d'Hygiène, March 8, 1946, OIHP papers, microfilm, T 20, WHO Archive.

81. Biraud, notes on the debates of the Economic and Social Council on February 7 and 8, 1946, February 20, 1946, R 6150, 8A/42169/41755, LNA.

82. The OIHP director general Robert Pierret referred to Morgan as "my old friend." Pierret to Sawyer, December 7, 1944, OIHP papers, microfilm, T 19, WHO Archive; P. G. Stock, Ministry of Health, to Topping, UNRRA, November 9, 1944, OIHP papers, microfilm, T 19, WHO Archive.

83. Mackenzie, "Extracts from Medical Relief in Europe: Questions for Immediate Study," *Royal Institute of International Affairs*, 1942, 62–66, R 6150, 8A/41755/41755, LNA.

84. Owen, draft of memo, Foreign Office, November 2, 1944, FO 371/40864, PRO.

85. Memo, Foreign Office, October 20, 1944, FO 371/41206, PRO.

86. Memo of conversation, Foreign Office, October 20, 1944, FO 371/41206, PRO.

87. Foreign Office to H. M. Embassy in Washington, DC, draft cable, undated, FO 371/41206, PRO.

88. Winslow, "International Organization for Health, Commission to study the organization of peace," April 1944, R 6150, 8A/42169/41755, LNA.

89. Subcommittee on Education and Labor, report to accompany Joint Senate Resolution 89, "Formation of an International Health Organization," undated, brought before Congress in August 1945, R 6150, 8A/42169/41755, LNA.

90. H. M. Embassy, Washington, DC, to Foreign Office, November 18, 1944, FO 371/41206, PRO; H. M. Embassy, Paris, to Foreign Office, November 23, 1944, FO 371/41206, PRO.

91. See Gautier-Cumming correspondence, throughout 1945, R 6061, 8A/4922/985, LNA.

92. Gautier, *For Whom the Bell Toils*, August 15, 1944, R 6150, 8A/42474/42474, LNA.

93. Gautier, *For Whom the Bell Toils*; Gautier to Madsen, November 12, 1945, R 60601, 8A/3931/985, LNA.

94. Biraud to Stouman, October 23, 1945, R 6150, 8A/41755/41755, LNA.

95. Cf. Stouman to Biraud, November 14, 1945, R 6150, 8A/41755/41755, LNA.

96. Goodman, *International Health Organizations*, 152.

97. Biraud to Gautier, April 3, 1945 and April 14, 1945, R 6159, 8A/42169/41755, LNA.

98. Madsen to Gautier, October 29, 1945, R 60601, 8A/3931/985, LNA.

99. Correspondence, R 6062, 8A/13441/985, LNA.

100. Biraud to Parisot, May 28, 1945, R 6062, 8A/13441/985, LNA; Gautier to Madsen, July 24, 1945, R 6061, 8A/3931/985, LNA; Gautier to Parisot, July 31, 1945, R 6062, 8A/13441/985, LNA; Gautier to Boudreau, November 30, 1945, R 6150, 8A/41755/41755, LNA.

101. Gautier to Madsen, November 12, 1945, R 6061, 8A/3931/985, LNA.

102. Gautier to Madsen, November 12, 1945, R 6061, 8A/3931/985, LNA.

103. Parisot to Gautier, August 20 and October 2, 1945, R 6062, 8A/13441/985, LNA; Gautier to Parisot, September 8 and October 26, 1945, R 6062, 8A/13441/985, LNA.

104. Gautier to Madsen, November 12, 1945, R 6061, 8A/3931/985, LNA; Gautier to Parisot, December 7, 1945, R 6150, 8A/41755/41755, LNA. Governor Lehman refused to open the Singapore office, claiming there was not enough time left before the planned end of UNRRA.

105. See "Projet de Constitution de l'Organisation Internationale de la Santé Publique," September 27, 1945, R 6150, 8A/41755/41755, LNA; for Gautier's

strategy, see Gautier to Cumming, October 24, 1945, R 6150, 8A/41755/41755, LNA.

106. See Gautier to Parisot, October 26, 1945, R 6150, 8A/41755/41755, LNA.

107. Gautier to Madsen, November 12, 1945, R 6061, 8A/3931/985, LNA.

108. See correspondence in R 6150, 8A/41755/41755, LNA; Stouman gave the draft to Louis L. Williams, the chief adviser for health affairs in the State Department; Stouman to Biraud, November 14, 1945, R 6150, 8A/41755/41755, LNA.

109. See, for example, Biraud to Cumming, October 16, 1945, R 6150, 8A/41755/41755, LNA.

110. Gillespie, "Social Medicine," 222–23; Gautier to Madsen, November 12, 1945, R 6061, 8A/3931/985, LNA.

111. Cumming to Gautier, October 25, 1945, R 6061, 8A/4922/985, LNA.

112. Deutschman to Gautier, October 27, 1945, R 6150, 8A/43934/41755, LNA.

113. Gautier to Parisot, December 7, 1945, R 6062, 8A/13441/985, LNA; Biraud to Parisot, March 8, 1946, R 6062, 8A/13441/985, LNA.

114. Gautier to Parisot, "Suggestion Relating to the Constitution of an International Health Organisation, I.P.H.O." December 7, 1945, R 6062, 8A/13441/985, LNA.

115. Gautier to Madsen, November 12, 1945, R 6061, 8A/3931/985, LNA.

116. Biraud to Štampar, February 26, 1945, R 6150, 8A/43627/41755, LNA; Memo of telephone conversation between Biraud and Tomlinson, February 28, 1945, R 6150, 8A/43627/41755, LNA.

117. Biraud to Štampar, February 26, 1946, R 6150, 8A/43627/41755, LNA.

118. Ministre des Affaires Etrangères to Pierret, March 27, 1946, OIHP papers, microfilm, T 20, WHO Archive; Pierret to Chef du Service Technique des Conférences Internationales, April 1946 and October 15, 1946, OIHP papers, microfilm, T 20, WHO Archive.

119. Cf. Stouman to Biraud, November 14, 1945, R 6150, 8A/41755/41755, LNA.

120. Mackenzie now represented UNNRA. Cumming represented both the OIHP and the Pan-American Sanitary Bureau (PASB). Goodman, *International Health Organizations*, 152–54, 183–85.

121. Rajchman's draft was circulated but apparently received only limited attention. Gillespie, "Social Medicine," 223; Cf. Gautier to Madsen, April 13, 1946, R 6061, 8A/3931/985, LNA.

122. Commission Preparatoire Technique, Sous-Commission chargée d'étudier les Rapports entre l'Organisation future et tous autres organismes, March 29, 1946, OIHP papers, microfilm, T 93, WHO Archive.

123. WHO Constitution, July 22, 1946. Available at http://www.searo.who.int/EN/Section898/Section1441.htm (accessed September 14, 2007).

124. The governmental element was eventually somewhat weaker in the WHO than in Biraud's original draft, since the assembly was to consist of delegates—"preferably" but not necessarily representing their health administrations—whereas members of the executive board were to be merely "technically qualified." Ultimately, the position of the assembly was stronger than in Biraud's paper since it was officially responsible for determining WHO policies. However, as the executive organ, the

committee retained important rights, such as the right to propose a program, study questions within its competence, and institute committees. The Pan-American Sanitary Organization, whose fate had been the subject of so much controversy, was to be fully integrated into the WHO. Cf. Goodman, *International Health Organizations*, 186–200.

125. Goodman claims that the range was wider than that of LNHO, OIHP, and UNRRA put together. Goodman, *International Health Organizations*, 166.

126. Cf. Goodman, *International Health Organizations*, 169.

127. Goodman, *International Health Organizations*, 155–66. In this interim commission, Gautier served as a consultant. Later he continued to work in the WHO. N. Howard-Jones, *International Public Health between the Two World Wars: The Organizational Problems* (Geneva: WHO, 1978), 75.

128. Biraud to Lester, August 26, 1946, R 6150, 8A/43934/41755, LNA.

129. Correspondence, R 6150, 8A/44073/41755, LNA; Goodman, *International Health Organizations*, 99.

Chapter Five

Europe, America, and the Space of International Health

James A. Gillespie

The international sphere was radically reshaped in the aftermath of World War II. Having emerged as the dominant power, the United States used its new influence to construct a new world order—at least in the West—based on a global network of institutions covering most areas of economic activity, trade, and security. With the growth of a new and lasting space for international economic and political cooperation, relations among the industrial democracies were profoundly reshaped. As John Ikenberry has argued, this postwar settlement spawned a "managed order organized around a set of multilateral institutions and a 'social bargain' that sought to balance openness with domestic welfare and stability."[1] The new order survived the next half century. It had "constitutional characteristics": an industrial sphere "characterized by multilayered institutions and alliances, open and penetrated domestic orders, and reciprocal and largely legitimate mechanisms for dispute resolution and joint decision making."[2] Founded on new economic and security relationships, it involved a complex rethinking of the interactions between the space of the nation-state, based on established principles of national sovereignty, and a widening space of international action, resting on the new authority of international agreements and agencies.

The position of international health organizations and programs in this postwar restructuring was complex. As domestic conflicts over the reshaping of health and welfare systems in the developed nations intensified, considerable pressure was exerted by ministries of health to ensure that the prestige of the newly created World Health Organization did not become a force for radical change. This pressure led WHO to remove itself from major debates over health funding and social security from the 1950s until the late 1960s.[3] Instead, it moved into a field that international agencies had hitherto found difficult: improving the health status of the populations of the former European colonies. The space and boundaries of the "international" were reshaped from a central concern with the social structures and welfare states of the developed countries—particularly of Europe—to a singled-minded focus on the developmental problems of Africa and Asia. This shift had several contexts—not least the East-West conflicts of the cold war.[4] Along with this went the changing interests of the European colonial powers. Within a decade, international health agencies moved from threatening the legitimacy of colonial rule to taking up the responsibilities of the departing overlords.

These changes had wider implications for the definition of the legitimate scope of international health—its functions, its scope, and its character. According to one view, the scope of international health is set by primarily technical forces. Internationalization was a slow but inexorable process as new technologies of disease control and eradication were discovered. International organization naturally followed, driven by this generally accepted language of science.[5] Taking issue with the focus on the technical, the "constructivist" school of international relations has argued that international health organizations function primarily as teachers of norms of cooperation and altruistic social improvement, not as participants in a politics of competing national interests.[6]

Europe and the Space of International Health

During the interwar years, international health was constituted in a narrowly European frame. The failure of the United States to join the League of Nations made its involvement peripheral. The programs of the two major international health bodies, the Office international d'hygiène publique (OIHP)—Paris based and conducting all its affairs in French—and the Geneva-based League of Nations Health Organisation (LNHO), concentrated on issues defined by their European sponsors.

Dominated by chief health officers from the European powers, the OIHP focused its attention on the narrow task of administering the International Sanitary Conventions, established under the Agreement of Rome in 1907. The United States representative and U.S. surgeon general, Rupert Blue, reported after an OIHP meeting in 1922 that "all nations [represented] were convinced of the necessity of a line of defense between the Orient and Europe."[7] Although the OIHP moved toward some more innovative work on the regulation of air travel and on incorporating advances in vaccination into international quarantine, it remained dominated by the interests of the metropolitan powers.[8]

Historians have given us a more favorable image of the League of Nations Health Organisation, partly because of its charismatic secretary, Ludwik Rajchman. Lacking the settled functions in international law of the Paris office, the LNHO was forced to carve out a new space of international action in public health. Its focus was far less Eurocentric than that of the OIHP—it completed pioneering work in China, developed a critique of quarantine as a barrier against the diseases of the East, argued for a focus on destroying the threat of epidemic disease at its source, and developed strong national health services.[9] With the invitation of the Nationalist Chinese government, the League could work freely there and complete limited projects with colonial health officials, such as developing the pioneering Rural Health Conference at Bandung in the Dutch East Indies in 1937. When nutritional problems were linked to restrictions on world trade in agricultural commodities, the LNHO's activities were expanded to attack a protectionism that restricted trade from primary producers. In the wake of the Bruce Report (1939), the LNHO's health and social activities were reorganized in an attempt to assume an expansive mission informed by the broader agendas of social medicine. In Bruce's view problems of health had a social origin, shaped by the "inability of classes and individuals to adjust themselves to the world in which they live." Outside Europe and North America, especially in the less developed nations, the task of international health was no longer to be carried out by the "old methods of imperialism" but by more altruistic international cooperation.[10]

There were clear limits to these attempts to reorient international health from its Eurocentric focus. Under Rajchman, the LNHO developed extensive advisory programs in China, but his open sympathies with Chinese nationalism led to deep suspicion from successive secretaries general of the League of Nations. The Japanese saw technical assistance by the LNHO, including its health programs, as an affront. These tensions reached their height in the late 1930s, when Joseph Avenol, the League's director general, argued that Rajchman's programs and Chinese sympathies were undermining attempts to lure Italy and Germany, Japan's allies, back into the League. The priorities of European power politics limited the LNHO's Asian activities and played a part in Rajchman's dismissal in 1937.[11] The LNHO hit a sanitary Monroe Doctrine when it attempted to expand its activities in the Americas. When Rajchman initiated an American Rural Health Conference in 1937, the Pan-American Sanitary Bureau, effectively funded and controlled by the U.S. Public Health Service, made it clear that the LNHO's presence was not welcome.[12]

UNRRA and the Reconstruction of Europe

Planning for the postwar world began early. Long before hostilities ceased, the memory of famine and epidemics and their contributions to political instability after World War I lent urgency to advocates of a massive aid and reconstruction program for the occupied nations. Great Britain set up the Inter-Allied Committee on Postwar Requirements (the Leith-Ross Committee), which listed the emergency supplies that liberated Europe would be likely to require, but had no funds to start practical work. The United States took a more activist approach. The Office of Foreign Relief and Rehabilitation Operations (OFRRO) was set up in late 1942, with a mandate to move beyond emergency relief into planning the first stages of the rehabilitation of shattered economies and systems of social support.[13] In November 1943, forty-four Allied nations, including representatives of occupied Europe, established the United Nations Relief and Rehabilitation Administration (UNRRA) with a mission "to help liberated territories to secure those supplies and services which are essential for the health and stability of their populations and which cannot be provided by other means." UNRRA was to provide emergency food, clothing, and medical supplies as soon as military operations ceased: "Long range reconstruction and production for war purposes will not be its task."[14]

In postwar history, UNRRA has been relegated to a footnote, written off as a temporary experiment in internationalist enthusiasm, of interest mainly as the site of some of the opening maneuvers of the cold war. If it is mentioned at all in general studies of postwar reconstruction, UNRRA makes a fleeting appearance as the unsuccessful precursor of the Marshall Plan.[15] At worst, historians have portrayed it as a grand failure of internationalist-minded American liberalism—"a bandage applied to a gunshot wound"[16] by naïve devotees of the more radical side of Roosevelt's New Deal, who set out with ambitious goals for remaking a liberal, internationalist world, but failed from a lack of "realism and drive."[17]

At the time, its planners took a more grandiose view of their position. Charles-Edward Winslow, a leader in American public health, argued, "Relief inevitably merges into rehabilitation, rehabilitation into reconstruction, and reconstruction into the welfare of the permanent society of autonomous, democratic cooperating peoples which is the object of our postwar planning."[18] UNRRA's early leaders, such as Philip Jessup and Herbert H. Lehman, its first director general, argued for the need to "think big," to convince Roosevelt that "UNRRA is the model for the postwar organization . . . not merely another technical international committee."[19] If UNRRA fell short of some of these more ambitious objectives, especially in economic reconstruction, its relief activities of shipping food, clothing, and essential medical supplies to the former occupied territories of Europe and Asia provided an unprecedented model in multilateral emergency aid. Between 1944 and 1947, when UNRRA was dissolved, it spent almost US$4 billion on aid. Almost 90 percent of that amount came from Anglo-American sources; three-quarters of the total was voted by the U.S. Congress. UNRRA's field operations, especially in health, drew on models developed by the Rockefeller Foundation's

International Health Division during the interwar years and became the progenitor of fieldwork in the UN system.[20]

In 1947, the director of medical services of UNRRA, Dr. Wilbur Sawyer, declared that his organization was "by far the largest international health organization which the world has yet seen." UNRRA's Health Division was the theater for a complex battle over the future direction of international health work. Selskar Gunn, one of its main architects, argued that the basic purpose of the new organization was to "build up an organized world society," taking existing areas of health cooperation and extending these into "a world system."[21] UNRRA employed 1,288 health professionals, including 488 medical practitioners, predominantly in Germany (in the camps), China, Greece, Austria, and Italy. At its height, in 1946, it spent $14 million on its health division and another $68 million on medical and sanitary supplies.[22]

With over 80 percent of its funding and supplies coming from the United States government, UNRRA's planners accepted without demur the call of Thomas Parran, the U.S. surgeon general, for a health organization that could provide not only emergency services, such as disease control and relief from malnutrition, but also "the re-establishment of medical services, hospitals, dispensaries, sanatoria, health centers, laboratories, environmental sanitation, control of endemic diseases, and other essentials for health." Parran added: "A constant objective of the health program [of UNRRA] should be to demonstrate the effectiveness and need for international collaboration in public health. In so doing it will facilitate the later development of a permanent worldwide health organization."[23]

UNRRA's first focus was the liberated areas of Europe. Although European governments welcomed the prospect of material aid for reconstruction, they had considerable reservations about an internationalism that carried conditions as to how the assistance would be applied. A "debtors' war" broke out over the terms of postwar assistance as the United States Treasury, the State Department, and the Office of Lend-Lease Administration attempted to impose strict conditions on economic and other aid.[24]

In this fiscal politicking, UNRRA was an anomaly, caught as it was between European suspicions of American intentions and the U.S. Congress's increasingly cool view of multilateral commitments. At least nominally, UNRRA's spending policies were set by a council that broadly represented donor nations, but most of its funds were voted by—and dependent on the sympathy of—Congress. It received its strongest support from the British Foreign Office, which saw it as a vehicle for leveraging its own limited resources: with minimal contributions of their own, the British could influence the shape of United States aid for postwar relief. Whereas the European allies suspected that UNRRA would be merely "a tool of the American department of state" or, at best, an Anglo-American venture, the view from Capitol Hill was radically different. Many members of Congress were still not ready for such an open-ended commitment to international action—as the "general impression on the Hill . . . [is] that UNRRA is out to rebuild the whole world."[25] Funding was assured only after frantic lobbying and assurances that the new organization was not out to "feed the world."[26] Even so, the program faced continual congressional interference.[27]

Relief was to go primarily to European nations and to China (which had a quite separate program). Only the Allies or neutral countries that had been occupied by the Axis powers were eligible. France, Belgium, the Netherlands, Denmark, and Norway made an early judgment that the terms of UNRRA assistance were too demeaning and that their political leverage or their foreign reserves would enable them to do better elsewhere. Jean Monnet, the Washington representative of the Comité français de libération nationale (CFLN), developed direct relationships with Washington-based supply agencies and access to scarce shipping, bypassing UNRRA. A U.S. survey of the impact of UNRRA's programs in northwest Europe found that the "demands for safeguards and guarantees" accompanying its programs made "the offers useless."[28]

UNRRA's planners soon realized that they faced a cool welcome in northwest Europe. Raymond Gautier of the League of Nations Health Section warned that "relief action will, at the beginning at least, be mainly an Anglo-Saxon concern. Other countries will come in with whatever meagre resources they may have. They will, therefore, be handicapped from the outset. Would it not be better to sever relief from planning and to consider the latter on a basis of complete equality between nations?"[29] Recently, Daniel Fox has argued, "Practitioners of U.S. foreign policy during the Cold War appear to have learned from the implementation of the Marshall Plan in Britain to keep their opinions about the health and social policies of other countries, especially essential allies, to themselves."[30] The same lesson had been learned by their UNRRA predecessors, who soon abandoned grandiose plans of international reconstruction in Europe and moved their activities to apparently more tractable—and needier— regions. The proper sphere of international health shifted from the questions of reconstruction—especially the issues of social security and health services that preoccupied northern Europe—to interventions focusing on infectious diseases in the less-developed Mediterranean countries. International health became one arm of the struggle by the United States and its allies to build stable, politically sympathetic regimes on the periphery.

UNRRA, International Health, and the Cold War

From the beginning, there was a conflict between UNRRA's missions as a supplier of emergency relief and as a leader in the broader goal of reconstruction. This second role was ill defined: did it mean rebuilding institutions and economies, or funding temporary assistance until local elites could take full control? Wilbur Sawyer argued that UNRRA's significance lay more in "bridging the war-caused gap in the evolution of international health organization than . . . [in] its relief operations of a purely emergency kind."[31]

This conflict over objectives became even more confused as wartime alliances broke down. UNRRA's relief operations in Eastern Europe came under hostile U.S. congressional scrutiny, ultimately leading to a cutoff of funding and to closure in 1947. At the same time, the Soviet Union and its allies, though desperate for UNRRA supplies, were deeply suspicious of its ambitions. Under these political constraints, UNRRA's operations were reshaped from attempts at rebuilding health services—with their constant political pressures and the threat of falling into the quagmire of cold war conflicts—toward more narrowly focused, vertical disease-eradication projects. New technologies, such as DDT spraying, offered quick, measurable returns with minimal dependence on local cooperation and resources. Successes in deploying these methods helped reshape the focus of international health, reinforcing other pressures that removed contentious issues of health service organization from its agenda.

With its northern European operations limited to refugee relief, UNRRA found that the devastated regions of Eastern Europe were eager for supplies, but Charles-Edward Winslow's program of a progression "from relief to rehabilitation to reconstruction and permanent welfare" proved more difficult. UNRRA's operations had commenced at the high point of Allied cooperation, effectively providing a continuation of Lend-Lease aid to those Eastern European nations judged allies or victims of the war. Soviet officials played an active role in administering the distribution of UNRRA aid, encouraging its relief supply programs, but resisting more activist interventions.[32] UNRRA's Prague office was run by the Russian R. I. Alexeyev, and there were frequent reports that UNRRA supplies were being relabeled as Russian aid or diverted to the Red Army.[33] The new Czechoslovak government responded by restricting UNRRA's work, insisting that in future no UNRRA officers could operate "unless they are virtually appointed by and responsible to the Czech government and of Czech nationality"—that is, the Czechs would accept UNRRA aid, but would in future keep distribution in their own hands.[34] In the Balkans, UNRRA met with suspicion. In Albania, the government of Enver Hoxha never got over its suspicion that UNRRA was "simply a front for some nefarious Anglo-American purpose." The Yugoslavian government, led by Marshal Josip Broz Tito, was primarily interested in supplies and hostile to supervision of distribution. It allowed some small antimalaria and typhus programs in Macedonia.[35] These programs, however, became victims of the hardening terms of the cold war. When the Yugoslavs requested aerial spraying with DDT, on a model that had proved successful in Greece, UNRRA refused on the grounds that "the planes would have been used for military purposes." The sanitary engineers who attempted to work in Yugoslavia faced a wall of suspicious obstruction.[36]

Italy, newly liberated by the Anglo-American armies, offered fewer of these political obstacles and became the first real proving ground for UNRRA as a service agency. Despite British and Soviet objections to UNRRA's aiding a former enemy, the United States used its financial domination to force a policy change.[37] The Italian mission caught UNRRA in a familiar dilemma: should UNRRA confine its activities to temporary relief, or set out to rebuild Italian society? Dominated by "a forlorn band of liberals who hoped to implement the philosophy of the New Deal in the reconstruction of Italy," this aspect of the Italian mission quickly fell afoul of powerful elements within Italian conservatism and of the United States embassy.[38]

UNRRA's Italian supply operations concentrated on a massive feeding program for mothers and children.[39] It soon extended to the control of infectious disease, reviving prewar cooperative projects to control malaria, working closely with Italian malariologists such as Alberto Missiroli of the Institute of Hygiene—an easy exercise, as both sides were familiar with each other from prewar Rockefeller programs.[40] On the basis of these control methods, by the end of the summer of 1944, the UNRRA-funded malarial control program had "effectively kept this disease in check throughout the liberated provinces."[41]

Building on this success, UNRRA began work with the Rockefeller Foundation on an even more ambitious program in Sardinia to eradicate the malarial anopheles mosquitoes from the island. The campaign suffered from divisions over objectives and local suspicions that UNRRA was a tool of wider political projects. Although the incidence of malaria declined, vector eradication remained elusive. In spite of these problems, the project set the pattern for much international health action over the next two decades: massive, military-style vertical campaigns led and driven from the outside that focused on less-developed nations or regions.[42]

Greece and the Cold War

UNRRA's health objectives in Greece went well beyond "relief." As Edward Stettinius, the U.S. secretary of state, warned in late 1944, "It was possible for a short time after liberation to prevent 'disease and unrest' with minimum food and medical supplies. Now something more is required. The alternative would appear to be persistent disorder and delay in the firm establishment of democratic forms of government in these countries."[43] The focus of UNRRA and its concept of the scope of international health shifted to the most devastated—and powerless—of the former occupied nations.

UNRRA's Greek operations began in the shadow of the civil war fought between the communist-led partisans of the National Liberation Front–National Popular Liberation Army (ELAS-EAM) and the British- and American-supported government in Athens. Open warfare led to the evacuation of

UNRRA's staff to Cairo barely a month after starting operations. The short period of relative social calm after the Varkiza Pact of January 11, 1945 allowed field operations to recommence. By mid-1946, the Greek mission employed thousands of Greek workers and professional staff and seven hundred foreigners (mainly British and American); 191 of the latter were health professionals. However, UNRRA remained in an uncomfortable position. From the start the Greek mission complained of being "unavoidably associated with a regime of force and discrimination." Its public health workers met with continual accusations of leftist sympathies. At the same time, its work was central in building the social and economic stability that would aid the anticommunist cause.[44]

In its efforts to bring services "to the standards both in function and equipment of a modern western nation," the UNRRA Health Division encountered a variety of obstacles. Some problems were national—corruption and nepotism in government employment, excessive centralization in Athens, and reluctance to delegate power to local authorities. As James Miller Vine, UNRRA's medical director in Greece, put it, "We were of the firm opinion that no efficiency could be achieved in medical services in Greece while these methods were in force. We never hesitated to proclaim this and while we met with full agreement from responsible officials and politicians, we cannot pretend that we have had any success in altering the present and time-honoured systems."[45] Several UNRRA leaders had worked in the Rockefeller Foundation's abortive prewar Greek program, retaining bitter memories of failures in the absence of a trained workforce and infrastructure and the obstacles to reform posed by weak, highly politicized, and frequently corrupt local authorities.[46] UNRRA responded by asserting greater direct control of operations, including the antimalaria program. By September 1945, the Greek operations were reported as "happier and more inspiring" than those in Italy, largely because "the complete incompetence and corruption of the Greek Health administration as compared to the Italian" had forced UNRRA to take complete control.[47]

Vine, for one, argued that the goal was to ignore local capacities (and wishes) and inscribe a "first best" health system, proudly proclaiming that "some of those projects may in the end be too costly for Greece to maintain up to the almost ideal standards we are setting, but they will have such standards always before them."[48] In private, Vine's views were less sanguine. He noted the incompetence of public health administration from the (frequently changing) minister down to the regional offices, "hopelessly overstaffed with incompetents from Athens and the big cities. . . . We came to Greece to fight against disease, distress, poverty and the other expected aftermaths of war. We found that we had as well to fight against laziness, inertia, self-interest, corruption, venality, on the part of many of those who had the direction of this nation." He warned that "Greece was presented with a system of Public Health Administration and Function with all the modern practice and that having trained Greeks in their methods, the foreign organisation withdrew and the local skeleton fell back into its cupboard to moulder on and ruminate on its temporary disinterment."[49]

Vine argued that UNRRA's successes would come through avoiding such problems. If a competent civil public health authority could not be constructed, mosquito control through engineering works or even local spraying would be too difficult. It was difficult to hire and retain competent local staff. Transportation in the remote northern areas of Thrace and Macedonia was primitive and dangerous. Politics was also a problem. Local teams of sanitary workers were suspected by the Athens government of leftist sympathies—to the extent that UNRRA briefly withdrew its operations in Crete in protest over arrests of Greek medical workers. Despite continual problems with supplies, "No one denies the fact that it was the work of the planes that rounded out the over-all result, taking the country as a whole." The pilots and mechanics were based on the regular air force, bypassing the "determination on the part of the Ministry of Health, aided and abetted by professional jealousy [from Greek malariologists] . . . to completely disrupt the organization."[50]

Aerial spraying with the new insecticide DDT offered a technological alternative that sidestepped local politics. DDT was still a new compound. The Tennessee Valley Authority had sprayed malarial swamps from the air successfully; several UNRRA engineers had participated in this work. Although the first U.S. Army reports advocating widespread spraying warned, "Personnel must not consider an effective insecticide like DDT as a substitute for sanitation and preventive medicine," UNRRA's workers in Greece were strongly tempted to rely on this technological fix.[51] The "lack of discipline and cooperation in the civilian population made [it] difficult [to spread] mosquito awareness in public health education." Despite the reluctance of Greek malariologists to embrace aerial spraying, Vine and other UNRRA medical staff were confident that "malaria could be controlled by DDT alone." The work could accept political realities and remain Athens based. A team of American sanitary engineers loaned by the U.S. Public Health Service was assisted by Greek malariologists, engineers, inspectors, and foremen trained in mixing and spraying.[52]

Despite (or because) of these problems, Greece became the prime site for the gospel of DDT. The elimination of household insects, bedbugs, and flies as well as mosquitoes won local support, or at least compliance. In 1946, when this work was expanded with airplanes, the ability to sidestep local administrative problems increased. At the program's height, ten aircraft were in regular use, some flown by the Royal Air Force, but most with Greek pilots and crews, some trained in the United States in aerial-spraying techniques. One UNRRA sanitationist proclaimed, "Airplane work alone, if done systematically and under proper supervision in the lowlands and coastal area, could eliminate mosquitoes in many areas, and in others keep the density so low that malaria would cease to be a problem . . . [It is] the answer to a sanitarian's prayer."[53]

But UNRRA's work was cut short by a U.S. Congress alarmed at its lack of direct control over the agency's activities. Its residual funds went largely to the new United Nations Children's Emergency Fund (UNICEF), its activities to the infant World Health Organization. Both became direct legatees of UNRRA's reformulation of international health, which became defined as primarily a problem of the control of infectious diseases in less-developed countries, supplanting broader aims of reconstruction and welfare. We have seen how the institutional politics of European reconstruction shaped this shift in priorities. Northern and Eastern Europe states resisted UNRRA as a vehicle for Anglo-American hegemony. In southern Europe its successes and failures were also shaped by the vicissitudes of state building during the early cold war. As Europe recovered, UNRRA's successors in the new United Nations agencies turned their focus toward Asia and Africa. These regions posed more severe problems of international public health. Again, international interventions were shaped by the new forms of state that emerged during the protracted and uneven process of decolonization in the postwar decades.

The Colonial Question: Europe beyond Its Shores

As the European states emerged from the war, they moved to reclaim their colonial territories. Postwar political history is commonly written in domestic terms—with decolonization seen as an inevitable and peripheral sideshow to the construction of welfare states and moves toward European unity. But recent histories of both the metropolitan powers and their colonies have emphasized the impossibility of such a neat separation. As Frederick Cooper has noted, "It is not terribly demanding to ask historians of Europe to acknowledge that colonies mattered. It is another thing to ask them to rethink the narrative of the growth of the nation state." In the case of France, "it is far from clear when and to what extent the nation-state clearly differentiated itself from the empire-state until the era of decolonization."[54]

This ambiguous and uneven record of withdrawal has implications for our understanding of the formation of international health in the foundation years of the World Health Organization (WHO). The colonial powers initially saw multilateral agencies as part of a broader threat to their sovereignty. At the same time, through the United Nations they faced new scrutiny of their fulfillment of promises of broader social development in colonial possessions, development that none could afford to finance by itself. These contradictory pressures became the framework within which international health made its slow, final shift from identification with the interests of developed Europe. The new international agencies started with sweeping plans to realize the visions of interwar social medicine. Political reality soon tempered these dreams. Like UNRRA, WHO and UNICEF struggled to adapt their policies to fit the agendas of suspicious recipient nations and new models of political and economic development that gave little space to the claims of public health.[55]

The Western powers had emerged from World War II with a renewed determination to retain most if not all of their colonial possessions. Although Britain now acknowledged the loss of India as inevitable, it did not see the decline of the remainder of its tropical empire as fated. Indeed, the expansion of the trustee system, rather than self-determination, emerged as the dominant theme of the new United Nations Organization. Instead of decolonizing, the European powers attempted to modernize labor systems and administration in a self-conscious attempt to impose European models in colonial territories. The meeting of French colonial administrators in January and February 1944 at Brazzaville in French Equatorial Africa was part of a "quest for progressive imperialism" for the postwar era. The French did not question their presence in Africa; the progressivism of Brazzaville lay in a politics of development that accepted metropolitan France as the standard of the future.[56] From Brazzaville on, the French remained concerned lest American support for "trusteeship" become a basis for interference in the operations of territories. This concern led France to embrace the principle that the relief of the conditions of indigenous peoples justified continued metropolitan control.[57] In the French colonies, the Fonds pour l'investissement en developpement économique et sociale (FIDES) assumed that developing colonial economies—and the social and health infrastructure this required—would produce dividends for the French economy. In the British case, the Colonial Development Act of 1940 brought with it a rhetoric of "junior partnership" and "welfare imperialism."[58] The Belgians, often regarded as the laggards in colonial development, set up a rurally focused Development Fund for the Indigenous Population (FOBEI) in 1947.[59]

Committed to the long term, the European powers were wary about outside intervention in what they conceived as their domestic affairs. They were concerned that the legitimacy of colonial rule would suffer if it appeared dependent on aid from the United States or international organizations. Health issues saw a move toward "technical" cooperation around disease-eradication programs, although in practice the cooperation focused on low-cost programs. However, with the competing demands of metropolitan reconstruction at home, few resources were actually available to build the broader capacities of colonial health systems. Weak finances meant limited action. British initiatives in community development in Kenya responded to the social upheavals caused by the reabsorption of returning African troops, but were quickly abandoned in the face of opposition by local European elites and lack of money. Despite later attempts by the Colonial Office to extend community development programs based on the doctrine of international agencies such as the

International Labour Organization (ILO), such programs foundered on the realities of colonial power relationships.[60] Not only were resources limited, but development programs aimed at native populations—particularly if they involved local participation—quickly raised the ire of white settler groups, who were fearful of any concession to local rule.

Both the United States and the Soviet Union, although from radically different perspectives, were openly critical of the survival of the imperial system. U.S. dominance over the new multilateral agencies heightened suspicion that their operations in Africa and other colonized areas would be driven by a new fervor for decolonization. At the same time, the financially exhausted European powers looked gratefully to international agencies that could relieve their increasingly onerous responsibilities for the welfare of colonized peoples.

The European powers made it clear that UNRRA was to keep its distance from their colonial possessions. Despite the desperate needs of the Asian colonies occupied by the Japanese, UNRRA's aid was galling to national pride. As the British Foreign Office warned, the "US Govt and public would think and say that if we cannot provide relief for our colonies we have not the slightest moral claim to retain them. Indeed I would not put it past the US Govt to make the giving up of the colonies a condition of their financial assistance to us, if once we supported this idea by asking an international body to relieve them."[61] As reports of the terrible Bengal famine (in part caused by the diversion of food to the needs of the war) arrived, the U.S. Congress persuaded the UNRRA Council to extend its brief to "any area important to the military operations of the United Nations which is struck by famine or disease." But this "India clause" remained a dead letter, as the Indian government refused to request emergency assistance.[62]

Again, UNRRA's American architects learned to temper their ambitions for UNRRA as an agent of serious reform. When U.S. forces entered French North Africa, the Americans received a hint of what was to come. Dudley Reekie, a medical officer from the Office of Foreign Relief and Rehabilitation Operations, the agency coordinating U.S. aid for reconstruction, warned that "this is not an occupied country but is Allied, and French prestige is the key to the situation. The French do it or it is not done. What one thinks of the French is neither here nor there."[63] Other colonial powers shared these misgivings even as they reluctantly accepted aid. The Netherland government allowed a UNRRA mission to visit the Dutch East Indies, but warned that the colonial power did not need "outside assistance" to fulfill its obligations. Health was an area where external advice was welcome—as long as it was limited to technical questions, such as the establishment of central agencies for serum production.[64]

However, impoverished European powers faced a real dilemma, seen in an anguished counterargument in the British Foreign Office that it was "absurd that we can go on pretending to be rich when we are really poor." The Colonial Development and Welfare Act 1940 had pledged Britain to a vast increase in health and welfare expenditures; by the end of the war these costs eating up almost one fifth of colonial budgets. The Foreign Office warned that if Britain failed to get UNRRA funds for Burma and Hong Kong (eligible for UNRRA aid as both had been occupied by the enemy), whereas China was lavishly funded, the colonial power would forfeit its moral claim to continued authority.[65] This debate remained unresolved. William Hasler, one of the strongest supporters of UNRRA within the Foreign Office, characterized British policy as "100% unilateralism with perfunctory hat raisings to combined machinery and internationalism."[66]

These fears intensified as international health organization moved from UNRRA to more genuinely multilateral forms. From the British Ministry of Health, Melville Mackenzie warned that "it is impossible to expect the countries well developed technically to be overruled by the vote of nations less developed from a Public Health and Medical point of view."[67] Independent colonial representation was a threat. The Colonial Office strongly opposed direct colonial representation at the 1946 conference to establish the World Health Organization, warning that if any such representative attended "it will be extremely difficult to avoid including something in the [WHO] constitution to perpetuate this system."[68]

There were three external challenges to the hegemony of the European colonial powers over the colonies. Each challenge initially met strong resistance. The first was the attempt of the International Labour Office (ILO) to build on its prestige as the only significant survivor from the wreckage of the League of Nations to become the main international force in social and health policy. With a strong prewar record of support for reform of labor conditions in dependent territories, the ILO argued that the new standards of "social security" developed for postwar Europe and America must apply equally in their colonial possessions. A similar impulse governed debates over the structure of the World Health Organization. Supporters of a strong regional organizational structure for WHO—largely drawn from Latin America and the Middle East, with support from independent India after 1948—threatened to mobilize forces that would undermine the control of colonial health administrations. The third challenge came from the United States and other primarily noncolonial supporters of a postwar liberalization of trade. An attack on the closed trading relations of the British and French empires extended to the remnants of sanitary protectionism. According to the new approach to international public health associated with the American architects of WHO, the first tactic against disease was eradication at its source. International quarantine, with its restrictions on movements of people and commerce, must finally be supplanted by programs that drew on UNRRA's experience—namely, vertically driven disease-eradication programs that were only minimally constrained by respect for national boundaries or sovereignty.

The ILO and the Social Mandate

The most determined effort to internationalize the colonial question came from the International Labour Organization. The ILO had been the most forceful of the League of Nations agencies in pursuing colonial questions. The Forced Labour Convention (1930) was widely ratified and was followed in 1936 and 1939 by instruments protecting the rights of indigenous workers. Great Britain accepted these ILO initiatives, but they met with "serious attack" from other European powers, which resisted the regulation of forced labor as an imposition of the views of outsiders on sovereign colonial governments. They drew on the more novel emphasis on colonial development, to argue that seemingly just labor market reforms would have the perverse effect of restricting economic growth.[69]

The war years saw the ILO push its claims for a program of comprehensive social security that would be built on universal compulsory insurance for health, sickness, unemployment, and old age. The ILO then extended this rousing agenda to full support for the rights of the peoples of "dependent territories." The 1944 Philadelphia Conference marked the zenith of the ILO's campaign to place comprehensive social security, including universal access to medical care, at the heart of postwar planning. The radicalism of the Declaration of Philadelphia was matched by the ILO's Recommendations on Social Policy in Dependent Territories, which called for the "metropolitan" powers to extend similar rights to workers in dependent, non-self-governing territories. In 1947, these recommendations developed into a sweeping Convention on Social Policy in Non-Metropolitan Territories, which asserted the rights of the people of dependent territories to play a leading role in devising social policies, called for adequate technical and financial assistance, and promoted improved standards in public health and employment. The convention's central principle was embodied in the declaration, "Any expansion of production, or even any new social service, which is dictated from above and does not attempt to obtain indigenous support, will prolong the frustrations that may be felt by indigenous peoples."[70]

The ILO moved from the "protection of dependent peoples" to treating labor in the dependent territories as subject to the same norms as in developed countries, thus replacing implicit benevolent prewar paternalism. Based on the "framework of an international order," the 1947 ILO convention singled out public health, nutrition, and medical care as responsibilities of the "metropolitan" powers.

The ILO's timing was propitious. Frederick Cooper has argued that the response of the colonial authorities to this challenge was both technical and moral, an attempt to depoliticize a set of problems—especially around the continued use of forced labor, which had become an international embarrassment.[71] For the moment, Britain and France still believed that retaining colonial power was both a duty and a vital precondition for rapid economic recovery at home. The political stability and economic growth of the colonies in turn required modernization of colonial labor and social conditions. At the same time, the leading colonial powers accepted a moral challenge, the conviction that the new emphasis on social rights and citizenship could be a vehicle to relegitimize their rule. These responses proved fraught with danger. Modernization on these terms required both a political and a financial commitment. Both proved to be fragile. But failure would leave colonial administrations open to internal challenge and international scrutiny. The same fears that had blocked UNRRA's activities in the European colonies were now focused on its successors, the United Nations technical organizations: WHO, the Food and Agricultural Organization (FAO), and UNICEF. The colonial authorities coveted the funding that these agencies could tap through U.S. aid budgets. For the moment, the lure of an internationalization of health and welfare was balanced by the dangers that such internationalization opened for colonial rule.

The Regional Question

The ILO may have exposed the limits of imperial welfare, but deeper challenges were presented by regionalism—led by Latin American members of WHO.

The future of the Pan-American Sanitary Bureau (PASB) assumed a central role in the planning of WHO. On one side, many Latin Americans saw a sinister, possibly Soviet-led, conspiracy to undermine the "sanitary sovereignty of the Americas" by weakening (or even abolishing) the autonomy of PASB and centralizing power in Geneva.[72] For their part, the British were highly suspicious of the regional model, whose cause was not helped by the emergence of a Pan-Arab Sanitary Bureau with links to the Arab League. The Colonial Office feared the Pan-American Sanitary Bureau was part of a "pan American machinery of political influence," aimed at weakening British and French colonial powers. The PASB excluded from membership all non-self-governing territories, including British and French possessions in the Caribbean. "If only the epidemiological intelligence fund was in question, this would not greatly matter. But if the regional bodies were to be endowed with a wide range of functions, particularly as regards positive health work, this might not be a happy position, looking even to the use made by the United States of the PASB as an instrument of penetration in Latin America."[73]

The British government began a campaign to include its West Indian possessions in the Pan-American Sanitary Bureau, notwithstanding the strong opposition of anticolonialist Latin American powers. The Latin countries imposed humiliating terms, in particular the insistence that delegations be led by "native" medical practitioners. The British protested both the exclusion of self-governing colonies from access to international agencies and their resources—on the grounds that they were not formally independent—and what they regarded as an unwarranted interference in the affairs of those still governed from London.[74] These contradictory pressures helped shape policies in the new international organizations. The Colonial Office pushed for a strongly centralized WHO, opposing any body based on "a loose federation of virtually autonomous regional agencies" in order to prevent the organization's balance from being "distorted to the great disadvantage of the United Kingdom and more especially the Colonial Empire."[75]

If the potential for "interference" from regional organizations was blunted by centralizing power in Geneva, a second response was to control any interventions in the colonies. Opinions varied: as with UNRRA, an influential part of British official opinion held that international programs, if properly controlled, provided an opportunity to relieve the British treasury and local budgets. Other colonial powers were more hostile to outside intervention. The French and Belgian governments initiated the Combined Commission for Technical Cooperation in Africa South of the Sahara (CCTA) in January 1950, drawing in the British, South African, and Portuguese governments. Liberia was admitted rather reluctantly on Franco-British insistence, on the grounds that inclusion of the only independent black African state would legitimize the CCTA as a barrier to the "political interference" of international agencies such as the ILO and WHO. France and Belgium saw the CCTA as an alternative model of international cooperation, evolving into an Inter-African Medical Committee dominated by colonial medical services, which might eventually enter into a loose relationship with WHO. Such a development would remove the threat of a WHO regional office and prevent any colonial power from cooperating with UN technical agencies behind the backs of its fellows. (Britain was the prime target of suspicion.) Though cooperating with the other colonial powers for the moment, the British remained more skeptical, warning that critics would justifiably paint the CCTA as a "white man's club" that was interested mainly in the health problems of expatriate Europeans or the economic effects of ill health.[76] These fears had a basis. Although the CCTA launched campaigns against the tsetse fly and trypanosomiasis, it remained trapped in the colonial dilemma: how the "metropolitan" powers could meet the demands, external and internal, for development while struggling to fulfill their domestic fiscal obligations. In an effort to keep the initiative and credit in imperial hands, the CCTA attempted to become the intermediary for programs initiated by WHO and other UN technical agencies under the largely U.S.-funded expanded technical assistance program.[77]

The CCTA was never very robust. The French and Belgians wanted it to become the intermediary for all specialized agencies in sub-Saharan Africa—viewing "the establishment of new bodies in terms, not of producing results in Africa, but of preventing other organizations obtaining a foothold in the colonies."[78] But starved for funds, the CCTA gradually lost its political backers. The Colonial Office saw it as a vehicle for grand, but empty, projects initiated by the French to keep the UN at bay, whereas France was suspicious of tepid British feelings about cooperation. The CCTA's conferences, including two on malnutrition and infant feeding, raised problems of protein malnutrition and kwashiorkor as central questions of infant health. However, in both instances leadership came from WHO and FAO experts. By 1956, the British had largely given up on the agency, recognizing that without generous funds it could provide no competition for the UN agencies.[79]

Liberalism, Trade, and Quarantine

The final blow to any thought of excluding agencies such as WHO from "interference" in colonial affairs came with a fundamental shift in the focus of international health. The interwar years had seen a slow abandonment of the old restrictive, quarantine-based approaches to disease control. The revisions to international sanitary codes made by the Office international d'hygiène publique (OIHP) in the light of modern aviation had marked a turning point in an otherwise conservative agency. During the postwar years, observers combined the liberalism promoted by the United States and its allies with newer and more aggressive approaches to public health in a critique of the notions of national sovereignty that underlay the hostility of the colonial powers to outside scrutiny.

The rhetoric of the early postwar years was marked by an intensified celebration of the possibilities in a new liberal era of open exchange of peoples and trade. Frank Boudreau (president of the Milbank Memorial Fund in New York, but previously a pioneer of the League's Epidemiological Intelligence Service), warned the U.S. Congress that the only alternative to joining WHO was "building our own dykes"—but even this was no solution, as aircraft can fly over dykes. Boudreau stated, "The World Health Organization will enable national health departments to cooperate effectively together for the prevention of disease. . . . [I]t will clear disease at the source, in the places and countries in which it arises." Although the League of Nations had built up an effective alarm system, epidemiological intelligence of the highest order was useless if the national health services in affected nations were weak.[80] Boudreau echoed the dominant group of public health officers in the United States, who drew on the interwar experiences of the League of Nations and the Rockefeller Foundation, as well as of UNRRA's later work to conclude "the control of epidemic disease depended not solely—or even primarily—on barriers at a national frontier, but on the stamping out of foci of infection within the country where such foci existed."[81] UNRRA's Greek antimalaria campaign had its apotheosis in the campaigns led by WHO and UNICEF in the 1950s: vertical campaigns focused on single diseases.

In the face of these challenges, by the mid-1950s the postwar colonial project was looking less rosy. The European powers were facing greater resistance to their continued rule from colonial populations and increasingly strong domestic economic arguments against those continued commitments. Jacques Marseille has pointed to the change in French official views: once regarded as an essential basis for economic recovery, colonial possessions were now seen as a burden, delaying rather than supporting the recovery and modernization of the metropolitan power.[82]

One effect of this change in attitude was the rapid disappearance of the suspicion of the anti-imperial intent of international agencies. As early as 1950, Britain had broken ranks with fellow CCTA members and welcomed the prospect of a WHO African Region. Although other powers remained hostile, the Colonial Office argued that representation from Southern Rhodesia and South Africa would easily outweigh the only independent African voice, impoverished Liberia.[83] When the 1952 ILO Convention on Social Security (Minimum Standards) was extended to nonmetropolitan territories, the metropolitan powers offered little resistance, although some quietly failed to ratify.[84]

The colonial powers abandoned the welfare promises of the 1940s and clearer lines developed between Europe and the colonies, especially in the least developed African regions. As the reach of Europe returned to its historic boundaries, openings in the former colonies for WHO and other international agencies widened, especially in technical areas. Instead of constituting dangerous outside interference, these programs became a cheap way of meeting obligations and deflecting criticism from the growing band of newly independent nations in the United Nations. In both French and British African colonies, the costs of development were well outside the ability, or political will, of the metropolitan powers. The early negotiations to form a European Economic Community were bedeviled by France's insistence on bringing its remaining colonies into "association" with the EEC—an insistence resisted by West Germany and the Netherlands as thinly disguised subsidies for French colonial policy.[85] The involvement of international agencies became more attractive as self-governing regimes, such as preindependence Ghana, preferred WHO and the ILO to the financially straitened CCTA. The most attractive alternative became a transition to local rule—a reshaping of territorial power that relieved the former colonial powers of their dilemma.[86]

Notes

1. G. J. Ikenberry, *After Victory: Institutions, Strategic Restraint and the Rebuilding of Order after Major Wars* (Princeton, NJ: Princeton University Press, 2001), 184–85.

2. Ikenberry, *After Victory*, 210.

3. J. A. Gillespie, "Social Medicine, Social Security and International Health, 1920–1960," in *The Politics of the Healthy Life*, ed. E. Rodríguez-Ocaña, 227–35 (Sheffield: EAHMH, 2002).

4. R. Packard, "Visions of Postwar Health and Development and Their Impact on Public Health Interventions in the Developing World," in *International Development and the Social Sciences*, ed. R. Packard and F. Cooper, 96–113 (Berkeley: University of California Press, 1997).

5. R. Cooper, "International Cooperation in Public Health as a Prologue to Macroeconomic Cooperation," in *Can Nations Agree? Issues in International Economic Cooperation*, ed. R. Cooper, 178–254 (Washington, DC: Brookings Institution, 1989).

6. M. Finnemore and M. Barnett, "The Power of Liberal International Institutions," in *Power in Global Governance*, ed. M. Barnett and R. Duvall, 161–75 (Cambridge: Cambridge University Press, 2005); M. Finnemore, *National Interests in International Society*, 69–88 (Ithaca, NY: Cornell University Press, 1996).

7. R. Blue, Report of the October Meeting of the Office International d'Hygiène Publique, October 20–November 2, 1922, RG90, Group 12, Box 1 (hereafter RG90/12/1), United States National Archives (hereafter USNA), College Park, MD.

8. *Vingt-Cinq Ans d'Activité de l'Office International d'Hygiène Publique* (Paris: OIHP, 1933), 69–71, 106–9.

9. League of Nations, *The Prevalence of Epidemic Disease and Port Health Organization and Procedure in the Far East: Report Presented to the Health Committee of the League of Nations by F. Norman White* (Geneva: League of Nations, 1923), 31.

10. F. Boudreau, "Memorandum on the Reorganization of the Health, Opium, and Social Sections," C-E. A. Winslow Papers, 749/81/1274, Sterling Library, Yale University (hereafter Yale).

11. C. Thorne, *The Limits of Foreign Policy: The West, the League, and the Far Eastern Crisis of 1931–33* (London: Hamish Hamilton, 1972), 377; M. Balinska, "Le 'Plan Mandel': Georges Mandel, Ludwik Rajchman et l'aide à la Chine à la veille de la deuxième guerre mondiale," *Revue d'Histoire Diplomatique* 14 (1997): 22–24, 33.

12. Memo, H. Cumming to Secretary of State [Cordell Hull], May 18, 1937, Parran Papers, 90/F-14 FF 115, Hillman Library, University of Pittsburgh (hereafter HLUP).

13. C. Hull to F. D. Roosevelt, May 5, 1942, President's Official File, OF 4966 UNRRA 1942, Franklin D. Roosevelt Presidential Library, Hyde Park, New York (hereafter FDRPL).

14. Edward Stettinius (Secretary of State) Memorandum on the Scope and Operations of UNRRA, September 10, 1943, President's Official File, OF 4966 UNRRA 1943, FDRPL.

15. Even those who stress the importance of international institutions in reshaping the European political and social order have ignored UNRRA. See, for example, B. Eichengreen, "Mainsprings of Economic Recovery in Postwar Europe," in *Europe's Postwar Recovery*, ed. B. Eichengreen (Cambridge: Cambridge University Press, 1995), 5–6; M. Hogan, *The Marshall Plan: America, Britain and the Reconstruction of Western Europe, 1947–1952* (Cambridge: Cambridge University Press, 1987), 29–31.

16. J. E. Miller, *The United States and Italy, 1940–1950: The Politics and Diplomacy of Stabilization* (Chapel Hill: University of North Carolina Press, 1986), 64.

17. F. S. V. Donnison, *Civil Affairs and Military Control: North West Europe 1944–1946* (London: HMSO, 1961), 345.

18. C.-E. A. Winslow, *International Organization for Health* (New York: Commission to Study the Organization of Peace, 1944), 14.

19. Philip C. Jessup to H. Lehman, June 22, 1943, Jessup Papers, A150, Library of Congress, Washington, DC (hereafter LC).

20. W. Sharp, *Field Administration in the United Nations System: The Conduct of International Economic and Social Programmes* (London: Stevens and Sons, 1961), 22.

21. S. Gunn, "United Nations Relief and Rehabilitation Administration: Proposed Health Program and Organization," April 6, 1943, Winslow Papers, 749/100/1786, Yale.

22. W. Sawyer, "Achievements of UNRRA as an International Health Organization," *American Journal of Public Health* 37 (1947): 41.

23. G. Woodbridge, *UNRRA: The History of the United Nations Relief and Rehabilitation Administration* (New York: Columbia University Press, 1950), vol. 1, 434; United States Office of Foreign Relief and Rehabilitation Operations (hereafter OFRRO), Committee IV, Sub-committee 2, Preparations for Atlantic City Council, Minutes, November 15, 1943, PAG-4/1.3.1.5.0.0:3, United Nations Archives, New York City (hereafter UNA); "Report of the Subcommittee on Policies with Respect to Health and Medical Care," *UNRRA Journal: 1st Session of Council, Atlantic City, 10 November to 1 December 1943* (Washington, DC), 1947, 94.

24. R. Clarke, *Anglo-American Economic Collaboration in War and Peace, 1942–1949* (Oxford: Clarendon Press, 1982), 24–25.

25. OFRRO, Committee IV, Preparations for Atlantic City Council, Relations with Congress and Public, Minutes, October 27, 1943, Jessup Papers, A150, LC.

26. S. Marble, "What Has Happened to UNRRA?" *Christian Century*, February 21, 1945, 239; F. B. S. Sayre to Roosevelt, August 10, 1943, Francis B. Sayre Papers, Box 12, file Correspondence 1943, LC; memo of conference with Sol Bloom, Chairman, House of Representatives Foreign Affairs Committee, August 30, 1943, Francis B. Sayre Papers, Box 12, file Correspondence 1943, LC.

27. In contrast, later U.S. food relief programs, firmly under U.S. control, were conducted with wide executive discretion. L. Martin, *Democratic Commitments* (Princeton, NJ: Princeton University Press, 2000), 113.

28. M. Margairaz, *L'État, les finances et l'économie: Histoire d'une conversion 1932–1952* (Paris: Comité pour l'histoire économique et financière de la France, 1991), 2:756–64; S. Rosenman, "Report to the President of the United States on Civilian Supplies for the Liberated Areas of North West Europe" (Washington, DC: Committee on Foreign Relations, House of Representatives, 79th Congress, 1st Session, 1945), 205–11.

29. R. Gautier, "The Future Health Organisation," May 31, 1943, PAG-4/1.3.1.50.0:3, UNA.

30. D. Fox, "The Administration of the Marshall Plan and British Health Policy," *Journal of Policy History* 16 (2004): 207.

31. W. Sawyer, "Achievements of UNRRA as an International Health Organization," *American Journal of Public Health* 37 (1947): 45.

32. L. Martel, *Lend Lease, Loans and the Coming of the Cold War* (Boulder: Westview, 1979), 150.

33. A. Teichova, "For and Against the Marshall Plan in Czechoslovakia," in *Le Plan Marshall et le Relèvement économique de l'Europe*, ed. R. Girault and M. Lévy-Leboyer (Paris: Ministère de Finances, 1993), 112; W. Ullmann, *The United States in Prague, 1945–1948*, East European Quarterly Monographs, no. 36 (Boulder, 1978), 36–37.

34. Memo, Col. Delshaye, June 7, 1944, John Alexander-Sinclair Papers, ms. ENG.C.4655, Bodleian Library, Oxford (hereafter BLO).

35. Woodbridge, *UNRRA*, vol. 2, 145–46, 174.

36. H. Stanley Banks in "Discussion of the present status of infectious disease control in continental Europe," *Proceedings of the Royal Society of Medicine* 40 (February 28, 1947): 628; L. Killen, "Politics and the Rockefeller Foundation in Postwar Yugoslavia," *East European Quarterly* 28 (1994): 297–302.

37. Stettinius to Kirk, October 10, 1944, U.S. State Department, *Foreign Relations of the United States, 1944* (Washington, DC: U.S. Government Printing Office, 1967), 2:347.

38. Miller, *United States and Italy*, 207.

39. Delegazione del Governo Italiano per i Rapporti con l'UNRRA, *I risultati di una inchiesta sui consumi alimentari nelle convivenze assistite dall' UNRRA* (Rome, 1947), iii, 73; UNRRA, European Regional Office, Division of Operational Research, Operational Analysis Paper no. 6, *UNRRA's Welfare Program in Italy: Supplementary Feeding of Mothers and Children* (London: UNRRA, 1946), 23–24, 28.

40. D. Stapleton, "Internationalism and Nationalism: The Rockefeller Foundation, Public Health and Malaria in Italy, 1923–1951," *Parissitologia* 42 (2000): 127–34; S. Litsios, "Malaria Control, the Cold War and the Postwar Reorganization of International Assistance," *Medical Anthropology* 17 (1997): 255–61.

41. H. Kumm, "Malaria Control West of Rome during the Summer of 1944," Rockefeller Foundation Archives, RG 1.2, Series 700, Box 12, Folder 102 (hereafter RF 1.2/700/12/102), Rockefeller Archive Center, Pocantico Hills, New York (hereafter RAC); P. Russell, Allied Control Commission, Public Health Sub-commission, Malaria Control Branch, "Memorandum on malaria and its control in liberated Italy, 1 January–30 September, 1944," RAC 1.2/700/12/101.

42. J. Farley, "Mosquitoes or Malaria? Rockefeller Campaigns in the American South and Sardinia," *Parassitologia* 36 (1994): 165–73; J. Logan, *The Sardinian Project: An Experiment in the Eradication of an Indigenous Malarious Vector* (Baltimore: Johns Hopkins University Press, 1953); J. Farley, *To Cast Out Disease: The History of the International Health Division of the Rockefeller Foundation, 1913–1951* (Oxford: Oxford University Press, 2004), 145–50.

43. Stettinius to Roosevelt, December 15, 1944, U.S. State Department, *Foreign Relations of the United States, 1944*, 2:324–25.

44. Woodbridge, *UNRRA*, vol. 2, 98–100; vol. 3, 421.

45. J. Miller Vine, "Historical Notes, UNRRA Greece, Health Division," [1947], PAG-4/4.2:35, UNA.

46. D. Giannuli, "'Repeated Disappointment': The Rockefeller Foundation and the Reform of the Greek Public Health System, 1929–1940," *Bulletin of the History of Medicine* 72 (1998): 47–72.

47. N. Goodman to W. Sawyer, September 29, 1945, PAG-4/1.3.1.5.0.0:10, UNA.

48. J. Miller Vine, "UNRRA's Health Campaign in Greece," *Lancet* 247 (1946): 790.

49. Miller Vine, "Historical Notes."

50. C. Damkas et al., "Final Report: UNRRA Greece Mission Northern Region," Salonika, November 1946, 568, PAG-4/4.2:36, UNA; UNRRA, "The Program of Insect Control on Crete," [1946], 2, PAG-4/4.2:36, UNA; D. E. Wright (USPHS), "Report on the Activities of the Sanitation Section of Health Division UNRRA from Nov. 1944 to Dec. 1946," 13, PAG-4/4.2.135, UNA.

51. G. Smith (UNRRA Balkan Mission), "DDT for Relief and Rehabilitation," December 1944, PAG-4/1.3.1.5.0.0:12, UNA; P. Noel (U.S. Army), "DDT Insecticide," August 11, 1944, PAG-4/1.3.1.5.0.0:8 DDT, UNA.

52. J. Miller Vine, "Malaria Control with DDT on a National Scale: Greece 1946," *Proceedings of the Royal Society of Medicine* 40 (1946–47): 841–48.

53. P. S. Robinson, "Malarial Control at Araxos," PAG-4/4.2:35, UNA; G. E. Smith, "Preliminary report on the uses of DDT in Greece—1946," August 31, 1946, PAG-4/4.2:35, UNA; D. E. Wright, "Report on the Activities of the Sanitation Section," PAG-4/4.2:35, UNA.

54. F. Cooper, "Decolonizing Situations: The Rise, Fall and Rise of Colonial Studies, 1951–2001," *French Politics, Culture and Society* 20 (2002): 65–66.

55. S. Amrith, "Development and Disease: Public Health and the United Nations, c. 1945–55," in *Worlds of Political Economy*, ed. M. J. Daunton and F. Trentmann, 217–40 (Basingstoke: Palgrave, 2004).

56. F. Cooper, *Decolonization and African Society: The Labor Question in French and British Africa* (Cambridge: Cambridge University Press, 1996), 177–82; M. Shipway, "Reformism and the 'Official Mind': The 1944 Brazzaville Conference and the Legacy of the Popular Front," in *The French Colonial Empire and the Popular Front*, ed. T. Chafer and A. Sackur (London: Macmillan, 1999), 145–47.

57. H. Michel and B. Mirkine-Guetzévitch, eds., *Les idées politiques et sociales de la résistance* (Paris: PUF, 1954), 339; D.-C. Danielle, "Les Problèmes de santé à la Conférence de Brazzaville," in *Brazzaville: Janvier–février 1944, Aux sources de la décolonisation: Colloque organisé par l'Institut Charles de Gaulle et l'Institut d'Histoire du Temps Présent*, 157–69 (Paris: Plon, 1988).

58. Cooper, *Decolonization and African Society*, 204–5; M. Havinden and D. Meredith, *Colonialism and Development: Britain and Its Tropical Colonies* (London: Routledge, 1993), 206–35.

59. J. G. Janssens, "Comparative Aspects: I. The Belgian Congo," in *Health in Tropical Africa During the Colonial Period*, ed. E. E. Sabben-Clare, D. J. Bradley, and K. Kirkwood (Oxford: Clarendon Press, 1980), 221–22.

60. J. E. Lewis, "The Ruling Compassions of the Late Colonial State: Welfare Versus Force, Kenya, 1945–1952," *Journal of Colonialism and Colonial History* 2 (2001).

61. Letter, S. D. Waley to J. M. Keynes, January 15, 1945, FO371/51354 12706, Public Record Office, London (hereafter PRO).

62. M. S. Venkataramani, *The Bengal Famine of 1943: The American Response* (Delhi: Vikar Publishing, 1973), 53–56.

63. Letter, D. Reekie (OFRRO) to T. Parran, May 27, 1943, Parran Papers, 90/F-14 FF 1047, HLUP.

64. Letter, E. N. Kleffens (Netherlands Foreign Office, London) to H. Lehman, November 24, 1944, FO371/51354 12706, PRO.

65. Minute, P. J. N. Stent, January 22, 1945, FO371/51354 12706, PRO.

66. Memo, D. Ogilvy to W. Hasler, March 20, 1945, FO371/51354 12706, PRO.

67. Minute, M. Mackenzie, September 21, 1943, CO859/66/114 XC3668, PRO.

68. Minute, A. H. Poynton, March 13, 1946, CO859/110/2, PRO.

69. International Labour Office, *Social Policy in Dependent Territories* (Montreal: ILO, 1944), 54–55.

70. ILO, *Social Policy in Dependent Territories*, 49–60, 140–41, 134.

71. Cooper, *Decolonization and African Society*, 216–17, 220.

72. C. E. Paz Soldan, *La OMS y la Soberanía Sanitaria de las Américas* (Lima: Instituto de Medicina Social de la Universidad Mayor de San Marcos, 1949), 35–58.

73. "'UK objects in international health organization': Notes by the Ministry of Health," FO371/57071 XC3430, PRO.

74. "Note by Colonial Office," August 1947, CO857/156/1 XC3668, PRO.

75. Memo, K. Robinson (Colonial Office) to Goodwin (Foreign Office), September 12, 1946, FO371/59619 XC3502, PRO.

76. D. G. Pirie, "Minute," May 24, 1950, CO936/64/5 XC4387, PRO.

77. Memo, D. G. Pirie to M. Hepp, March 8, 1950, CO859/216/2 XC4173, PRO; Memo, Wilson Rae, February 10, 1950, CO936/64/5 XC4387, PRO.

78. J. Kent, *The Internationalization of Colonialism: Britain, France and Black Africa, 1939–1956* (Oxford: Clarendon Press, 1992), 269.

79. Colonial Office, *Malnutrition in African Mothers, Infants and Young Children: Report of the 2nd Inter-African (CCTA) Conference on Nutrition, Gambia 1952* (London: HMSO, 1954); Kent, *The Internationalization of Colonialism*, 273–85.

80. U.S. House of Representatives, Foreign Affairs Committee, *United States Membership in the World Health Organization, Hearings June 13, 17 and July 3, 1947* (Washington, DC, 1947), 70.

81. Commission to Study the Organization of Peace (CSOP), *Uniting the Nations for Health* (New York: CSOP, 1947), 12. This report was drafted by a committee that included the leading public health figures Winslow and Boudreau.

82. J. Marseille, *Empire colonial et capitalisme français* (Paris: Albin Michel, 1984), 348–49.

83. "Brief on the possible establishment of an African Region," 1950, CO936/64/5 XC4367, PRO.

84. Cooper, *Decolonization and African Society*, 362–63.

85. L. Sicking, "France and the Colonial Dimension of the European Economic Community," *French Colonial History* 5 (2004): 215.

86. Cooper, *Decolonization and African Society*, 430–32.

Part Three

Preserving the Local

Chapter Six

Designs within Disorder

International Conferences on Rural Health Care and the Art of the Local, 1931–39

Lion Murard

"Public health, like government, must be 'of all the people' and 'by all the people,' as well as 'for all the people.'" This statement by C. E. A. Winslow, professor emeritus of public health at Yale University, to the Fifth World Health Assembly in 1952, outlines a grassroots, developmentalist program of public health that he hoped would not be "sold as a finished product of expert thinking" but would instead be "planned to meet the needs of a particular locale."[1]

A legacy of the League of Nations Health Organization (LNHO), Winslow's call included three essential components: (1) the equation of public health with social improvement; (2) a move away from top-down, large-scale crash programs offered by outsiders; and (3) a deep sensitivity to the peculiarities of local, "vernacular" cultures. As early as 1936, the elite among transnational experts were claiming that "the best health program is to raise the standard of living of the people."[2] In arguing for the importance of avoiding community health organization "imposed by fiat from on high," Winslow was mirroring their reservations about the "standard" solutions and other prepackaged projects that American philanthropy deployed between the wars to almost every European locale.[3] Andrija Štampar , Bela Johan, Ludwik Rajchman, Frank G. Boudreau, Edgar Sydenstricker and John A. Kingsbury as well as Selskar M. Gunn, Jacques Parisot, René Sand, John B. Grant, and Berislav Borcic: all of these tough-, like-minded professionals had been won over to the principle of a locally democratic path to root-and-branch reform. The disenchantment with cookie-cutter solutions was rife even inside the Rockefeller Foundation. Persuaded that it was neither possible nor desirable "to have a policy which will work well in both France and Turkey," some mercurial officers had, by the mid-1920s, started disowning the long-entertained illusion of a popular mobilization from above.[4]

Gradualist, indigenous development was the new fetish endorsed by the "epoch-making" European conference on rural hygiene (held in Geneva in 1931).[5] Concern with what would work in each locale caused the LNHO to convene "regional gatherings" in far-flung corners of the world.[6] Among these meetings were the Pan-African Health Conference (Johannesburg, November 20–30, 1935).[7] Others were the Conference of Far Eastern Countries on Rural Hygiene (Bandung, August 3–17, 1937) and the conference of American countries devoted to the same topic (scheduled for November 10, 1938 in Mexico City but canceled).[8] This worldwide, all-out drive targeting downtrodden villages marked a "decisive watershed" in the politics of disease prevention.[9] Long dedicated to the *classes laborieuses, classes dangereuses* (calling attention to income differentials), social medicine now tilted toward agrarian societies (noting ethnic-geographic differentials). By the eve of the canceled European Conference on Rural Life (scheduled for the summer of 1939), discussions of disaggregating health questions from locality had been relegated to the wastebasket. Lifting peasants out of poverty required capturing their life conditions in minute detail.

In public health circles, there was much excitement about garnering "spontaneous" village community support.[10] Bottom-up participation, public health professionals assumed, would have a quick health payoff. This hoped-for participation and "local ownership," watchwords of the 1930s, are the subjects of this article.

Prologue: Health Demonstrations

The chief lesson that John Grant, the Rockefeller Foundation's self-styled "medical Bolshevik," learned from his first assignment in Puerto Rico in 1919 was that "you couldn't secure implementation unless you had a technical health consciousness among the consumers."[11] Health demonstrations were the chosen vehicle for developing such technical consciousness. To ensure reliable services, the demonstrations strove to determine the cost of an adequate program and the feasibility of community support. Arguably, the most important overall achievement of the flagship Framingham tuberculosis demonstration, launched during the spring of 1917,[12] was not so much the development of a series of well-rounded health activities in this Massachusetts city as the "stimulation of public sentiment in favor of them."[13] The hope was to make "believers . . . out of cynics."[14] "This is the real point," the head of the Commonwealth Fund stated. "If we can prove that public health is not only purchasable but worth purchasing, then the cost will take care of itself."[15]

One of the first attempts to elicit taxpayers' support dates from the early 1920s, when the Committee on Administrative Practice (CAP) of the American Public Health Association, chaired by Winslow, calculated the "earnings on the dollar expended" for health care.[16] The CAP's appraisal forms for expressing public health achievements fitted the complex reality of local health work into a Procrustean bed of numerical targets. And yet these "forays into a mathematical never-never land" did not become irrelevant.[17] However debatable the assigned monetary values might be, such numerical ratings did allow for comparison from town to town. The "Framingham yardsticks" and other science-based performance standards provided "a common denominator, a uniform basis of comparison for local health work regardless of variations in size, population, budget, or health problems of the different counties."[18] Moreover, such comparisons led to an "automatic self-standardization" of the localities concerned.[19] Numerical scores did not merely classify communities according to their ability to purchase health protection; the boosting of intercommunity competition spilled over from the local to the national level.

"Framinghaming" was the neologism coined to refer to this determination to rationalize administrative health practices by turning a hodgepodge of local, fortuitous happenings into a concerted national program.[20] For its part, the Milbank Memorial Fund continually called for communities to "repeat the Framingham demonstration on a larger scale," and to transpose the experience thus gained into general practice.[21] In assessing the three New York Milbank demonstrations in the late 1920s, Winslow conceded that their objective was "not to help Cattaraugus County, Syracuse and Bellevue-Yorkville, but to use them as levers to change health practice in the United States."[22]

Success stories did not provide a simple blueprint for imitation. Scoring health practices tended toward overstandardization, "which is one of our characteristic national vices," according to Winslow.[23] It pushed local authorities to think in terms of standard patterns rather than local needs: 30 nurses per 100,000 inhabitants, 8 visits for each and every case of whooping cough, and so on. Although the program's "modules" could be easily deployed in nearly any locality, they tended to be blatantly indifferent to the specific logic of *place*.

Reproduce, Imitate, Copy

"With God's help," an unvarnished Midwestern senator exulted in 1940, "we will lift Shanghai up and up, ever up, until it is just like Kansas City."[24] Although spokespeople for "philanthropic globalism" after World War I would have voiced that cliché more tactfully, their reasoning was much the same. The Rockefeller Commission for the Prevention of Tuberculosis in France guaranteed officially that tuberculosis could be brought under control "only by French agencies rooted in life and tradition of the people."[25] In private, however, it was "anxious to extend our work [. . .] while we would have a greater influence than if we came to the game later, after the French had taken the initiative."[26] Was this doubletalk? Not at all. Pointing out the "right way" to Europeans would spare them "the mistakes that we made in the United States twenty years ago."[27] With the world's nations arrayed in marching order, it was enticing to "teach French doctors American methods,"[28] apply American standards to British nursing,[29] and plant in Hungary the precept, "brought from America," about the "absolute indispensability of public health nurses."[30] Health demonstrations were seen as setting a "standard for all to follow."[31]

Imbued with a millennial-utopian vision of applied science uniting a divided world, the Rockefeller Foundation International Health Board transferred holus-bolus the practices and standards designed in the American South (or British Guiana).[32] It swore "to avoid the impression that foreigners are coming in to assume functions which belong to the French."[33] At the same time, it relished the fact that the antituberculosis organization offered to the French was "more or less like the one that exists in America."[34] How ironic were these unswerving efforts to redesign the Old World in an endlessly replicated image of the New and, simultanenously to claim that this image was intensely localized! The campaign against malaria designed by an American transplant in Rome, the Rockefeller Foundation–sponsored "*stazione sperimentale*," was presented from the mid-1920s onward as a "distinctly Italian enterprise."[35]

But the well-worn positivist faith in an unforced universalization of best practices was waning. "Are we not dogmatists and too much sold on our dogma?" the more sensible Rockefeller field officers were asking.[36] The Rockefeller Foundation's Paris office had already intimated as much in 1921: disinclined to judge others by the extent to which they contrived to be like themselves, it was satisfied in Prague "to combine the best of American and Czech."[37] This attitude signaled a break with the easygoing "culture-free" model of health. In 1927, Selskar M. Gunn led a charge: "Americanizing European public health, herein lies the greatest danger in the future for our work in Europe."[38] This was a witty remark by a man who, a short time before, had been delighted with the eventual "de-Austrianization" of the successor states (first of all, Czechoslovakia). "They want to make their country a small United States, and are looking in our direction," Gunn breezily reported after returning from Prague in June 1919.[39]

In this trip to Prague, the first visit by a Rockefeller official to central Europe, Gunn reached the self-satisfied conclusion that a "strong demand for adequate health service will have to be created."[40] Alas, we have already seen this movie. How could an elite-guided, U.S.-style community experiment "create" a sound, intelligent public opinion abroad? The belief that persuasion and education would bring the desires of the population in line with the plans of experts was a fable that James Scott has rightly called the "populist technocrat's creed."[41] Rockefeller philanthropy had just suffered a blow in France, where the biggest antituberculosis campaign ever conducted in the world had targeted 1.25 million adults and 1.5 million children, but with no real success.[42] "There is much interest in France concerning tuberculosis, infant mortality and venereal diseases," Gunn complained in February 1919, "but as far as a conception of public health as a whole is concerned, there are not many signs of activity."[43] This was a major disappointment and, in fact, a "repeated" one.[44] But should we be surprised that a revolution from above failed to mobilize the grassroots and encountered trouble building up its own popular base? No amount of rhetoric can obscure the contradictions.

What had changed on the cusp of the 1930s was that Europe now claimed to have its own indigenous methods for bringing in (mobilizing) the local population. Danish folk high schools, Italian *bonifiche*, the Hungarian Green Cross, Croatian rural health centers, the Bavarian *Zweckverband-System*—these stellar, influential showpieces and pilot schemes set the stage for a recontinentalization of health models. One thing was certain: social medicine in Europe had begun to tilt away from urban settings. Not only did its welfare commitments appeal to the rural masses, but its particular, intensely communal achievements drew the real map of European health care.

The First International Conference on Rural Health Care, 1931

The test case for public health, both to gain a foothold in the European hinterland and to take off as a popular movement, was to be the 1931 Geneva conference. At a time when postwar mass democracy failed to consolidate itself in central and eastern Europe and the socialist parties turned against the new and popular agrarian groups, the LNHO-sponsored gatherings on rural hygiene extended a hand to peasant organizations and solicited their involvement in opening equal access to health. Ludwik Rajchman and his associates admitted that these meetings had a political tone. Unable to cure the working class movement's "incredible folly," which David Mitrany has judged a "central factor in the making of the Second World War,"[45] Geneva redoubled its efforts to break the stranglehold over the rural masses and their dedicated leaders.

Attended by delegates from twenty-three countries in Europe and observers from the United States, Mexico, China, India, and Japan, the first International Conference on rural health care (from June 29 to July 7, 1931 in

Geneva) aimed at crafting a "charter for the peasantry."[46] "Rural populations have as good a right to health as children or urban populations" was the official motto.[47] Following a Spanish initiative, agronomists, architects, hygienists, and engineers met with representatives from public hospitals, illness insurance funds, farmers' associations, and the medical corps, set the minimum standards for rural health administration and, even more important, drew attention to using health as an elixir for socioeconomic development.

The bold decision was geared to the principle of "adapting to local conditions."[48] How could health officials set up operations in villages without learning, as pioneers in social medicine in South Africa stated clearly, "what the community feels, thinks and does about its health needs?"[49] The best solution might turn out to be a subterfuge, such as that created by Bela Johan, director of the Hungarian State Institute of Hygiene, to soothe perennial tensions between farm and city. As he would recall some years later, deep-seated, almost ingrained hostility toward government bureaucracy made attendance at the health centers on the vast Putza region a distant dream. Johan's strategy for getting mothers to bring in their poorly fed infants was to secure forty wagonloads of sugar and then spread the word that any child examined by a doctor would receive two pounds per month of this hotly demanded, expensive foodstuff. Soon after, Johan got the idea of using the same sort of incentive to gain compliance from pregnant women, who were "rather resistant to this sort of visit."[50]

The 1931 conference recognized that culture and politics could be formidable impediments to rural public health. Lifting those impediments with the help of food, lectures, traveling exhibits, lantern slides, and photographs was the everyday task of the statesmen of the public health: "What is essential is to obtain the collaboration of the population *by any and all means.*"[51]

Health as a Means of Wealth Creation

Public health professionals marshaled European expertise to take up the challenge of rousing the country folk and obtaining their backing. For years, "cooperative Denmark" had been a second home for health educators,[52] an agrarian commonwealth where the "best health propaganda work is done by dairies."[53] "I am still under the charm of your country," Ludwik Rajchman, the League of Nations medical director, wrote in 1925 to his close friend, Thorvald Madsen, president of the Health Committee. "[George E.] Vincent [the Rockefeller Foundation president] fully shares our admiration of everything Danish."[54] Everything? The word is strong, since it is hard not to have reservations about a nation governed by the single idea of its homogeneity, a peasant-based democracy that tended to instill in the poverty stricken, the weak, and the deviant a "fear of a loss of civic status" with, as a consequence, negative eugenics.[55]

Folk high schools, a hotbed of politics and of the cooperative movement, were at the center of this adulation.[56] Older than farm cooperatives, whose cultural adjuncts they were, the *folkehøjskoler* taught in a summer term a curriculum that combined Nordic myths, old heroic poetry, and biblical history with singing and gymnastics, the universal vernacular for bogus nationalisms.[57] Dairying and bookkeeping were not overlooked, nor were the diseases of livestock and the scientific treatment of cows as milking machines. However, youngsters were protected from too much bookishness. Education was not an alternative term for schooling, Nicholai Grundtvig, "the Prophet of the North," pronounced dogmatically. Therefore, the folk high schools used very few textbooks, assigned no lessons, had no examinations, and did not "graduate" anybody.[58] As with the Russian populists, on-the-ground learning was the watchword.

By the mid-1920s, a number of "physicians and statesmen of public health" had bought into this approach. The laws of health and farmhouse sanitation woven into the fabric of rural folkways instead of being "sold" by experts or leaders, this was the Danish record. As American progressives pointed out with admiration, the teacher in a folk high school or an agricultural experiment station "must be willing to *learn* his community before he dares of *teaching* it anything."[59]

Education Is Not Enough

Without a genuine populist movement, a locally democratic path to a "national-social-and-health" renaissance was very unlikely. Apart from Denmark, the poster child for popular participation was the Yugoslavia of Andrija Štampar .[60] The son of a village schoolmaster, Štampar drew on the vitality of "peasantism" in the newborn Kingdom of Serbs, Croats, and Slovenians to build from scratch a truly national health service. "You are veritably a magician who waves a wand and polyclinics, sanatoria, institutes, malaria stations and health houses spring from the ground," the Rockefeller Foundation's president, George E. Vincent, told the "Balkan bear" in the mid-1920s.[61] Even more telling was Štampar's "peaceful conquest of a whole population through health work," the LNHO marveled.[62] The LNHO's medical director urged eastern European administrators to attend Štampar's lectures and emulate his consensus-building qualities. "Learning his doctrines" might endow central Europe with a common idiom.[63]

Indeed, transnational experts viewed Štampar's land as a crucial testing ground for widening the reach of social medicine. "He has completely won the confidence of the peasantry," Selskar Gunn stated in 1924.[64] Štampar, who headed the Health Ministry's Department of Hygiene and Social Medicine (May 28, 1919–May 20, 1931), chose in that very year a dozen villages to make a general demonstration of a safe water supply, the cleaning of gutters, the removal of manure, and the whitewashing of homes inside. In each locale, a salubrious house, a school of home economics, and a small health center were to be built. Villagers would come to expect increasing returns on invest-ment in cleanliness, and "their cooperation will be easily won," predicted the Vienna-trained doctor.[65] As he probably realized, the official advisory commit-tees (made up of the mayor, the priest, the teacher, and one or two promi-nent citizens) who were to oversee the nurse's and doctor's jobs, were hardly representative. Pilloried as "ratifying public bodies" whose role was to grant populist legitimation to decisions made elsewhere, the advisory committees hardly set the stage for the form of rural government Štampar sought—a gov-ernment, as he confided to Gunn, "which would take in consideration all the social needs of the community."[66] Such well-schooled committees were clearly out of touch, not only in Yugoslavia, but also in Poland, where a petted and compliant local elite "did not wait long before resigning."[67]

And yet, as a whole, Yugoslavia (Croatia above all) avoided this detestable model of "participatory autocracy." "Imaginative nationalisms" were resusci-tated from the previous organs of peasant self-government. A spiritual driv-ing force in the day-to-day business of cooperation, the Croat Peasant party's cultural branch reanimated music societies, rediscovered long-forgotten folk costumes, and coped with adult illiteracy "not through professional teachers but by a kind of self-help among the villagers themselves."[68] These "invented traditions" were the attraction of Stjepan Radic's peasantism.[69] In his mem-oirs, David Mitrany, a British scholar of Romanian origin, recalled observing, as he traveled from one hamlet to the next in the land of the southern Slavs in 1924 "the most impressive experience of what a down-to-earth movement could achieve when bent upon inner development, almost wholly through cooperatives, including cultural and health cooperatives."[70]

Ethnic Polarization

Of course, ethnic politics metastasized through the Rockefeller-sponsored Zagreb School of Public Health—now called the Andrija Štampar School—which Radic inaugurated on October 3, 1927 in the presence of the League of Nations Health Committee's leading members.[71] Štampar, a Croat of Ger-man lineage, fell into line with the dour but honest Christian leader described by Rebecca West: "Radic was the spit and image of Tolstoy," a poster image whose name was synonymous with Croatdom: "Not even Gandhi had more magnetic effect on his followers."[72] As the exalted expression of a "peasant civilization" antipathetic to urban life, the Zagreb School was quite different from its sister institutions elsewhere in Europe, precisely because it aimed to spread "knowledge of health among the peasants" and thus involve them in growth-creating policies. Peasants "often realize their own needs better than do people who come from the cities," Štampar claimed.[73] Thus, the school targeted young rural inhabitants, who, in groups of thirty to forty, attended its Danish-style "Peasant University" courses.[74] These included cooking, homemaking, childrearing, tending to the sick, weaving, and embroidery for girls (three months); and farm machinery, cooperatives, infectious diseases, privies, and spittoons for boys (five months).[75] The nine hundred young people selected by their villages from 1926 to 1937 were not deaf to the call of Croatian nationalism, since they came from the very districts where "there has existed for many years an exceedingly strong peasant movement."[76] After swearing to stay away from depraved town life and to be teetotallers, these young catechists went back home to initiate others to temperance, dig public wells, and establish health centers.[77]

More important than the particular courses, hearts and minds in the villages were being remolded by the "teacher-propagandists" trained in rural hygiene at the Zagreb School. Armed with lecturing materials, portable projection equipment, and slides, the propagandists each moved through twenty or thirty localities during the winter, dispensing courses with a show of support that came from the attendance of Economic Concord's (the Radic party's cooperative branch) farm and veterinary inspectors. The climax of the visits was the formation of village-based associations that competed in draining marshes, erecting manure storage tanks, or cleaning houses and streets. The inspectors paid attention to layouts for cheap housing, especially the proper places for bedrooms, outhouses, cesspools, and manure pits of the "Kentucky-type." Mraclin, a village 20 miles (32 kilometers) from Zagreb, was transformed into a "model health demonstration center," an idyllic museum showpiece with fourteen hundred inhabitants.[78] Many local health centers emulated its example in what the Rockefeller Foundation enjoyed calling "Dr. Štampar's realm."[79]

Carrying the Message to the People

Where peasants were "convinced that hygiene pays,"[80] a positive-feedback loop occurred. This reassuring mantra of the 1930s encapsulated the concept of "hygienic-economic object" so dear to Belgrade's Union of Health Cooperatives. At the instigation of the Serbian Child Welfare Association of America and its active chairman, John Kingsbury (the executive secretary of the Milbank Memorial Fund from 1921 to 1935), the Belgrade Union in 1929 called for every "health *zadruga*" to install one such object: refuse and dung bins, school latrines, sanitized wells, stables, and so on.[81] Out of the approximately fifty cooperatives involved in Serbia and elsewhere (in particular among the German minority in

Voyvodina), only one mountain village (Slavkovica, near Ljig) showed much interest in home sanitation.[82] Expert workmen under the supervision of an engineer were sent there to attack infection at its sources in the water supply, toilets (or rather their absence), and manure piles: "It was a real practical school which was visited by the larger part of the village; and, after the work was complete, many of the villagers began to erect individually similar objects in their own households."[83] Slavkovica soon became a "model village," the Serbian counterpart of Mraclin in Croatia. Coop members in the neighborhoods volunteered to dig public wells, sanitize stables and pigsties, and pave the village square.

Local ownership was crucial for producing concrete, visible outcomes, for which individuals were accountable. Štampar's quick fix—"*Kittel Schule*, short courses for peasants, a good field staff, experimental agricultural stations and laboratories"—was geared to delivering results rather than plans.[84] Indeed, it squared fairly well with the incentive-based views of growth that the Rockefeller Foundation's General Education Board had tried in the boll-weevil-infested American southern states, through Seaman Knapp's farm demonstrations.[85] "From farmer to farmer through emulation, rather than from expert to farmer through education," the "Knapp ethos" turned out to be remarkably pervasive.[86] It suffused, for instance, the boys' corn, poultry, or tomato clubs and the girls' gardening or canning clubs that evolved into the nationwide 4-H Clubs for the development of Head, Hand, Heart and Health. In Yugoslavia too, the Young Farmers' Clubs found themselves coopted into the day-to-day business of improving the country's diet.[87] The goal was to *show* villagers the advantages they might reap from encouraging advances in health. Decades of rhetoric about participation had failed to leave much of a mark. Merging financial and health interests, officials assumed, would create a sense of stable expectations. As a result, locals would take over the whole matter and promote their own agendas.

Were these discrete showcases of "correct" sanitation transferrable? The basic recipe for a demonstration to be convincing and, in Kingsbury's words, "compel imitation," called for the audience to compare what it was seeing with its own living conditions.[88] Adopted not as something foreign but as the right way to do things, it would keep going beneath a "native mask." "Ocular demonstrations" using motion pictures, posters, and photographs, Štampar argued, provided the best results when the clothing and general looks of the characters closely corresponded to the audience's.[89] How to present showers, model toilets, and proper bedding to village youngsters? The actors should wear traditional dress, the action should take place *in situ*, and the story should be written by a local writer.[90] Folkways thus became the "fixative" that helped each of these sparsely settled, self-sufficient "model units" to stand on its own.

And yet the model units' radiating, capillary influence transcended spatial location. For they managed to be both distinctive and, at the same time, highly adaptable to foreign "contamination" if it was brought to the country folk in the right way. As a *nativistic movement,* each unit articulated the particular culture in which it remained embedded; as a nativistic movement *of foreign kindling,* they fitted into a continuum ranging between the purely local at one end to the purely Danish, or American, at the other. Grown from the outside in as well as from the inside out, they were in dire need of further "contamination" in order to survive.

Americanization or Americanism

The opening of the John Kingsbury Health Home at Pranjane in November 1930, to which "people traveled half the night, some of them coming from thirty-five kilometers away, on foot," is a good case in point. Four priests conducted religious services, which were followed by festivities drawing more than "a thousand peasants, boys and girls, young and old, dancing the kolo hand in hand on the green lawn."[91] In this memorable scene, we catch a glimpse of something rare: an American scheme that took hold from the bottom up. Countless U.S.-style projects in France and elsewhere perished, we might say, from an excess of imitation. In Pranjane, however, a highly original mixture of an indigenous "Americanism" (local, not alien) was manufactured/concocted.

This Americanism—or the dissemination of a common language both flexible and serviceable in local forms—contrasts with the prior Americanization that superimposed alien ways on native ones.[92] Geneva was not unaware of the role of the Rockefeller philanthropies in the accomplishments of the 1920s. The American member of the League's Health Section stated with self-satisfaction on the eve of the 1931 meeting, "The permeation of European health practice by American influences [runs so deep] in the smaller countries of central and eastern Europe [that] American public health practice is almost idealized."[93] But Europe slowly found its own voice. Livingston Farrand, the first director of the Rockefeller Mission for the Prevention of Tuberculosis in France (1917), candidly admitted his intent to "gather the results of the work done in different places in America during the last fifteen or twenty years and apply them in concentrated form."[94] Aware that a recipient community aims at reasserting its altered or shattered cultural identity without "subservience" to the donor,[95] Elisabeth Crowell claimed in 1926 to be offering the southern Slavs the "result of our American experience plus a digest of our various European experiences."[96]

This seismic shift recalls the one made in the Pacific where, captured by local interests, the static, freeze-frame Rockefeller models "swiftly dissolved during implementation."[97] Far from imposing external and noninvolving "appropriate" practices, as James Gillespie asserts about Australia, officials redefined health priorities depending on the context so as to "advance quite distinct political and administrative projects."[98] This shift had far-reaching consequences, since the very plurality of experiments—more or less combinable, and sometimes incommensurable—dealt a fatal blow to the prevailing diffusionist viewpoint. "I am far from convinced that American methods are necessarily the best for European countries," Gunn declared outright from his Paris headquarters. "There exist men and women who have a better understanding of the local problems and the means to be used to meet them than we have."[99]

Localness, plasticity, an awareness of the contextual and the vernacular: these watchwords constitute a real departure from American "export models," Winslow reported with admiration while touring the Balkans in the summer of 1929: "Štampar has been wise in attacking the first problems first (lack of fundamental decencies, virulent scarlet fever, anthrax, rabies) and not attempting to transport advanced procedures into a primitive country."[100] This is no surprise, since Štampar had turned away from forced-march modernization. Public health as a politicized form of culture was the new catchphrase of a Danish-style plan that "the people in general, and the peasantry in particular, are backing more and more."[101] Patience with local peculiarities earned loyalties.

In sum, the 1931 European conference epitomized the LNHO triple commitment to (1) putting a premium on the recovery of a mass peasant-class constituency; (2) increasing health and wealth in tandem; and (3) knitting together a continental "unity" of nested, interlocking modules that could also be springboards for further influence.

Bandung, or the "Reconstruction" Method, 1937

The Geneva gathering was not yet a distant memory in 1932, when with China's support the Indian delegate asked the LNHO to convene a meeting for the Far East similar to the one for Europe (or even more ambitious). Accepting a Dutch invitation, thirteen Far Eastern governments sent delegations to Java in August 1937 to promote rural hygiene,[102] with the full realization that the conference "will extend into the general field of rural reconstruction."[103]

The Ambiance of Social Medicine

Full-tilt rehabilitation spelled the end of the "disease-oriented" approach. Building on the assertions of 1931 that long-run development could be tackled only if health activities went "hand in hand" with education, agriculture, veterinary science, home industry, and the like,[104] and those of 1937 that "the problem of hygiene is often one of indigence,"[105] public health was now considered a vehicle for holistic "community-oriented" programs.[106] By 1930, Selskar Gunn had seen the handwriting on the wall. During a meeting with Rockefeller trustees, officers, and directors, he urged satisfying the "full needs of the community rather than an isolated need such as public health."[107]

The Commission on Rural Revival and the Collaboration of the Population was obviously the "keystone," to borrow Rajchman's word, of the Bandung gathering.[108] At the time, in newspapers from Bombay to Jakarta, from Hanoi and Manila to Colombo, no plea was more familiar than "rural uplift" (or "rural welfare"), and no call more repeated than for villages to have installed whatever would make them "more attractive": a health center, library, school, cooperative, veterinary service, home gardens, and family industries started from scratch.[109] Demands were even raised for land reform to become part of the state agenda lest pump-priming be "fatally ephemeral."[110]

"Know your area, and know your people": so went the slogan of Rockefeller health units in Ceylon.[111] In contrast, the small League's Committee, chaired by the malariologist E. J. Pampana, which was preparing the Bandung meeting, faced enormous indifference during its trip through India in April 1936: "A great ignorance of the villager's life appears generalized. No survey of nutrition, no survey of the causes of death in rural areas has ever been made."[112] Still, convincing natives to keep their environment from being a mudpile or instilling "healthful habits of life" was fully feasible, as the Poerwokerto health unit on Java was demonstrating.[113] An equivalent of the Polela center in South Africa, Mraclin in Croatia, or Gödöllö in Hungary, the Dutch East Indies model unit received young mothers with their babies in a humble peasant house with bamboo walls, an earthen floor, coarse mats, and rudimentary furniture of the sort "to which villagers are accustomed"; even the material used by visiting nurses (the local *mantris*) suggested the interest in "taking sides with simplicity."[114] Making home visits routine and conducting, house by house, a village sanitary census required consensus-building qualities.

Again, there was no single recipe: "Any attempt to proceed on standardized lines would be disastrous."[115] As Gunn warned in his (unsigned) introduction to the Far East conference's report: "It is vain to implement programs that do not correspond to the population's customs and level of education."[116] By this time, fact-finding (the size of farms, productivity of the soil, literacy) could not be divorced from "Asian" values. Born in India, where "islands of rural reconstruction" had been initiated on a demonstration basis in Madras,[117] Travancore,[118] and the Punjab,[119] the Better Village Movement amounted to "an Oriental manifestation of social planning."[120]

For all its efforts to steer clear of ethnic pride, the League's premium on indigenous takeoff bore the fruit of nationalist fragmentation. For Štampar, Croat peasants were the "standard-bearer of national and political ideas."[121] In a similar vein, for Rabindranath Tagore, "Villages can be likened to women, they are the cradle of the race."[122] Once on this path, social medicine increasingly nurtured the Third World aspirations that had become molded into an ideological hunger for nationhood.

A Threatening West and the Trauma of Contact

Could transnational expertise assist slow-moving societies to recover a sense of their own national identity? The emblematic case here is Nationalist, Guomindang China from 1929 to 1937, to which the League dispatched twenty-seven tough-minded professionals (hydraulic and road engineers, British economists, Italian sericulturists, and Croatian sanitarians such as Štampar and Borcic) as part of a grand global scheme for which Ludwik Rajchman had cleared the way as liaison officer.[123] "Intimately associated" with T. V. Soong and Jean Monnet's (never-reached) objectives,[124] Rajchman strove to give statelike coherence to a centuries-old empire "that he was pained to see disorganized, at the mercy of the Japanese aggression."[125] Plagued by poor administration, stultification, and warlordism, mainland China was still competing for the record for the longest period of misgovernment. The National Quarantine Service (July 1930), the National Economic Council (August 1931) and the "three-year plan for the development of the health services, conceived as an instrument of rural reconstruction," all were engineered to prevent China's flimsy structure from falling apart.[126]

The key to a "true collaboration" with Nanking—as opposed to "international control"—was willingness to adapt to "Chineseness."[127] On his visit to the young, unruly republic in June–July 1931, Gunn shrewdly reported, "Western civilization is under fire in China."[128] Shoehorning the latter into received models was no longer on the agenda. Not surprisingly, the Rockefeller Foundation's multidisciplinary China Program (1935) departed from its preset (and grandiose) goals. While standards of excellence were abruptly abandoned, the Foundation changed its approach to "Chinafy" narrow, monitorable objectives "involving local government, security, education, livelihood and public health" that required only meager existing financial resources.[129] Giving super-medicine to China fell out of favor. Thus, artificial transplants, such as the Peking Union Medical College (PUMC), the "Johns Hopkins of China," found their influence nullified.[130]

Hence, aid agencies remained content with backing Chinese efforts that were "60% efficient rather than Western ones that were 100%."[131] Attention was drawn to ham-handed, fragile experiments of the sort designed by the

Mass Education Movement at its demonstration center in Tinghsien (Ding-xian), Hopei (Hebei) Province. An instant hit, as Gunn noted, this "village self-government organization" sparked unequaled enthusiasm, for talented PhDs "actually ended up being students of the peasants rather than their leaders."[132] Plainly, Tinghsien was an unconventional, home-grown success, failing to follow any Western blueprint for how to be modern.

The Tinghsien Educational Movement

From the grand tour he made in 1935 at the League's expense, C. C. Chen, the doctor in charge of the rural health station in Tinghsien, returned home stirred by Berislav Borcic's Zagreb Institute of Hygiene which, "not unlike the [Chinese] Mass Education Movement, advocated an integrated approach for solving rural problems." Of what he had seen in India ("a disappointment"), in the Soviet Union, Austria, Poland, and ("much more interesting") Croatia, he was "most impressed with the work being done among the peasants in Yugoslavia."[133] Andrija Štampar , Chen's elder by fifteen years and one of the brightest intelligence gatherers on rural China, where he and Borcic had spent several years as the League's "men on the spot," repaid the compliment in 1936. Tinghsien, 83 percent of whose population of four hundred thousand was illiterate, was "the experimental district which impressed me most favorably," Štampar noted: one hundred thousand medical consultations per year, fifty thousand persons attending educational discussions of health, smallpox eradicated.[134]

It was not immediately apparent how the complex pieces of the puzzle of poverty, disease, ignorance, and misgovernment fitted together. In its native, didactic form, "Tinghsienism" pursued obsessively a single goal: literacy.[135] It had its roots among the tens of thousands of needy "coolies" whom the British had displaced en masse from Shantung to war factories in France during World War I: an uneducated, toiling mass to whom the American YMCA dispatched the best on its Christian, liberal Chinese staff. At the head of this good-hearted team was Y. C. James Yen (1893–1990), a young graduate of Yale (1918), who labored in Paris to draw up a vocabulary of one thousand characters for publishing the *Hebdomadaire de l'ouvrier chinois*. Back in China (1921), Yen founded a popular library with a thousand works, concise and instructive, and launched the National Association of Mass Education Movements (1923, henceforth MEM).

One of Yen's first articles—"How to Educate China's Illiterate Millions for Democracy in a Decade"—underscores the gradual transformation of a nationwide federation of literacy movements into an all-inclusive reconstruction agency on the road to making "the primitive peasant not merely a scientific farmer, but a progressive citizen of the Chinese republic."[136]

Thanks to the Milbank Memorial Fund, which he approached through a former Yale classmate, Edgar Sydenstricker, the highly regarded statistician of the U.S. Public Health Service, Yen obtained funding for a "Chinese Cattaraugus County."[137] He set up MEM's national headquarters in Tinghsien, a six-hour train ride from Peking. MEM was given control over the local government. This move to Tinghsien—"a 'Sinification' of liberalism," to borrow Charles Hayford's phrase—brought PhDs and long-gowned scholars face to face with village China; each changed the other.[138]

Yen was not alone in disregarding Westernized education for proud, inward-looking societies. His right-hand men (including Chen, in charge of MEM's public health department), the Rockefeller "men on the ground" (first among them, John B. Grant, the head of PUMC's public health department) and a steady succession of League pundits—starting with Rajchman, the "most listened-to political advisor in Nanking"—were equally skeptical.[139] Just as in India, where the British empire was satisfied with creating a class of people "Indian in blood and color, but English in taste, in opinions, in morals and in intellect,"[140] the $12 million that the U.S. Congress had allotted for Chinese higher education in 1908 as an indemnity for the Boxer Rebellion bred "cultural mongrels."[141] Stifled by the bookish education that they imbibed abroad, they were "better qualified to handle the social problems of Germany and America than those of China." Coming primarily from urban, coastal China, the medical graduates in particular "had no idea of what the villages of their own country looked like."[142] Not surprisingly, League planners called for removing "all signs of European and American influence,"[143] an injunction in line with the dictum of Richard Tawney (the author of *Land and Labour in China*, 1932): "To look at the shelves in a university and see the acres of American textbooks is absolutely nauseating. More nationalism is badly needed."[144]

What was afoot in Tinghsien was "ventriloquism." While drawing on the Japanese New Village Movement's pastoral socialism, Yen's ten-year plan (1929) had "much in common with the one suggested by Štampar for Yugoslavia."[145] But the desire to have something really Chinese (and to set China itself against a wider world) waxed all the stronger. Tinghsien's mission statement prevented it from rehashing simplistic external answers; instead, it groped toward something distinctive: the use of unpaid, summarily trained village farmers as "medical helpers." Although the concept failed in India where it had been introduced—"perhaps because the health workers had been selected by the physicians rather than by a peer group within the village"[146]—under the Tinghsien self-referential model, lay personnel were held accountable to the top village organization, namely, the "alumni" association of the "people's school" for adults. By 1930, MEM's quick fix for growth no longer lay in "kill fly" days, "better home" clubs, tree planting, or road improvement, but in the assignment of its 423 "people's schools" (with more than ten thousand students) to create an elite from scratch.

A cohesive village self-organization formed from among the alumni was mandated to spearhead the "four fundamentals" of rural uplift: cultural education, economic betterment, public health, and citizenship training. Elected by fellow members, the key figures of an idyllic peasant republic—the demonstration farmer, the coop organizer, the "little teacher," and the village health worker— would spring up for the first time from within the village itself.

Plainly, Tinghsien's (and Bandung's) enduring contributions were related to health economics.[147] The data collected from 1926 to 1933 by MEM's department of social survey under Sidney Gamble—*Ting Hsien, a North China Rural Community*—painted a bleak picture: mud often used at childbirth to stanch bleeding from the umbilical cord, unboiled water drunk from wells only a few feet from open latrines, rampant diarrhea, tetanus, dysentery.[148] As C. C. Chen wrote about the abysmal record of infant mortality (199 per thousand live births), "Our first responsibility was to prevent communicable and infectious disease."[149] His preoccupation with cookie-cutter solutions led him to champion specificity rather than universality. In charge of the Tinghsien program from January 1932 to July 1937 (after a year of graduate work in 1930–31 at the Harvard School of Public Health, at Yale with Winslow, and at the Reichhaus für Hygienische Volksbelehrung in Dresden), this superb professional supported the suggestion of John B. Grant, his former professor at PUMC, to keep high-tech medicine at bay.[150] Even by pooling resources, no village was able to support a modern physician. Private medicine, despite its appeal, appeared mismatched, as would its *feldscher* variant suggested by Julius Tandler for training Chinese medics in two years.[151] Emphasizing the immediacy of the need, Chen chose to train village aides for a mere ten days.

The mantra, "economic practicability," led simultaneously to a socialization and deprofessionalization of medicine.[152] But Tinghsien was not mere bricolage. The peasant-medic was the capstone of a three-tier health service. At the pyramid's apex was the district health center; by 1935, it had three doctors, thirteen nurses, a dentist, a pharmacist, and a sanitary inspector to staff a fifty-bed hospital. At the base, in each constituent locale (average population eleven hundred), a full-time farmer elected from the graduates of the people's school recorded births and deaths, vaccinated against smallpox, and rendered simple treatments from the contents of a first-aid box. The fulcrum of community medicine was the middle, supervisory level: the subdistrict health station with its full-time physician, committed to providing the "barefoot doctor" the immense gratification of being needed. At regular meetings at the station—a market town encompassing twenty-five to thirty villages—"medical knowledge would filter downward while medical cases would be referred upward."[153] Though fragile as spider's web, this three-level machinery paralleled the Croatian health centers as one of the world's first integrated village-based health systems.

En Route to the Tennessee Valley

Out of the single, mesmerizing model of Tinghsien arose the concept of coordination favored in Miguel Bustamante's Mexico and Jacques Parisot's Lorraine.[154] Tinghsien also inspired a rare piece of high-profile, collaborative action—the North China Council for Rural Reconstruction, targeting 2, perhaps 10 million people.[155] Consisting of MEM, the Shantung provincial government, and five well-regarded university colleges, the North China Council—which was the major institutional accomplishment of Gunn's New China Program (1935)—refrained from siphoning one million Rockefeller dollars for a high-powered training institute in plant breeding, veterinary medicine, pest control, and rural sociology, or some other grand global demonstration. Instead, this multimember vocal body (of which John B. Grant was the only Western member) used aid resources to connect *already successful* programs, such as those implemented by its founding fathers in social medicine, local government, civil administration, rural engineering, and literacy. Pooling "several fragmentary native efforts into a united movement to improve the lot of the Chinese peasant" was all the rage.[156]

First impressions, in effect, were somewhat depressing. "Plenty of plans, mostly on paper," as the economist and political scientist Leonard S. Hsü put it.[157] Perhaps rehabilitation was indeed "the most pregnant of all the political phenomena in the Far East."[158] But its heavy-handed implementation required revision. Take the much-abused example of the community-based welfare centers in Kiangsi (Jianxi). Unlike MEM's private endeavor, the muscular Kiangsi Rural Welfare Service fitted into Chiang Kai-shek's (Jiang Jieshi's) strategy of exterminating the Red Army through road construction, water conservancy, and improvements in sericulture. Its inception dated to a November 1933 LNHO mission headed by Andrija Štampar . He reported that "the chief link of unrest" in a province just cleared of soviets was "the tenancy system."[159] Besides bold land reform, the envoys urged the creation of wide-ranging powerhouses of "welfare" (and not health) that, paired with agricultural stations, were to shelter a "team of builders of rural civilization" (doctors, midwives, teachers, and coop and home-industry technicians).[160]

The hoped-for rehabilitation came at a price. Launched in conjunction with Chiang's "New Life Movement," much of the work was useful, but "everything, from the building of roads to the spectacular removal of five thousand latrines, has been done by compulsion."[161] For its part, Robert Haas, secretary of the League's Council Committee on Technical Cooperation with China, noted that the locals were "*probably forced* to improve the conditions of hygiene in their dwellings."[162] So much for a plan loaded with Yugoslavian experience.[163] Indeed, the welfare activities in Kiangsi "fell grotesquely short" of L. Rajchman, T. V. Soong, and J. Monnet's confidence in civic training and a merit-based civil service as a panacea for growth.[164] After six years in Nanking, Borcic, "the uncrowned prince of the Chinese health service,"[165] complained in July 1936, "To drift on as we are now doing makes our work here extremely difficult and, in my opinion, useless."[166]

Doubtless, Borcic's frustration reflected the four and a half days he spent in November 1935 in the Tennessee River Valley with Jacques Parisot, Frank Boudreau, and other LNHO representatives.[167] "The granddaddy of all regional development projects" (as well as a fair prototype for international action),[168] the TVA brought together seven states for soil erosion control, better agricultural practices, and rural sanitation in pursuit of a "valley development in its entirety."[169] Working shoulder to shoulder with the ARC, the Rockefeller Foundation, the U.S. Public Health Service, state and local health officials, and even the federal Department of Agriculture, the TVA's Health Section triggered a united stand against malaria.[170] Like the National Tuberculosis Association, which, thirty years earlier, had stirred the public with the traveling exhibits that it kept on the road indefinitely,[171] the Health Section used demonstration farms as classrooms, set up mobile library units, and placed educational manuals in the hands of community leaders.

The European visitors showed zest for what they knew might await them, from regional planning to the gradual renewal of a sense of community.[172] An unexpected beacon in the decade's darkness, the TVA took over the development process in neglected villages "more bleak than anything to be met in the worst parts of the Balkans."[173] By dint of its efforts, the TVA aroused an all-important "malaria consciousness."[174] Like all awakenings, the new consciousness rested on local believers. It was little wonder that top emissaries of the LNHO made much of the way southerners got *interested* in biology, malariology, and engineering. The officials' narrative captured the flame of an experience that made severly tested people into stakeholders, often enthusiastic ones, in the meliorist project. Treating the rural masses as willing collaborators, "an auxiliary and not just a simple beneficiary," soon became the LNHO's paramount concern.[175]

Toward a European Conference on Rural Life, 1936–39

More than "going local" was at stake in the all-embracing European conference on rural life (instead of "rural hygiene," as in 1931) that the League of Nations Health Committee's Bureau plotted during its Moscow (June 22–28) and Paris (October 29) 1936 sessions. What occurred was the "truly amazing extension" of the international health agenda.[176] In a world of shrinking horizons, the prospect of pioneering the largest-ever gathering on vaccines, food supplements, improved seeds, roads, waterpipes, and nurses was irresistible to the LNHO. We may note the baffling range of topics on the checklist penned by Jacques Parisot (soon to be president of the Health Committee):

I. The rural ambiance: peasant culture, art and folklore, farm loans, agrarian reform, the cooperative movement, rural development, community planning, transportation, electrification, local administration;

II. Food and produce;

III. The rural house and its outbuildings;

IV. Peasant education: general, technical, hygiene, homemaking;

V. Peasants at work: new farming methods, rural industries;

VI. Peasants at rest: libraries, radio, cinema, *dopolavoro;*

VII. Medical and social policies: maternal and child care, birth control, nurseries and kindergartens, malaria, alcoholism, health personnel, midwives, *feldscher*... [177]

The timing of the LNHO's decisive expansion of its global reach is intriguing. Much of Europe was in a state of massive "involution." "Low-pressure" states and sluggish economies were the current situation. Political "downsizing" was in force, with large areas of the continent closing in on themselves. Still, Geneva increasingly indulged in grand spatial analysis.

Democracy's Rise and Fall

Bread-and-butter issues shaped the geopolitics of the decade. At a time when "green" (that is, central and eastern) Europe was caving in under wheat surpluses, the need to "start up, back up and speed up" domestic recovery held center stage.[178] Faced with deprivation, aimless fragmentation, and toxic politics, the LNHO could no longer "pull apart the sanitary, economic and social aspects" of peasant malaise.[179]

Geneva's vade mecum on consumer economics was Wallace Ruddell Aykroyd and Etienne Burnet's proto-Keynesian report, "Nutrition and Public Health" (June 1935). In line with the Australian economist Frank McDougall (the future director general of the Food and Agricultural Organization), who campaigned for "a deliberate association of the agricultural and health problems,"[180] the writers suggested that the secret of health as well as of growth and productivity lay in a good diet.[181] Such ideas had an impact on world affairs as vitamins turned into "political facts."[182] Disputes raged about calories and nutrients, food budgets, and home economics, elating nationalist leaders (in particular Mahatma Gandhi).[183]

"Economic appeasement"—to quote McDougall's memorandum of December 21, 1936—was the (ambiguous) byword for contentment. It reflected the democracies' commitment to preclude the establishment of the entire continent as a single *Grossraum* and to reassert themselves through "the backing of the masses."[184] Fascist welfare states taught democrats that granting individual liberties was not enough to secure people's loyalties. It was no surprise that phrases such as "marrying health and agriculture" (September 1935) or tackling "the wider problem of the standard of living" (September 1937) surfaced again and again in the League Assembly's debates.[185] Hitler's grip on crisis-torn Europe provided the rationale for discretionary national policies to move in more interrelated directions.

Chief among these desperate, last-minute League attempts to rally popular support was the European Conference on Rural Life. Although its driving impulse flowed from the truly Hobbesian state of fear that prevailed in 1936–38, the conference actually smoothed the way for embattled Europe to restyle itself as "socially concerned" and for country folk to see state agendas "clearly related" to welfare.[186] As Ludwik Rajchman confided to Rockefeller officials before leaving for Moscow on June 1, 1936, this meant that "the future of the League no longer turned on secondary issues such as health work, but must rest on the major issue of prevention of war."[187] All LNHO policy after 1936 was a footnote to Rajchman's statement.

Bailing out Eastern Europe

To realize these goals, the conference laid its "chief emphasis" on "the eastern European peasantry."[188] "Well-being as a whole"—the very purpose for convening the meeting—could hardly be entertained unless anything resembling convergence emerged.[189] This hoped-for betterment was presented less as "a means of general relaxation of political tensions" than as an incentive for a regional rapprochement among contending nations.[190] In fairness, there was no way that the League could neutralize polarized politics, let alone deter would-be continental hegemons.

In fact, however, developmental similarities increased as direct political connections diminished. At a May 1930 meeting in Paris, the director of the Johns Hopkins School of Hygiene was dazzled to discover how tight a group his European colleagues were and how amenable to "the rather extraordinary world influence" of the League's Health Section: "The directors of the continental European schools seemed to rely for guidance upon the officers of the Secretariat."[191] For their part, the Rockefeller-sponsored institutes and schools, established during the mid-1920s as a fractal set of hierarchies, had grown in power, numbers, and ambitions. Acting as regional beach-heads for the LNHO's authority, they maintained a surprising degree of interconnection with each other. The Health Section, relying on the directors of institutes and schools, was now taking a chance to push for a much wider "interconnectivity."

Was Geneva tilting toward some Austro-Hungarian pattern in health matters? One thing is certain: the "Habsburg" tint of the countless committees convened on the eve of the conference. One example was the "Consultation on Medico-Social Policy at the Countryside" that brought together on the shores of Lake Geneva in mid-October 1938 (a few days after the Munich Agreement) such enterprising "Zwischeneuropäers" as Andrija Štampar , Berislav Borcic, Bela Johan (Budapest), Martin Kacprzak (Warsaw), Dimitri Combiescu (Bucharest) and Ion Balteanu (Iasi).[192] Notwithstanding the general "abatement" of the age, much of the LNHO's health work was kept going "horizontally" through the aggregation and collaboration of influential experts of the same stripe. Geopolitical evidence of this continuation is to be found in the core group of countries that declared a resolve to experiment with a system of health indicies "for rural uses" (November 1937, eight nations out of the twenty-eight to take part in the Conference) and to produce a monograph on the health status of their rural populations (May 1938, twelve nations out of the twenty-eight). In addition to French-speaking nations, these "core countries" were Hungary, Poland, Czechoslovakia, Yugoslavia, and Romania.[193] Empire was back with a vengeance, as its less-than-robust successors were rife with divisions.

Relocating the Countryside

With regard to Western Europe, uplifting the countryside was hardly distinguishable from relocating it. Had not the absence of relations been the fundamental, underlying constant in the relation between town and village? To span the rift between town and countryside, the Geneva conference focused on an amphibian creature, "the industrial-rural worker."[194] Recall the camps set up by Franklin D. Roosevelt's Civilian Conservation Corps and subsistence homestead projects, or, earlier, the archetypal *Randsiedlungen*, the Weimar-sponsored shantytowns of semisubsistence that workers erected on the cities' rims. With urban areas awash in crises of relief and unemployment, the recession provided the spur for a revival of rural crafts, family industries, forestry and public works.[195]

Of course the tide of farm-to-city migration would be stemmed only when the two "civilizations" reached the same level. Echoing the director of the Warsaw School of Hygiene, who said, "We have forgotten the countryside by leaving it to its fate,"[196] the entrepreneurial Parisot, from his chair of social medicine in Nancy, assumed that his work on milk or typhoid fever, "by rendering service to the peasants, attracted their confidence."[197] Electricity and running water did play a role in stopping the "exodus" and "paved the way for a return to the land."[198] By this time, welfare policies had become equated with population policies: by addressing itself in a holistic fashion to the myriad problems still plaguing the rural masses, social medicine had an impact on territorial distribution. In the process, the "people's war for health" turned a wretched humanity from "passive or reluctant on-lookers" to "the best craftsmen of their own improvement."[199]

Social Economics at the LN

Dispatched to Paris in February 1939 to secure the conference on rural life, which was still in the works, Pietro Stoppani, the head of the League's Economic Section, was welcomed by the French minister of agriculture, ethnologists enthralled by an exhibition on folklore, and Selskar Gunn, who was back from a tour of Yugoslavia, Czechoslovakia, and Hungary. Stoppani was struck by the depth of the craze for "the social, intellectual and I would even say, the sentimental aspects of the life of peasants."[200]

To some extent the new marching orders had grown out of the depression. The storm brewing on the continent was inevitably reflected in the League's romance with development economics. As Gunn remarked in early 1939, at the end of his just mentioned trip to a hard-pressed central Europe, "With the topsy-turvy conditions of the world, there is developing a growing feeling that the rural populations, with their conservatism and stability, may play an important role in the ultimate development of national sanity."[201] But, then, too, the much-needed village uplift had its own momentum. Charles-Edward Winslow's comment in 1918—"The rural problem is of course the great unsolved problem of public health"[202]—was relayed to the other shore of the Atlantic, where many a tear was shed because of this "astonishingly deadly plague of rural tuberculosis."[203]

These rising perils fueled the completion of workable, implementable standards for medical services, housing, and nutrition. Yet the Sisyphean efforts at reviving and reassuring traditional farming societies resulted in a *sui generis* phenomenon, rather than an ephemeral artifact of Nazi Germany's ascendancy. Danish folk high schools; Croatian health centers; and medical helpers in the Dutch East Indies, India, or China did not rise from the depression like newly hatched chicks; instead, they were links in a chain of inventions, each one based on its predecessor. "Penetrating the very intimacy" of rural life had become an international byword for rerooting democracy.[204]

Conclusion

Whether crises ultimately help or hinder the institutionalization of collaborative international mechanisms is an open question. The 1930s rural conferences, Rajchman's brainchildren, were an attempt to take over and coordinate activities hitherto under the aegis of the nation-state. When in the summer of 1938 Rajchman prompted the Health Committee to "orient rural life" in Europe as had been done in Asia and would be done in America, might he have been thinking of remaking the LNHO into a functional supranational authority—an outsized replica of the Tennessee Valley Authority?[205] The TVA—a template for interstate transformation and an undisputed prototype of task-oriented agencies that turned from an overt political approach to an indirect welfare one—promoted the view of national problems as "the municipal sections of international problems."[206] Convinced as he was of the importance of gradual reforms, incremental improvements and experimental probing, Charles-Edward Winslow did not shy away from the complacent fantasy of an overarching body. The ideal type of organization, he wrote in the WHO's *Chronicle* in the 1950s, was "a series of regional TVA's," if not a single worldwide TVA.[207]

Just how quickly that sun will rise is disputed. Universal though it claims to be, public health is not a unitary, still less a uniform, endeavor. The health demonstrations of the 1930s were outcroppings in a flattened landscape. The links among the outcroppings—which spanned large distances—gave a sense of (scale and) unity to reform-minded healers. But diversity, not unity, was the hallmark of the age. All roads led to Geneva, but the local reigned supreme.

Notes

1. C.-E. A. Winslow, "The Economic Value of Preventive Medicine," *Chronicle of the World Health Organization* 6 (1952): 195–97.

2. "Report by Dr. A. Štampar on his missions to China," October 15, 1936, CH1220, 20, League of Nations Archives, Geneva (hereafter LNA).

3. C.-E. A. Winslow, *The Price of Sickness and the Cost of Health* (Geneva: WHO, 1951), 57.

4. S. M. Gunn to R. B. Fosdick, October 6, 1926, Record Group 3, Series 900, Box 17, Folder 122 (hereafter 3/900/17/122, RAC), Rockefeller Archival Center, Tarrytown, NY.

5. J. Parisot, "L'œuvre poursuivie et à poursuivre dans le domaine de l'hygiène rurale," Report to the Health Committee Bureau, Moscow, June 1936, 2, CH1218, LNA.

6. A. Loveday, "Les travaux de la 5è réunion du Bureau d'hygiène," January 4, 1937, R6103, C17.1937.III, LNA.

7. H. Tilley and R. J. Gordon, *Ordering Africa: Anthropology, European Imperialism, and the Politics of Knowledge* (Manchester: Manchester University Press, 2007).

8. Requested on September 30, 1936 by thirteen Latin American delegations along with Spain and the Netherlands; the opposition by the United States won out at the very last minute.

9. F. Konrich, Germany's delegate, on July 7, 1931, in *Conférence européenne sur l'hygiène rurale*, II, *Procès-verbaux* (Geneva: Société des Nations [hereafter SDN], 1931), 73.

10. "Résolutions de la Conférence intergouvernementale des pays d'Orient sur l'hygiène rurale," December 1937, 1311, *SDN, Journal Officiel* (hereafter *JO*), C473. M.202, LNA.

11. "The Reminiscences of Doctor John B. Grant [1961]," Glen Rock, NJ, 1976, 86–87 (microfilm).

12. A total of eleven thousand persons, or close to the two-thirds of the population, received complete medical examinations. Between 1917 and 1923, the infant mortality rate fell by 40 percent and tuberculosis deaths by 68 percent.

13. L. I. Dublin, *A 40-Year Campaign Against Tuberculosis* (New York: Metropolitan Life Insurance Company, 1952), 92.

14. W. Rose [1917], quoted in J. Farley, "Mosquitoes or Malaria? Rockefeller Campaigns in the American South and Sardinia," *Parassitologia* 36 (1994): 165.

15. Barry C. Smith, quoted in *Health Demonstrations in the United States*, Supplement to the *American Journal of Public Health*, February 1927, 21.

16. H. F. Vaughan, "Local Health Services in the United States: The Story of the CAP," *American Journal of Public Health* 62 (1972): 95–111; L. Murard, "Atlantic Crossings in the Measurement of Health: From American Appraisal Forms to the League of Nations' Health Indices," in *Medicine, the Market, and the Mass Media: Producing Health in the Twentieth Century*, ed. V. Berridge and K. Loughlin, 19–54 (London: Routledge, 2005).

17. J. Farley, *To Cast Out Disease: A History of the International Health Division of the Rockefeller Foundation, 1913–1951* (Oxford: Oxford University Press, 2004), 37.

18. W. S. Rankin, "Report of the secretary of the North Carolina State Board of Health," March 6, 1924, 5.3/236/64, RAC.

19. C.-E. A. Winslow, "The International Appraisal of Local Health Programs," *Milbank Memorial Fund Quarterly* 15 (1937): 4.

20. J. A. Kingsbury to L. R. Williams, December 7, 1921, Kingsbury Papers (hereafter JAK), Part II, Box 23 (hereafter II/23), Manuscript Division, Library of Congress, Washington, DC (hereafter LC).

21. C.-E. A. Winslow, *Health on the Farm and in the Village: A Review and Evaluation of the Cattaraugus Health Demonstration with Special Reference to Its Lessons for Other Rural Areas* (New York: Macmillan Company, 1931), 38.

22. C.-E. A. Winslow to J. A. Kingsbury, November 30, 1928, Winslow Papers, 749/222/81/1283, Sterling Library, Yale University (hereafter Yale).

23. C.-E. A. Winslow, "Administrative Practice," *American Public Health Association Yearbook 1930–1931*, Supplement to the *American Journal of Public Health* 21, 1931: 66.

24. Senator Kenneth S. Wherry of Nebraska, quoted in K. Hildebrand, *German Foreign Policy from Bismarck to Adenauer: The Limits to Statecraft* (London: Unwin Hyman, 1989), 155.

25. L. Farrand [1917], 1974, 900/Hist.1/8, RF History, RAC.

26. L. R. Williams to W. Rose, July 2, 1920, 1.1/500T/26/259, RAC.

27. L. R. Williams to V. Heiser, October 13, 1919, 1.1/500T/26/258, RAC.

28. "Report of the XIXth arrondissement (Paris)," September 18, 1919, 1974, 900/Hist.1/8, RAC.

29. A. M. Rafferty, "Internationalising Nursing Education during the Interwar Period," in *International Health Organisations and Movements, 1918–1939*, ed. P. Weindling, 266–82 (Cambridge: Cambridge University Press, 1995).

30. S. M. Gunn, "Public health in Hungary," 1924, 163, 1.1/750/4/38, RAC.

31. Winslow, *Health on the Farm*, 8.

32. R. E. Kohler, "Science and Philanthropy: Wickliffe Rose and the International Education Board," *Minerva* 23 (1985): 85. Developed in British Guyana (1914), H. H. Howard's "intensive method" became "the basis of the RF's International Health Board hookworm campaign elsewhere." See J. Gillespie, "The Rockefeller Foundation, the Hookworm Campaign and a National Health Policy in Australia, 1911–1930," in *Health and Healing in Tropical Australia and Papua New Guinea*, ed. R. M. MacLeod and D. Denoon (Townsville: James Cook University, 1991), 75.

33. G. E. Vincent to Mrs. Bliss, July 11, 1917, 1.1/500T/25/249, RAC.

34. L. R. Williams, "La Fondation Rockefeller pour la lutte contre la tuberculose en France. Son action pendant et depuis la guerre," *La Revue du Musée Social* 2 (1922): 5.

35. L. W. Hackett [1924], quoted in G. Donelli and E. Serinaldi, *Dalla lotta alla malaria alla nascita dell'Istituto di Sanita Pubblica. Il rulo della Rockefeller Foundation in Italia: 1922–1934* (Roma-Bari: Laterza, 2003), 64.

36. S. M. Gunn to G. E. Vincent, May 16, 1927, 3/900/21/159, RAC.

37. B. B. Page, "First Steps: The Rockefeller Foundation in Early Czechoslovakia," *East European Quarterly* 35 (2001): 287.

38. S. M. Gunn to G. E. Vincent, May 16, 1927, 3/900/21/159, RAC.

39. S. M. Gunn, "Report of a visit of investigation in Czechoslovakia, 1–14 June 1919," quoted in B. B. Page, "The Rockefeller Foundation and Central Europe: A Reconsideration," *Minerva* 40 (2002): 270.

40. S. M. Gunn [1919], quoted in Page, "First Steps," 280.

41. J. C. Scott, "The Tennessee Valley Authority: U.S. High Modernism Undone," an unpublished part of J. C. Scott, *Seeing Like a State: How Certain Schemes to Improve the Human Condition Have Failed* (New Haven: Yale University Press, 1998). Thanks to Scott for permission to use this material.

42. A. Bruno, "Contre la tuberculose: La Mission américaine Rockefeller en France et l'effort français, 1917–1925" (PhD diss., Faculté de Médecine, Paris, 1925).

43. S. M. Gunn to W. Rose, February 14, 1919, 1.1/500T/26/257, RAC.

44. N. White [1934] quoted in D. Giannuli, "'Repeated Disappointment': The Rockefeller Foundation and the Reform of the Greek Public Health System, 1929–1940," *Bulletin of the History of Medicine* 72 (1998): 47–72.

45. D. Mitrany, "The Making of the Functional Theory: A Memoir," in *The Functional Theory of Politics* (London: London School of Economics and Political Science, 1975), 58.

46. W. Chozko, *Conférence européenne*, II, *Procès-verbaux* (1931), 74, LNA.

47. *Conférence européenne*, I, *Recommandations* (1931), 14, LNA.

48. Health Section (O. Olsen) to Dr. W. Krul (Netherlands), July 23, 1931, R6045, LNA.

49. G. W. Gale [c. 1951] quoted in S. Marks, "South Africa's Early Experiment in Social Medicine: Its Pioneers and Politics," *American Journal of Public Health* 87 (1997): 453.

50. B. Johan in "Consultation sur la politique médico-sociale à la campagne," Geneva, October 10–14, 1938, R6104, CH1374, LNA.

51. A. Štampar, "Méthodes les plus effectives pour organiser les services d'hygiène dans les régions rurales," *Conférence*, I (1931), 33, LNA.

52. D. T. Rodgers, *Atlantic Crossings: Social Politics in a Progressive Age* (Cambridge, MA: Belknap Press, 1998), 354–58.

53. M. Kacprzak, *Conférence*, II (1931), 53, LNA.

54. L. Rajchman to T. Madsen, Paris, July 20, 1925, R905, 12B/33149/31035, LNA.

55. J. Kuhn, "L'assurance-maladie facultative au Danemark" (1927), quoted in J. Parisot, "Les Assurances sociales en France: Les enseignements de l'étranger," *Revue d'hygiène et de prophylaxie sociales* 9 (1930): 83; B. S. Hansen, "Something Rotten in the State of Denmark: Eugenics and the Ascent of the Welfare State," in *Eugenics and the Welfare State: Sterilization Policy in Denmark, Sweden, Norway, and Finland*, ed. G. Broberg and N. Roll-Hansen, 9–76 (East Lansing: Michigan State University Press, 1996).

56. F. C. Howe, *Denmark: A Cooperative Commonwealth* (New York: Harcourt, Brace & Co., 1921), 96.

57. E. C. Branson, *Farm Life Abroad: Field Letters from Germany, Denmark, and France* (Chapel Hill: University of North Carolina Press, 1924), 183–84.

58. J. K. Hart, *Light from the North: The Danish Folk High Schools, Their Meanings for America* (New York: Henry Holt, 1927), 29.

59. Hart, *Light from the North*, 149.

60. P. Zylberman, "Fewer Parallels than Antitheses: René Sand and Andrija Štampar on Social Medicine, 1919–1955," *Social History of Medicine* 17 (2004): 77–91.

61. G. E. Vincent [1926], quoted in Z. Dugac, "New Public Health for a New State: Interwar Public Health in the Kingdom of Serbs, Croats, and Slovenes and the Rockefeller Foundation," in *Facing Illness in Troubled Times: Health in Europe in the Interwar Years, 1918–1939*, ed. I. Borowy and W. D. Gruner (Frankfurt am Main: Peter Lang, 2005), 294.

62. L. Bernard, "Conférence tenue à l'occasion de l'inauguration des écoles d'hygiène publique de Budapest et de Zagreb," October 27, 1927, 11è session du Comité d'hygiène, Geneva, 28 octobre–3 novembre 1927, C579 M3205, 142, CH661, LNA.

63. L. Rajchman, "Système de liaison avec les administrations sanitaires," November 1, 1927, 11è session, 144–45, CH670, LNA.

64. S. M. Gunn, "Public Health in Jugoslavia," 1924, 54, 1.1/710/1/4, RAC.

65. S. M. Gunn, "Jugoslavia," 1924, 236–38, 1/710/1/4, RAC.

66. S. Litsios, "Selskar Gunn and China: The Rockefeller Foundation's 'Other' Approach to Public Health," *Bulletin of the History of Medicine* 79 (2005): 308.

67. M. Kacprzak, "Commission pour l'étude des Centres de santé ruraux," Geneva, April 28–30, 1931, R5927, LNA.

68. D. Mitrany, *Marx against the Peasant: A Study in Social Dogmatism* (Chapel Hill: University of North Carolina Press, 1951 [1927]), 239–40. Mitrany reports

a membership of three hundred fifty thousand in 1939 for Peasant Concord, the Croat Peasant Party's cultural branch.

69. M. Biondich, *Stjepan Radic, the Croat Peasant Party, and the Politics of Mass Mobilisation, 1904–1928* (Toronto: University of Toronto Press, 2000), 62–90.

70. Mitrany, *Functional Theory*, 62–64.

71. M. D. Grmek, ed., *Serving the Cause of Public Health: Selected Papers of Andrija Štampar* (Zagreb: University of Zagreb, 1966), 31.

72. R. West, *Black Lamb and Grey Falcon: A Journey Through Yugoslavia* (Edinburgh: Canongate, 2001 [1942]), 101, 597.

73. A. Štampar, *Public Health in Jugoslavia* (London: School of Slavonic and East European Studies in the University of London, 1938), 23–24.

74. According to Štampar, the School in Zagreb is "following the example of peasants' universities in Denmark": Grmek, *Serving the Cause*, 114.

75. A. Brenko, Z. Dugac, and M. Randic, *Narodna Medicina: Folk Medicine* (Zagreb: Ethnographic Museum, 2001), 205.

76. Štampar, *Public Health in Jugoslavia*, 24.

77. Like Stjepan and Anton Radic, who made it a strict rule never to enter a café, Štampar was, according to Grant, "a rabid Socialist and looked very much askance on either smoking or drinking": "The Reminiscences of Doctor J. B. Grant [1961]," 329–31.

78. C. Prausnitz, "L'Enseignement de l'hygiène en Yougoslavie," in *Rapport sur les travaux des Conférences des Directeurs d'Écoles d'hygiène tenues à Paris, du 20 au 23 mai 1930, et à Dresde, du 14 au 17 juillet 1930* (Geneva: SDN, 1930), 117–22, CH888, LNA.

79. G. K. Strode to C.-E. A. Winslow, June 11, 1929, Winslow Papers, 749/III/96/1672, Yale.

80. M. Kacprzak, *Conférence européenne*, II (1931), 53, LNA.

81. S. G. Solomon, "The Intermediary as Strategist: John A. Kingsbury, Soviet Socialized Medicine, and 1930s America" (forthcoming).

82. J. Tomasevich, *Peasants, Politics, and Economic Change in Yugoslavia* (Stanford: Stanford University Press, 1975 [1955]), 594.

83. B. Konstantinovitch and K. Schneider, *Principles of Rural Hygiene and Health Cooperatives* (Belgrade: Union of Health Cooperatives, 1931), 57–58.

84. Gunn's diary, February 15, 1928, quoted in Litsios, "Selskar Gunn," 305.

85. S. A. Knapp [1910], quoted in R. B. Fosdick, *Adventure in Giving: The Story of the General Education Board* (New York: Harper & Row, 1962), 54.

86. D. Fitzgerald, "Exporting American Agriculture: The Rockefeller Foundation in Mexico, 1943–1953," in *Missionaries of Science: The Rockefeller Foundation and Latin America*, ed. M. Cueto (Bloomington: Indiana University Press, 1994), 75.

87. M. Colombain, "L'hygiène rurale et les coopératives sanitaires en Yougoslavie," *Revue Internationale du Travail* 32 (1935): 35.

88. J. A. Kingsbury to Mr. A. Milbank, "Interoffice Memorandum, January 27, 1922," JAK, II/41, LC.

89. Štampar, *Public Health in Jugoslavia*, 26.

90. Prausnitz, *Rapport sur les travaux des Conférences des Directeurs*, 120.

91. G. Radin (November 14, 1930), quoted in V. O. Freeburg, "Yugoslavia Leads in Rural Health Centres," *Milbank Memorial Fund Quarterly* 12 (1934): 23.

92. For the classical distinction between Hellenization and Hellenism, see G. W. Bowersock, *Hellenism in Late Antiquity* (Ann Arbor: University of Michigan Press, 1996), xi.

93. F. G. Boudreau, "The European Conference on Rural Hygiene," memorandum transmitted by Arthur Sweetser to Raymond Blair Fosdick, February 24, 1931, 1.1/100/21/176, RAC.

94. L. Farrand, letter to S. A. Knopf about the 1917–19 campaign in France, in S. A. Knopf, *A History of the National Tuberculosis Association: The Anti-Tuberculosis Movement in the United States* (New York: NTA, 1922), 407.

95. G. Lafosse, "Le Centre d'hygiène et d'assistance médico-sociale de Vanves," *Revue philanthropique* (1929): 855–56.

96. E. Crowell to A. Štampar, March 9, 1926, quoted in L. Killen, "The Rockefeller Foundation in the First Yugoslavia," *East European Quarterly* 24 (1990): 356.

97. J. Gillespie, "The Rockefeller Foundation and Colonial Medicine in the Pacific, 1911–1929," in *New Countries and Old Medicine*, ed. L. Bryder and D. A. Dow (Auckland: Pyramid Press, 1995), 382.

98. Gillespie, "The Rockefeller Foundation in Australia," 87.

99. S. M. Gunn to R. B. Fosdick, October 6, 1926, 3/900/17/122, RAC.

100. C.-E. Winslow, "Malaria Control in Italy, Albania, and Macedonia," 2/1929/554/3729, RAC; C.-E. A. Winslow to F. F. Russell, September 4, 1929, 2/1929/554/3729, RAC.

101. L. Mitchell to S. M. Gunn, September 17, 1926, quoted in Killen, "The Rockefeller Foundation," 353.

102. They were Birmany, British North Borneo, Ceylon, China, Fiji Islands, Hong Kong, India, the Dutch East Indies, Indochina, Japan, Malaya, the Philippines, and Siam.

103. A. S. Haynes (president of the preparatory committee), "Note in view of the conference on rural hygiene in the Far East," summer–autumn 1936, R6095, LNA.

104. A. Štampar, on the European Conference, in Grmek, *Serving the Cause*, 232.

105. P. M. Dorolle, "L'Organisation des services sanitaires et médicaux," Conférence des pays d'Orient sur l'hygiène rurale, Geneva, May 1937, 4, CH1253/1, LNA.

106. M. Cueto, "The Origins of Primary Health Care and Selective Primary Health Care," *American Journal of Public Health* 94 (2004): 1864–74.

107. S. M. Gunn [October 28–30, 1930], quoted in F. A. Ninkovich, "The Rockefeller Foundation, China, and Cultural Change," *Journal of American History* 70 (1984): 809.

108. L. Rajchman, "Exposé devant l'Assemblée annuelle du Conseil général consultatif" (LNHO–OIHP), Paris, May 19, 1938, R6145, 8A/33354/28671, LNA.

109. *Rapport de la Conférence intergouvernementale des pays d'Orient sur l'hygiène rurale* (Geneva: SDN, 1937), 54, A.19.1937.III, LNA.

110. "Résolutions," December 1937, 1313, *JO*, LNA; Rajchman, "Exposé," May 19, 1938.

111. S. Hewa, "Rockefeller Philanthropy and the Development of a Community-Based Approach to Public Health in Sri-Lanka" (unpublished paper, 2004).

112. E. J. Pampana to L. Rajchman, Benares, April 27, 1936, 8A/22509/8855, R6093, LNA.

113. J. L. Hydrick, *Intensive Rural Hygiene Work and Public Health Education of the Public Health Service of Netherlands India* (Batavia [Jakarta], 1937), 2.

114. P. M. Dorolle, "Commentaire sur l'œuvre d'hygiène rurale intensive à Java," an appendix in his translation of J. L. Hydrick, in *Hygiène rurale intensive* (Hanoi: Gouvernement général de l'Indochine, 1938), 67–68.

115. *Rapport de la Commission préparatoire* (Geneva: SDN, 1937), 80–81, LNA.

116. Introduction, in *Rapport de la Conférence intergouvernementale*, 27. On its authorship, see Litsios, "Selskar Gunn," 314, note 89.

117. "The Reminiscences of Doctor J. B. Grant [1961]," 562.

118. M. D. Spencer Hatch, "La Reconstruction rurale dans l'Inde," June 7, 1937, CH/Conf.Hyg.Rur.Orient/8, LNA.

119. The author of *Village Uplift in India* (n.d.), *The Remaking of Village India* (1929), *Up from Poverty in Rural India* (1932), and *The Better Village Movement* (n.d.), F. L. Brayne had the status of ad hoc Commissioner in the Punjab after starting "what is probably the first organized attempt of rural reconstruction in India" at Gurgaon; E. J. Pampana to L. Rajchman, April 27, 1936, R6093, LNA.

120. L. S. Hsü, "Rural reconstruction and social planning," May 11, 1937, 1, CH/Conf.Hyg.Rur.Orient/4, LNA.

121. A. Štampar, "Croat peasant literature," in *The Slavonic Year-Book, Slavonic and East-European Review* (1939–1940), 19: 293.

122. Quoted by Hsü, "Rural reconstruction," 1. See also Uma das Gupta, "Rabindranath Tagore on Rural Reconstruction: The Sriniketan Programme, 1921–41," *Indian Historical Review* 4 (1978): 354–78.

123. J. Osterhammel, "'Technical Cooperation' Between the League of Nations and China," *Modern Asian Studies* 13 (1979): 677.

124. "China in Evolution," *Economist*, May 5, 1934.

125. J. Monnet, *Mémoires* (Paris: Fayard, 1976), 130.

126. "Report of Dr. Rajchman on his mission in China," summarized in "Awakening China: A Nation Finding Itself," *The Times*, May 11, 1934.

127. L. Rajchman to J. Avenol and Lester, January 5, 1939, Avenol Papers, vol. 25, Ministère des Affaires Etrangères, Paris (hereafter MAE).

128. S. M. Gunn, "Report on visit to China, June 9–July 30, 1931," 1.1/601/12/129, RAC.

129. S. M. Gunn, "China Program," in *Annual Report* (New York: Rockefeller Foundation, 1935), 323.

130. S. Flexner [1915], quoted in Fosdick, *Story of the Rockefeller Foundation*, 86.

131. J. B. Grant [1922], quoted by M. B. Bullock, *An American Transplant: The Rockefeller Foundation and Peking Union Medical College* (Berkeley: University of California Press, 1980), 141.

132. S. M. Gunn, "Report on visit to China," 85. See also J. C. Thomson, Jr., *While China Faced West: American Reformers in Nationalist China, 1928–1937* (Cambridge, MA: Harvard University Press, 1969), 128.

133. C. C. Chen, *Medicine in Rural China: A Personal Account* (Berkeley: University of California Press, 1989), 103–4. On Chen, "the father of China's rural health care delivery system," see Bullock, *An American Transplant*, 163; Ka-Che Yip, *Health and National Reconstruction in Nationalist China: The Development of Modern Health Services, 1928–1937* (Ann Arbor: Association for Asian Studies, 1995), 28, 76–77.

134. "Rapport du Dr. A. Štampar sur ses missions en Chine," *Bulletin Trimestriel de l'Organisation d'Hygiène* 5 (1936): 1236.

135. E. Snow, "Awakening the Masses in China," *New York Herald Tribune*, December 17, 1933, quoted in C. W. Hayford, *To the People: James Yen and Village China* (New York: Columbia University Press, 1990), x.

136. J. Yen [1929], quoted in Hayford, *To the People*, 104.

137. "A Rural Health Experiment in China," *Milbank Memorial Fund Quarterly Bulletin* 8 (1930): 104. Edgar Sydenstricker, the Fund's head of epidemiology and a physician born in a missionary family in China, was the brother of the novelist Pearl S. Buck, who created America's image of China.

138. Hayford, *To the People*, 118.

139. M. Wilden, the French ambassador, to the minister of foreign affairs [Aristide Briand], Nanking, December 31, 1931, Asie 1918–1940, Chine 659, MAE.

140. E. B. Haas, *Nationalism, Liberalism, and Progress*, vol. 2, *The Dismal Fate of New Nations* (Ithaca, NY: Cornell University Press, 2000), 113.

141. J. K. Fairbank, *La grande Révolution chinoise, 1800–1989* (Paris: Flammarion, 1989 [1986]), 268–69.

142. C. C. Chen, "State Medicine and Medical Education," *Chinese Medical Journal* 49 (1935): 954.

143. C. H. Becker, M. Falski, P. Langevin, and R. H. Tawney, *La Réorganisation de l'enseignement public en Chine* (Paris: Institut international de coopération intellectuelle, SDN, 1932), 22.

144. R. Tawney to K. Zilliacus (secretary of the League's China Committee), June 3, 1931 Avenol Papers, vol. 23, MAE.

145. S. M. Gunn [1931], in Thomson, Jr., *While China Faced West*, 128.

146. Chen, *Medicine in Rural China*, 81.

147. L. S. Hsü, "Rural Reconstruction in China," *Pacific Affairs* 10 (1937): 257.

148. Originally published in three volumes in Chinese, these reports figure in S. D. Gamble, *Ting Hsien: A North China Rural Community* (with a foreword by Y. C. James Yen) (New York: Institute of Pacific Relations, 1954).

149. Chen, *Medicine in Rural China*, 74.

150. C. C. Chen, "Some Problems of Medical Organization in Rural China," *Chinese Medical Journal* 51 (1937): 804; J. B. Grant, "Public Health as a Social Service" [1940], in *Health Care for the Community: Selected Papers of Dr. John B. Grant*, ed. C. Seipp, 14–20 (Baltimore: Johns Hopkins Press, 1963).

151. J. Tandler [1935], quoted in Bullock, *American Transplant*, 186.

152. A. Štampar, quoted in "Reminiscences of Doctor Grant," 512.

153. Chen, *Medicine in Rural China*, 78. See also C. C. Chen, "Socialisation of Medicine in Rural China," May 1937, 15, CH1253/2, LNA.

154. A.-E. Birn, *Marriage of Convenience: Rockefeller International Health and Revolutionary Mexico* (Rochester, NY: University of Rochester Press, 2006), 144; L. Murard, "Health Policies Between the International and the Local: Jacques Parisot in Geneva and Nancy," in Borowy and Gruner, *Facing Illness*, 207–45.

155. Grant estimated at approximately "two million" the number of persons under the authority of the North China Council ("Organization and Training" [1953], in Seipp, *Health Care*, 164), even though, a few pages previously, he referred to "a ten million unit of population" ("Rural Reconstruction" [1950], in Seipp, *Health Care*, 152), a figure he also used for the Tennessee Valley Authority (in J. B.

Grant, "Philosophy of Rural Reconstruction in China," *Journal of the Royal Asiatic Society of Bengal* 6 [1940]: 132).

156. Fosdick, *Story of the Rockefeller Foundation*, 184.

157. Hsü, "Rural Reconstruction," 263.

158. G. E. Taylor, *The Reconstruction Movement in China* (London: Royal Institute of International Affairs, 1936), 2.

159. "Report by Dr. A. Štampar on his missions to China," October 15, 1936, 7, CH1220, LNA.

160. Chang Fu-Liang, *When East Met West: A Personal Story of Rural Reconstruction in China* (New Haven: Yale-in-China Association, 1972), 47.

161. G. E. Taylor, "Reconstruction After Revolution: Kiangsi Province and the Chinese Nation," *Pacific Affairs* 8 (1935): 306.

162. R. Haas, *Rapport présenté au Secrétaire général par le Secrétaire du Comité du Conseil sur sa mission en Chine, janvier-mai 1935* (Geneva: SDN, 1935), 18, C410 M206, LNA.

163. Yip, *Health and National Reconstruction*, 88.

164. Osterhammel, "Technical Cooperation," 676.

165. L. Rajchman, quoted in M. Balinska, *Une vie pour l'humanitaire: Ludwik Rajchman, 1881–1965* (Paris: La Découverte, 1995), 143.

166. B. Borcic, quoted by L. E. Eastman, *The Abortive Revolution: China Under Nationalist Rule, 1927–1937* (Cambridge, MA: Harvard University Press, 1974), 220.

167. "Hygiène publique et problèmes sociaux aux États-Unis. Rapport élaboré par les médecins hygiénistes qui ont pris part au voyage d'études . . . (4 novembre–7 décembre 1935)," *Bulletin de l'Organisation d'Hygiène* 5 (1936): 921–41.

168. Scott, *Seeing Like a State*, 6.

169. Roosevelt's phrase, quoted in D. E. Lilienthal, *Democracy on the March* (New York: Harper and Row, 1953 [1944]), 52.

170. E. L. Bishop, "The TVA's New Deal in Health," *American Journal of Public Health* 24 (1934): 1025.

171. R. H. Shryock, *National Tuberculosis Association 1904–1954: A Study of the Voluntary Health Movement in the United States* (New York: NTA, 1957), 102.

172. C. L. Hodge, *The Tennessee Valley Authority: A National Experiment in Regionalism*, 175–93 (Washington, DC: American University Press, 1938).

173. D. Mitrany, "The New Deal: An Interpretation of Its Origin and Nature" [1942], in *American Interpretations* (London: Contact Publications, 1946), 20.

174. E. L. Bishop, "Consideration of the Malaria Problem in the Tennessee Valley," *Southern Medical Journal* 30 (1937): 861.

175. J. Parisot, "Rapport sur le voyage collectif d'étude aux États-Unis d'Amérique," Minutes of the 23rd session of the Health Committee, Geneva, April 29–May 2, 1936, 7, CH/23è session/PV revisé, LNA.

176. E. F. Ranshofen-Wertheimer, *The International Secretariat: A Great Experiment in International Administration* (Washington, DC: Rumford Press, 1945), 159.

177. "Note du Pr. Parisot et du Directeur Médical [L. Rajchman] au sujet des études ultérieures sur l'hygiène rurale, 5è réunion du Bureau d'Hygiène, Paris, 29 octobre 1936," CH/Bureau/6, LNA.

178. League of Nations European Conference on Rural Life, "Report by the preparatory Commission on its first session, 4–7 April 1938," Geneva, May 13, 1938,

C161 M101, LNA. Published the same year as the Moscow meeting in 1936, J. B. Orr's *Food, Health and Income* (London: Macmillan, 1936) and P. de Kruif's *Why Keep Them Alive?* (New York: Harcourt, Brace and Company, 1936) (with headings such as "Should Children Eat?") stressed the acuteness of both nutritional underconsumption and agricultural overproduction.

179. "Commission préparatoire à la Conférence européenne sur la vie rurale, Juillet 1939. Aide-mémoire," Geneva, March 28, 1938, 4, R6103, CPVR/1(2), 8A/31762/8855, LNA.

180. W. R. Aykroyd, "International Health: A Retrospective Memoir," *Perspectives in Biology and Medicine* 11 (1967): 279; J. B. O'Brien, "F. L. McDougall and the Origins of the FAO," *Australian Journal of Politics and History* 46 (2000): 170; F. L. McDougall, "The Agricultural and the Health Problems," 1934, 4, RG3.1/D1, Food and Agriculture Organization Archives, Rome.

181. E. Burnet and W. R. Aykroyd, "L'alimentation et l'hygiène publique," *Bulletin de l'Organisation d'Hygiène* 5 (1935): 332.

182. H. Kamminga, "'Axes to grind': Popularising the Science of Vitamins, 1920s and 1930s," in *Food, Science, Policy, and Regulation in the Twentieth Century*, ed. D. F. Smith and J. Phillips, 91–96 (London: Routledge, 2000).

183. S. Amrith, *Decolonizing International Health: India and Southeast Asia, 1930–1965* (London: Palgrave, 2006); S. Amrith, "The United Nations and Public Health in Asia, 1940–1960" (PhD diss., University of Cambridge, 2004), 21–22.

184. See McDougall's memorandum in the League's *JO*, December 1937, Annexe 1681, 1222–9; S. Turnell, "F. L. McDougall: 'Eminence Grise' of Australian Economic Policy," *Australian Economic History Review* 40 (2000): 63.

185. S. M. Bruce on September 11, 1935, in the LN's *JO*, Supplément 138, Actes de la 16è Session Ordinaire, 53; F. L. McDougall, "Food and Welfare," *Geneva Studies* 9 (1938): 14.

186. F. L. McDougall, "The Origins of FAO," 1951 [typescript 5 f.], 1, RG3.1/D1, Food and Agriculture Organization Archives, Rome.

187. L. Rajchman, quoted in A. J. Sawyer's diary, June 1, 1936, 1.1/100/21/179, RAC.

188. L. Rajchman, "Note," January 25, 1938, R6103, 8A/31762/8855, LNA; J. Avenol, "Note" for Lester, Rajchman, Loveday, and Stoppani, January 19, 1938, R6103, 8A/31762/8855, LNA.

189. R.-H. Hazemann, LNHO, Sub-Committee of Experts on Rural Hygiene, Session from April 25th to April 27th, 1938, Summary of Proceedings, 8, R6103, 8A/31762/8855(3), LNA.

190. A. G. B. Fisher, "Economic Appeasement as a Means to Political Understanding and Peace," in *Survey of International Affairs 1937*, vol. 1, ed. A. J. Toynbee (Oxford: Oxford University Press, 1938), 64.

191. W. H. Howell to F. F. Russell, June 27, 1930, 1.1/100/21/175, RAC. Of course, the weaving of such a web was not to be ascribed to a single, all-absorbing center. Constant exchanges were quite as important as the occasional widely publicized moments of contact with Geneva.

192. "Consultation sur la politique médico-sociale à la campagne," Geneva, October 10–14, 1938, CH1374, R6104, LNA. The Preparatory Commission itself should have included Vladko Macek, Radic's heir at the head of the Croat Peasant party, but his name was ultimately deleted.

193. "Rapport sur la réunion des directeurs d'instituts et d'écoles d'hygiène tenue à Genève du 22 au 27 novembre 1937," *Bulletin de l'Organisation d'Hygiène* 7 (1938): 184; Health Committee's session, Paris, May 18, 1938, CH/18 mai 1938/PV révisés 4, LNA.

194. J. Parisot, "Past and Future Work of the League of Nations Health Organisation in the Field of Rural Hygiene," report to the Health Committee Bureau, Moscow, June 1936, 13–14, CH1218, LNA.

195. J. Parisot and G. Richard, "La Lutte contre le chômage," *Revue d'hygiène et de médecine sociales* (February 1933), 33–39; J. Parisot and G. Richard, "Contre le chômage: Le retour à l'artisanat rural par l'organisation de 'cours de dépannage,'"*Revue d'hygiène et de médecine sociales* (January 1935), 25–29.

196. W. Chodzko, "L'Assainissement de la campagne et l'organisation du service de la santé publique dans les campagnes," *Bulletin de l'Office International d'Hygiène Publique* 20 (1928): 1275.

197. J. Parisot to O. Olsen [handwritten card], March 23, 1934, R6045, LNA.

198. J. Parisot, "Past and Future Work," 1936, 13–14, CH1218, LNA.

199. Parisot, "Past and Future Work," 1936, 14.

200. P. Stoppani to the LN Secretary General, "Conférence européenne de la Vie rurale. Mission à Paris," February 9, 1939, Jacques Parisot Papers, Vandoeuvre-lès-Nancy (hereafter Vandoeuvre).

201. S. M. Gunn to R. B. Fosdick, March 6, 1939, 2/700/183/1317, RAC.

202. C.-E. A. Winslow to G. E. Vincent, June 15, 1918, Winslow Papers, 749/III/97/1691, Yale.

203. E. Leroy, "Prophylaxie de la tuberculose à la campagne," *Le Mouvement Sanitaire* 5 (1929): 554.

204. J. Parisot's words, Health Committee Bureau, June 22, 1936, 13, CH/Bureau/IV/Procès-Verbal, LNA.

205. L. Rajchman, Health Committee's 28th session, Geneva, June 30–July 2, 1938, 40–41, Vandoeuvre.

206. Mitrany, *Functional Theory*, 119.

207. Winslow, "Economic Value," 199.

Chapter Seven

Contested Spaces

Models of Public Health in Occupied Germany

SABINE SCHLEIERMACHER

The year 1945 and the end of World War II in Germany is often called the Stunde null, or "Zero Hour." According to this myth, following the liberation of the German population from fascism, Germany returned to democracy with the assistance of the Allies in the heart of Europe. Only the "Eastern Zone" under Soviet control maintained structures dating from the Nazi dictatorship. This account, however, is not supported by the historical sources. A study of the models of public health in occupied Germany shows that the governing authorities in both the Eastern and Western zones drew on traditions that dated back to the Weimar Republic and beyond, but emphasized different aspects of the traditions.

In the aftermath of the war, living conditions and the provision of medical care became increasingly precarious. The medical infrastructure had collapsed, resulting in catastrophic health conditions among the population. Many hospitals were destroyed, and medicines and medical supplies were scarce. A housing shortage, poor sanitation, and large numbers of refugees led to the spread of contagious disease and epidemics. The main goal of both the Allied authorities and the staff in the East and West German health administrations was to prevent an increase in infant mortality and to halt the spread of infectious disease and epidemics, including tuberculosis, typhus, dysentery, and sexually transmitted diseases. The Allied health-policy objective was to establish a medical, organizational, institutional, and legal framework to prevent the spread of diseases that would imperil the health of both the population and the occupying authorities.

The occupying authorities were largely helpless in the face of these challenges. Even though individual studies of the German social insurance and public health systems had been drawn up before the end of the war, and informational material preparing for a future occupational administration had been updated regularly since 1943,[1] there still was no overall concept for the reorganization of the health system in the zones of occupation.[2]

This chapter begins from the assumption that the objective of reorganizing German society as rapidly as possible led both the British and the Soviet occupation authorities to fall back on older structures within Germany. The governing authorities in the two zones faced a similar scarcity of resources and a comparable scope of difficulties, and both were guided by traditions that dated back to the Weimar Republic. Despite these similarities, however, differences in political orientation between the two governing authorities led the two emerging German states to embrace fundamentally differing visions of public health policy.

Health Care Administration in Germany before 1945

Health Insurance and the Medical Profession

In Germany, the system of social insurance introduced in the 1880s laid down legal regulations for the curative medical care of employed workers. In important ways, the evolution of the system of health insurance and its goals under the radically shifting political circumstances of the half century that followed shaped the administration of health care in Germany after World War II.

The urbanization and industrialization that occurred during the second half of the nineteenth century saw a marked decline in the social circumstances of broad elements of the population. Toward the end of the century, economic and social transformation and heightened internal migration made the establishment of a centrally regulated form of social insurance appear necessary even from the state's point of view. In the years that followed, accident, health, and disability insurance were introduced. These formed a unified program of social legislation within the framework of Bismarckian social policies of the 1880s. The objective was to provide material support to workers in case of disability within a system that would be financed mostly by the labor force. These state-prescribed social policies were characterized by several principles. First, insurance served as a countermodel to public welfare and assistance to the poor; second, insurance holders had a right to support in the case of disability; and third, insurance programs were organized in a decentralized fashion and managed by the workers themselves.[3]

In contrast to older forms of social insurance, these new models provided a legal right to support that liberated the insured from dependence on socially and politically discriminatory poverty assistance and strengthened their status as citizens of the state.[4] By 1911, the number of insurance providers totaled 23,159. The number of individuals (including family members) enrolled in statutory health insurance programs increased from 11 percent of the population during the German Reich to 55 percent during the Weimar Republic and later to approximately 70 percent of the population during the Nazi era.[5]

The development of health insurance in the Weimar Republic must be assessed against the backdrop of the consequences of World War I, which included the inflation of 1923 and the world economic crisis and resulting mass unemployment in 1929. Despite these severe economic limitations, the health insurance companies were enjoined to provide comprehensive medical coverage to the population under the newly formulated provision of Article 161 of the Weimar Constitution. In addition, the insurers were to establish a "comprehensive insurance program with the decisive participation of the insured."[6] This goal could only be realized with the assistance of a sophisticated welfare system that was largely supported by nonstate charitable organizations.[7]

The emergency decrees that the state issued during the global economic crisis adapted public health care and the relationship of the health insurance companies to the medical profession in response to the unstable economic conditions. The involvement of the state had an impact on the cooperative character of the health insurance system. The influence of employers on the administration and management of the health insurance system increased without a corresponding shift in the funding structure, but with a noticeable effect on the original cooperative principle.

In 1933, the National Socialist regime began to expand on the reforms and rationalization measures of the Weimar government. The Decree for the Reorganization of Health Insurance and fourteen additional later decrees expanded the Reich government's right to monitor insurance providers to "examine the utility and economic efficiency of their management."[8] State-appointed commissioners under the supervision of the Reich Ministry of Labor assumed control over the organization of the health insurance companies. The *Gleichschaltung* ("enforced standardization") of the statutory health insurance companies was accomplished by applying the Law for the Restoration of the Professional Civil Service of April 7, 1933 to health insurance company staff. Thirty percent of the employees of the Allgemeine Ortskrankenkassen (AOK), one of the largest workers' health insurance providers, were dismissed for their political beliefs, usually meaning SPD (Social Democratic party) or KPD (Communist party) membership. Ninety-five percent of the staff of the Berlin AOK was affected by this measure. Members of the Nazi party and its subsidiary organizations then assumed control over insurance administration. On July 5, 1934, the Law for the Reconstruction of Social Insurance inaugurated further reorganization of social insurance programs. Individual insurance branches were unified with the objective of "bringing social insurance into a closer relationship with the governance of the state." Supervisory control was centralized and more tightly organized and the influence of the medical profession was increased. In accordance with the Nazi *Führerprinzip* ("leadership principle"), new directors were appointed to head the insurance companies, effectively eliminating the self-administration of the statutory insurance companies.[9] The principle of individual health insurance increasingly shifted in favor of family insurance, which represented a culmination of developments that dated back to the Kaiserreich.[10]

Health insurance providers were now governed by population and health policy "community measures," including measures of "selection" and "elimination," preventive health care (social hygiene), and "racial hygiene." Health insurance paid for the preparation of "certificates of heredity" and for the forced sterilization of individuals deemed "inferior" under the Law for the Prevention of Hereditarily Diseased Offspring, enacted on July 14, 1933.[11] Germans who were defined as "Jewish" under Nazi racial legislation could be treated only by "Jewish" physicians and in "Jewish" hospitals. However, very few Jewish physicians obtained permission to practice as "therapists" (*Krankenbehandler*), and funding was withdrawn from "Jewish" hospitals. This effectively eliminated health services for the sick and disabled who fell under the purview of the National Socialist racial laws.[12]

The history of social insurance in Germany is deeply interwoven with developments in the medical profession and its organizations. The health insurance legislation of 1884 had not defined the occupation of physicians or the term *medical treatment*.[13] Until that point, health insurance providers did not permit free choice of physicians among the still comparatively small number of insured. Physicians employed by the health insurance companies were paid a yearly salary. This conjoining of professional and economic interests led to constant disputes between physicians and the health insurance providers. On December 23, 1913, the Berlin Agreement eliminated the health insurance providers' hiring autonomy, replacing it with a licensing commission. Henceforth only physicians listed with health insurance providers had the right to treat patients.[14]

The heightened control by health insurance providers and the fear that providers would increase monitoring and professional restrictions culminated in a general medical strike between November 1923 and January 1924.[15] As a result, many health insurance providers founded clinics in urban areas that were financed directly by the insurers. These clinics employed physicians from a wide range of specialties at fixed salaries.[16] In

1930, the Association of Health Insurers of Greater Berlin, which provided insurance to 1.163 million members, ran thirty-eight clinics that employed 196 physicians and 536 nursing and support staff. Although these clinics were in part the health insurance providers' response to the physicians' strike, they also were an advertisement for the health objectives of leftist political parties and physicians.

The majority of physicians were quite conservative, however, and proved receptive to National Socialism.[17] Physicians were amenable to a surprising level of accommodation, which culminated in a form of self-imposed *Gleichschaltung* and the entrance of many physicians into the Nazi party. (Forty-five percent of German physicians joined the party; in some regions this figure exceeded 60 percent.) Jewish and politically undesirable colleagues were expelled from professional organizations. "Non-Aryan" physicians and physicians who were engaged in medical activities deemed to be "communist in nature" were dismissed from physicians' administrative boards and committees.[18] The enactment of the *Führerprinzip* and the appointment of a Reich Physicians' Leader completely eliminated professional autonomy.

The National Socialists then restructured the health care system. Physicians politically affiliated with the workers' movement, only some of whom were members of the KPD and SPD, had contributed to the development of the Weimar health care system, which was influenced by principles of social hygiene. After the end of World War I, these physicians had participated in the reestablishment of public health services and the founding of clinics, cooperative health centers, and sex counseling centers.[19]

The Law for the Reconstruction of the Professional Civil Service initiated the expulsion of Jewish professors and physicians from universities, public hospitals, and the public health service. Another decisive step was the April 22, 1933 decree of the Reich Ministry of Labor, which withdrew health insurance licensure from Jewish physicians in private practice. The Fourth Decree to the Reich Citizenship Law of July 25, 1938 withdrew medical licensure for all Jewish physicians, which was effectively equivalent to professional disbarment. Only one third of the Jewish physicians who remained in the Third Reich were permitted to work as "therapists" to provide medical care exclusively to the Jewish population.[20]

With the start of the war, the Nazi regime enacted a prohibition on the establishment of new private medical practices and new fee scale regulations. The resulting decline in private income, which appeared to jeopardize living standards within the profession, led many physicians to develop a more distanced attitude toward the regime. By May 1940, two thirds of qualified physicians had been drafted to military service, which in turn meant that health care for the civilian population could no longer be assured. By 1942, the occupational health services had assumed the role of private medical care. Company physicians, of whom more than three quarters were Nazi party members, were charged with ensuring workers' "labor capacity." The principles of medical confidentiality and of free choice of physicians were both abandoned.[21]

Public Health Services and Social Hygiene

The public health service, which was an important component of the public welfare system, was institutionalized in the 1919 constitution of the Weimar Republic. Aimed particularly at those who did not have adequate claims to health insurance, the public health service presented itself as a supplement to the statutory health insurance programs.

The orientation of the German public health service was preventive. Spokesmen for the public health services emphasized the links between lifestyles and habits, living conditions, and disease, and worked to implement hygienic instruction and education on everyday health risks. In addition to this educational function, the public health services were supposed to provide health care and supervision to segments of the population identified as potential carriers of especially serious diseases and regarded as dangerous to public health. Therapeutic possibilities for treating "endemic diseases" (*Volkskrankheiten*) were still limited, and thus the prevention of disease was a matter of great public interest.

Community health care was based on principles of social hygiene. The key insight and message of social hygiene, formulated around the turn of the twentieth century in the wake of industrialization, was the link between the health status of specific elements of the population and their social circumstances. Recognition of this link resulted in the inclusion of social science insights and categories in medical research.[22] There were also practical ramifications: because social conditions influenced the development of disease, medical care was to be focused on areas where socially determined diseases arose and flourished.[23] Moreover, social hygiene prompted not only research into the origins of disease and disease prevention on the level of the individual, but also the political implementation of research findings in the form of health policy. Proponents of social hygiene, usually left-wing physicians, clamored for reforms in living conditions to promote the physical soundness and the personal well-being of the individual.

From the beginning, however, these reform ideas were also linked to attempts to encourage the individual to adapt to industrial society and its requirements. Social hygiene was thus located at the point of intersection between reform and accommodation. Moreover, the reestablished link between disease and physical constitution accorded new credence to theories of genetic disposition in the development of disease.

With the fall of the Weimar Republic, the field of social hygiene, which continued to be regarded as an oppositional science, abandoned its original social scientific orientation and adopted an increasingly biologistic mode of explanation. The monitoring of sociologically defined social groups was replaced with the perception of the *völkisch* whole as a socially undifferentiated population.[24] Many of the important legal decisions in the sphere of public health care had been issued after the end of World War I. The founding and the establishment of numerous welfare offices had led to the dismemberment of the local public health system. One of the objectives of public health policy of the period was to assemble these dispersed efforts and competencies under a central authority.[25] The regional health departments thus formed an organizational platform for the local public health system, which was headed by a physician.

In 1933, the new regime accomplished two long-standing goals: the centralization of health policy duties and the implementation of a racial-hygienic health, social, and population policy. National Socialist health policy was primarily conceived as a population and racial policy that would produce a "healthy body of the *Volk*." Nazi health and social policy was characterized by the indissoluble link between positive support and negative exclusion, the promotion of the "valuable" and the exclusion and annihilation of the "less valuable." Demands to implement eugenic and racial hygiene principles within in the public health system had existed since the Kaiserreich. However, because these demands had been legitimized within an economic mode of argumentation and explanation, they did not gain wide-scale acceptance until after the worldwide economic crisis.[26]

The "most important milestone in the development of the public health system," according to the statement of a leading medical official, was the Law on the Unification of the Health System, passed on July 3, 1934. This law focused on the establishment of state-controlled health departments.[27] The main objective of these health departments was implementing a health policy system founded on principles of racial hygiene.[28] Local health departments that agreed to follow these objectives and obtained state authorization were not disbanded. In addition, the confessional and party welfare organizations and the German Labor Front (*Deutsche Arbeitsfront*) were also preserved. The Reich Department of Health assumed control over state health departments. In this manner, the Nazi regime achieved a nationally unified health policy, a demand originally formulated under the Weimar Republic.

"Public Health" Policies in Germany after 1945

The health care systems in Britain and the Soviet Union, founded as they were on principles of state sponsorship, resembled one another structurally in many ways. Despite the similarities, as we shall see, the British and the Soviet occupation authorities established two quite dissimilar systems of health care in the German zones of occupation.

Health Policies in the British Zone of Occupation

The policies of the British public health officers who remained in Germany until 1951 were based on the maintenance of older structures of health and social insurance that originated in the Kaiserreich and were modified in later years. The principles of the British occupation, which had been formulated as early as October 1944, were undermined by the social and political realities of postwar Germany.[29] Confronted by the necessity to create a functional German health care system, the British authorities elected to leave existing structures in place. For example, in the choice between a decentralized and a centralized form of organization, the British authorities chose what they termed a "reasonable amount of central control."[30] The guiding principle behind British occupation policy was promoting the education of Germans by means of exemplary fellow citizens rather than by way of the British example. For this reason, the British encouraged the independent reorganization of the public health system by Germans. The British method of influence entailed using face-to-face consultation to guide the development of the public health system in accordance with its own vision.

The British authorities were not interested in forcing their vision on the German medical profession. Rather, they believed their role was to serve as a source of potentially useful knowledge.[31] The British authorities thus regarded their German counterparts as agents for enacting their vision. The report of a 1948 tour, for example, stated:

> Clearly it is no permanent solution of this problem to treat the German public health officers as subordinates and to leave all real responsibility in the hands of the Control Commission, that solution was discarded when public health was de-reserved. We assume therefore that the policy of H.M.G. is to encourage the Germans to produce an efficient public health service of their own and to help them with advice and example. We do not think that the most efficient public health service for Germany would be the most exact copy of the English system.[32]

On one point, however, the British authorities were in complete agreement and willing to advance a clear position: the health system was no longer to be organized along the model of a sanitation police. Instead, targeted "propaganda" and "personal contact" were to be employed to persuade the population to adopt appropriate health behavior. German physicians thus were encouraged to visit Britain and engage in independent study of the important elements of a different—in other words, British—public health system.[33]

There was no central public health authority within the individual zones or at the suprazone level until the founding of the Federal Republic (West Germany). The British military government created only two public health administrative organizations. The first was a zone advisory board with eleven subdivisions. This purely advisory body lacked executive authority. It was headquartered in Hamburg and met monthly in order to arrive at recommendations that were then passed on to the Health Branch of the Control Commission for Germany and Military Government. The second organization was a German Advisory Committee on Public Health within British headquarters that also had a solely advisory function. Its members also met monthly until fall 1946 in Bünde, Westfalia.[34] Comprising leading medical officials from the later Länder (Lower Saxony, North Rhine-Westphalia, Hamburg, Schleswig-Holstein) in the British zone, the German advisory committee did not address conceptual issues during the years 1945 and 1946. Instead, it focused on practical health policy issues such as the distribution of pharmaceuticals and efforts to combat infectious disease. A February 1947 Control Commission decree of the Länder in the British zone assigned legislative and the executive public health functions to the Länder.[35] The British authorities believed that one of the crucial "problems" was the municipalization of the health administration and the associated construction of a comprehensive public health system. However, the municipalization of the public health departments was not discussed openly by the British Public Health Advisor or the leading medical officials of the Länder.[36]

The British Public Health Advisor hoped to speed up the process of reestablishing the public health departments and public health officers and transferring authority from the Länder to the local level. The British authorities saw this as a way not only to facilitate more efficient health care, but also to achieve their vision of the democratization of public life more generally and the public health system in particular. However, the German ministerial officials in all of the Länder in the British zone opposed decentralization. The British authorities were themselves aware of the ambivalent reception of their plans. In a report on a tour of the British zone, two British officials wrote:

> The government of the Länder and their sub-divisions have to evolve a system of government. The former government was undemocratic and was highly centralized. There is a natural tendency to assume that it is democratic to decentralize, rather than to consider for each particular function what degree of centralization will be most efficient. This had led to a demand from the

politicians, resisted by public health experts, that the Kreis [district] should be autonomous in public health. Smaller authorities tend to under-insure against risks to public health and small communities find it difficult not to select their officers on political grounds.[37]

The British authorities again explicitly stated their hope that German public health officials would visit England. Another report thus remarked:

> The main problems in securing an efficient public health service in Germany are (i) to avoid politics in administration, and (ii) to substitute appropriate responsibility at each level for a system of direction from above. These are essentially problems of education. Education in principles of democratic local government should be supplemented by arrangements for suitable German public health officials to study the English public health system in action.[38]

However, the hope that acquiring a fresh perspective would influence the design of the public health system did not come to fruition. The British authorities soon realized that "the German Public Health organization was with few exceptions, a less flexible organization than its British counterpart."[39]

Adherence to National Socialist Structures

The statement issued in December 1944 by the Anglo-American headquarters, SHAEF (Supreme Headquarter Allied Expeditionary Forces) envisioned that the public health officers under subsequent occupation authorities would be "cleansed" of National Socialists and their sympathizers. However, there was also general agreement that the function of the health departments would be maintained. A later statement instructed that German public health service personnel should be "retained to the greatest extent possible."[40]

The denazification policy in the British zone of occupation was characterized by a high degree of pragmatism, and was limited to the dismissal of active National Socialists. Because denazification was less strictly implemented in Lower Saxony, many physicians hoped to be admitted there into private practice. Zone Executive Order No. 54, issued on November 30, 1946, ultimately established a unified denazification process for the British zone. In contrast to the practice in the American zone, this order called for a narrowly defined circle of individuals to be called before a denazification court. After undergoing denazification, even physicians who had been interned for political offences or had been removed from public office would still be permitted to go into private practice.

Those who framed these policies hoped that they would help ensure the availability of appropriately trained physicians and thus provide adequate health care for the population. Even though the plan had been to heighten measures to denazify physicians after the Nuremberg medical trial of 1946–47, many physicians who could prove they possessed special skills that would be difficult to replace were not dismissed.[41] Individuals who were classified as indispensable "experts" by the British authorities were exempted from denazification.[42] Preference was given to persons who were regarded as politically unblemished and who possessed administrative experience from the Weimar or the Nazi era.[43]

In this manner, representatives of National Socialist public health policy who had been involved in the formulation and implementation of genetic and racial hygiene legislation also influenced health policies in the British zone of occupation after 1945. For example, in Lower Saxony—which along with Schleswig-Holstein, Hamburg, Bremen, Westfalia, and parts of (west) Berlin was under British military control—health policy questions were handled in the German Ministry of Labor, Reconstruction and Health, later the Ministry for Health and Welfare.

Beginning in October 1945, the ministerial public health division was headed by the public health officer Otto Buurman. Buurman decisively influenced the postwar reestablishment of the health care system in Lower Saxony and the Federal Republic.[44] He was accorded a special intermediary role between the German and British authorities. Between 1927 and 1945, Buurman had acquired administrative experience in a number of public health organizations in the German Reich and in German-occupied eastern Europe.[45] The experience he acquired during the occupation of Poland was of particular importance to his postwar role in public health administration. As in postwar Germany, the population of occupied Poland was affected by resettlement, migration, and ghettoization, necessitating both medical care and efforts to prevent the spread of epidemics. From 1941 to 1943, Buurman was the leading medical official in the Krakow health administration.[46] He was also the deputy to Jost Walbaum, the head of the Department of Health in the Generalgouvernement.[47] Many of Buurman's assistants in Lower Saxony came from similar backgrounds and ranges of experience. In 1945, Franz Ickert was appointed Buurman's advisor. Ickert had worked from 1926 to 1932 in the health department of the Gumbinnen government, and worked for the government in Stettin from 1932 to 1945.[48] In 1948, Heinrich Ernst, who had known Buurman since 1938, was appointed his advisor.[49] Ernst had headed the health division at the Berlin Police Headquarters from 1933 to 1935. From 1935 to 1945, Ernst was advisor to the divisions of public health department and social insurance in the Reich Ministry of the Interior.[50]

In addition to preserving personnel, the British authorities also preserved important elements of National Socialist legislation. The Control Council Law No. 1 of September 20, 1945, annulled twenty-five Nazi laws, decrees, and ordinances with immediate effect.[51] However, these laws did not include a number of obvious racial hygiene laws such as the Law for the Prevention of Hereditarily Diseased Offspring of July 14, 1933, which authorized the forced sterilization program, and the Law for the Protection of the Hereditary Health of the German *Volk*, passed on October 18, 1935. The Law for the Unification of the Public Health System of July 3, 1934 and its implementation decrees, which must be regarded as one of the most important health policy decisions of the Nazi era, also were not annulled. These laws thus were one of the important lines of continuity from the Weimar Republic into National Socialism and the emerging Federal Republic.[52] The objectives and structures of the public health departments that were founded in Nazi Germany in conjunction with the Law for the Unification of the Public Health System were thus "preserved."[53] Because of the scarcity of economic resources, the public health administration was funded at the level of 1935.[54]

As already noted, the occupation authorities preserved the 1933 sterilization law and the "marital health law." However, the term *racial hygiene* was eliminated from everyday language, to be replaced by the word "eugenics" (*Erbpflege*). Beginning in 1945, a number of West German Länder attempted to apply the sterilization law.[55] However, the relevant laws and decrees varied widely across the zones of occupation, and they continued to be handled differently by the various Länder. The legal situation in the different regions was extremely complex, and many officials expressed the desire for regulatory unity. The activities of the existing hereditary health courts were limited to the "reopening of cases" that had been decided in the Nazi era. On February 20, 1946, the Allied Control Council issued a marriage law that called for the issuance of premarital marriage health certificates by the public medical officer once the law took force on March 1. In April 1947, the British occupation authorities endorsed the Nazis' 1935 Marital Health Law.[56] Although Lower Saxony and Schleswig-Holstein no longer adhered to the Marital Health Law, they were engaged in drafting new marital health legislation. In Hamburg, however, the Nazi Marital Health Law remained in force.

The Revival of Social Hygiene

The public confrontation over the revival of social hygiene and the strengthening of the public health system was accompanied by discussions on a number of issues that had their origins in 1948 in the public health committees of the Länder under British administration. These issues included the drafting of legislation for the reorganization of the public health system, the problem of neglect of the right to health in the Federal Republic's 1949 Basic Law, and the issue of health as a human right in the WHO's 1946 "Magna Carta." In 1948, the state secretary of Lower Saxony, Walter Auerbach, described the goals of public health administration at the founding of the Lower Saxony Health Council. Auerbach accorded special importance to the social hygiene objectives of the public health departments. The public health department was the lowest-level administrative authority that worked to "maintain and promote the health and labor force of the population." The goal of social hygiene, Auerbach believed, was the "care of those elements of the population who due to age, physical condition, or economic incapacity, were in need of special health services."[57]

According to Buurman's definition, social hygiene was directed toward the care of specific segments of the population. These included, for example, pregnant women, children, the disabled, and individuals with sexually transmitted diseases. In these instances, the physician assumed the mantle of state authority. As an "appointed servant of the state," the physician was obligated to serve not the welfare of the individual but rather that of the "general public."[58] Popular trust and approval, which had been damaged by compulsory vaccination programs, the threatened seizure of ration cards, and compulsory mass X-ray screenings for suspected cases of tuberculosis, was to be revived by the public health officer's trust-enhancing measures, including house calls and health education. If implemented, such measures would have led to an unprecedented expansion of the role of the public health officer. In addition, with the model of the British public health system in mind, there was discussion between Germans and British public health officers of training health inspectors, wardens, engineers, and welfare workers to assume public health functions. According to the German tradition of public health, these spheres of activity were confined to welfare workers.

According to Erich Schröder, a member of the Lower Saxony Health Council and a professor of social hygiene in Göttingen, public health functioned to guarantee the preservation of social "order." The purpose of health legislation was to preserve the health of the population and maintain its labor potential. The preservation of health was thus also an individual civic duty. The family as a "unit of social biology" was to be accorded particular attention within preventive social hygiene.[59]

Given the cost of reconstruction in the Federal Republic, the funds available for public health services were limited. Medical care remained largely the province of physicians in private practice and was curative in emphasis.[60] Following an October 25, 1945 recommendation by the German Health Services Advisory Committee in Bünde, Westfalia, the British

Control Commission founded academies for social hygiene in Düsseldorf and Hamburg on December 14, 1945. These academies were intended to address the scarcity of physicians for public health services.[61]

The academy for social hygiene in Hamburg trained public medical officers for Hannover, Schleswig-Holstein, and Hamburg, and later also for Berlin. The guidelines for the training of public health officers were based on the February 6, 1935 version of the Law for the Unification of the Public Health System and the February 13, 1934 regulations governing the training of public health officers. These Nazi-era laws and decrees, however, were to be implemented in accordance with the "elimination of National Socialist concepts from the curriculum." Although officials attempted to distance training regulations from National Socialist public health policies, the instructors were drawn from among the leading medical officers of Lower Saxony, Schleswig-Holstein, and Hamburg discussed above. In addition, the academies recruited individuals who were responsible for eugenic forms of social hygiene during the Weimar Republic, and who had participated in National Socialist racial policies after 1933.

Hans Harmsen was a prime example. Harmsen had been a leader in private welfare services within the fields of health care and population policy without interruption since 1926. During the course of these decades, he established a network of contacts on which he was able to draw in 1946. Harmsen advocated a eugenic form of social hygiene that when linked to *völkisch* ideology had proven compatible with the racial hygiene of the Nazi state.[62] From 1946 to 1956, 274 physicians (of whom thirty-nine were women) were trained as public welfare officials. They were appointed to the public health administrations in the Länder.

Public Health Policy in the Soviet Zone of Occupation (SBZ)

Whereas in the British zone of occupation the objectives of traditional health policy along with their modifications under National Socialism were preserved, the Soviets chose a different path in their zone of occupation. German health policy officials who were leftist in political orientation and affiliated with the workers' movement believed that the time had finally come to implement the reforms they had developed in the Weimar Republic, which had been abandoned following the political events of 1933. These officials found fruitful ground for their reformist visions within the Soviet Military Administration (SMAD), which was in the process of formulating similar objectives.

Even before the end of the Potsdam Conference, one of the Soviet Military Administration's first orders (No. 17, issued on July 27, 1945) established the two administrations that would be responsible for all issues of public health. The first of these departments was initially called the Main Administration and was later renamed the German Central Administration for Public Health (GCPH). The second department was the German Central Administration for Labor and Social Welfare (GCLSW).[63] The GCPH was responsible for the "public health system—for heading the departments of health care, the medical institutions and institutes for medical education, and the operations of the medical industry." The responsibilities of the central administration were governed by special SMAD "guidelines."[64]

Until the founding of the German Democratic Republic (East Germany) in 1949, all important public health decisions were made by the SMAD. On the German side, executive and legislative authority was initially held by the Länder and provincial governments. However, this authority could only be exercised on the express orders or with the agreement of the regional military administration. The SMAD thus needed to be a central coordinating authority. At first, the GCPH's function was expressly limited to advisor to the SMAD. All measures, whether on the level of the zone or on the level of the Länder and the districts, required the agreement of the proper SMAD representative. This was true especially for the employment of German officials in specific administrative and political positions. In such cases, the applicants were scrutinized to determine their degree of political culpability for actions undertaken in the Nazi era.

Paul Konitzer, a Social Democrat, was appointed president of the GCPH. Konitzer also had past administrative experience. From 1926 to 1933, he was head of the municipal public health department, a senator for health in Magdeburg, and a delegate to the Association of German Cities. At the end of the 1920s, Konitzer participated in public health administration reforms. As a member of the SPD, he was dismissed from office in 1933, arrested, and expelled from the city. Konitzer then entered private practice in Dresden. He was drafted into the German Wehrmacht in 1939, where he served as consulting hygienist beginning in 1942. In this capacity, Konitzer was also responsible for the medical care of Russian prisoners in the Zeithain POW camp. Despite his great success in reestablishing the public health system and his undisputed professional authority, the SMAD arrested Konitzer for his activities in Zeithain in February 1947.[65]

In August 1947, Karl Linser, who had no party affiliation, was appointed Konitzer's successor. Linser had been a dermatologist in private practice during Weimar and the Nazi era, and had little experience in public health policy. His delegates, vice presidents Alfred Beyer and Maxim Zetkin, had decisive influence on public health policy in the SBZ.

Alfred Beyer, who joined the SPD and the Union of Socialist Physicians in 1918, was active in a variety of functions in the Prussian Ministry of the Interior between 1919 and 1933, ultimately serving as the head of a ministerial department that addressed matters of public health policy and social insurance. From 1933 to 1939, he was unable to obtain permission to open a private practice as a physician. Beyer, an experienced administrator, was appointed head of a department in the GCPH from 1945 to 1946. From 1946 to 1949, he was deputy vice president and head of the department of social medicine in the GCPH.[66]

Maxim Zetkin, the son of Clara Zetkin, the influential socialist politician and fighter for women's rights, joined the SPD in 1902, the USPD in 1917, and the KPD in 1919. After his work as a military surgeon during World War I, he accepted an invitation to the Soviet Union and began working there as a surgeon. As a volunteer in the Spanish Civil War and a military surgeon in the Red Army, Zetkin was highly regarded for his medical competence and enjoyed the political trust of the SMAD.[67] Until he left what had become the Ministry of Health in the early 1950s, Zetkin influenced and at times participated in writing the actual texts of political decisions, laws, and decrees. The Soviet occupation authorities trusted Zetkin and assigned him responsibility for personnel policy decisions well beyond the sphere of the Central Administration. All new hires and dismissals required Zetkin's permission. Zetkin was also involved in "changes in the occupation of important posts in the Public Health Agency of the Länder, the provinces, and the universities" as well as in the "composition of committees, editorial boards, and the convening of consultations and meetings."[68]

Remigrants, or returning émigrés, were also important to the conceptual design of the public health system. Positions for physicians in the GCPH often remained empty for long periods due to the scarcity of suitable applicants.[69] In the first years after the war, remigrants thus assumed positions of leadership. Although they were only a small group within the total number of staff, the remigrants enjoyed disproportionate political influence. One example is Kurt Winter. In 1933, Winter emigrated to Palestine and then to Switzerland, where he passed his medical examinations in 1935, and received his doctorate in 1936. In 1937, Winter went to Spain to volunteer in the Spanish Civil War. In 1939, he worked as a refugee physician in Paris and Oslo. In 1940, he traveled on to Sweden, where he was interned. In 1943, he began to practice in the fields of psychiatry and social health. During his exile, Winter assumed positions in the KPD, and in 1945 he organized medical aid deliveries from Sweden to the SBZ. Winter felt indebted to the social hygiene and communist traditions. The Central Committee of the KPD planned to appoint him as public health officer in the GCPH. However, Winter initially declined the position in order to become a public health officer in Teltow in 1946, and the head of the Public Health Department of Brandenburg in 1947. From 1948 to 1949, Winter finally served as vice president and deputy director of the Central Agency for Health in the German Economic Commission. In his wide-ranging work, Winter helped preserve the tradition of social hygiene in the politics and science of the GDR.[70]

In its public health and social insurance programs, the GDR proceeded from a fixed canon of health policy decisions and objectives that had largely been established in the Soviet zone of occupation. The guidelines that shaped the reconstruction of public health in the GDR can be traced back to late nineteenth- and early twentieth-century workers' party programs.[71] The priority of public health care was prevention. Medical treatment had to be for all people at the same level. The state would need to assume overall responsibility for the medical care of its population.

Denazification

In the Soviet zone, the political cleansing deemed necessary by the Allies was carried out "more decisively" and in a "more consistent manner than in the Western zones."[72] The dismissal of physicians who had supported the Nazi regime from departments and positions and their legal prosecution had far-reaching consequences. The Länder were in charge of carrying out denazification. For example, Thuringia began the process of denazification with a Law on the Purging of Public Administration of Nazi Elements issued on July 23, 1945. The GCPH and SMAD did not issue guidelines for denazification until later that fall.[73] A nominal membership in the Nazi party was not sufficient grounds for dismissal as a public employee or for legal prosecution. These sanctions were limited to individuals who had held positions of authority in the party and in affiliated organizations or who had actively supported Nazi objectives. The political reliability of individuals who worked in the medical field and had contact with large segments of the population was deemed a matter of great importance. For this reason, physicians who hoped to assume leading positions were required to document their antifascist convictions. The Guidelines for the Purging of Nazi Elements from the Administration Serving the Health Care of the Volk,[74] issued by the GCPH on October 9, 1945, implemented a law issued by the SMAD on October 1, 1945 that "assigned priority to the denazification of the health administration from the very start."[75] This represented an attempt to "first establish uniform standards for all physicians."

However, these standards were "modified under the pressure of the personnel situation."[76] The GCPH did not possess legislative competence to enact uniform regulations for the Länder, which insisted on their right to democratic self-governance. For pragmatic reasons, the SMAD elected to endorse the interests of the Länder, permitting regulatory exceptions in light of the scarcity of physicians. The sanctions on physicians included the withdrawal of licensure, professional disqualification, a ban on the opening of a private practice, the seizure of office furniture and medical equipment, and requirements to practice in the sphere of public health. The latter could include an obligation to assume a position in a distant location, for example a rural region with a severe shortage of physicians. As a special "penance," physicians could be required to work in efforts to combat epidemics and in refugee health care. But even though it was implemented more extensively than in the Western zones, political cleansing in the GDR failed.

In spring 1946, the GCPH estimated that party membership ranged from 65 to 80 percent of doctors according to region. For physicians in private practice, the estimate assumed figures approaching 80 to 90 percent.[77] However, the manner and extent of political cleansing did not have the same rigor and consistency in the medical profession as in other professional groups. With the shortage of physicians to combat epidemics and provide medical care to camps and emergency shelters, the authorities were hard pressed to prevent the collapse of health care.[78] Moreover, as "qualified replacements for physicians who are slated for dismissal were lacking," local networks of elites tended to protect medical personnel from denazification. In the case of the physicians, permanent replacement was rare: even physicians who had been assigned to "penance duty" were usually only temporarily removed from their former positions.[79]

In the Soviet zone, the Law for the Prevention of Hereditarily Diseased Offspring was deemed a crime against humanity in accordance with Control Council Law No. 10. In the beginning, the SMAD intended to prosecute all physicians who had been involved in racial eugenic health proceedings. But after the intervention of German jurists, this plan was modified and only physicians who had been involved in forced racial and political sterilizations were prosecuted. The rationale was that "it is impossible to strip an entire zone of physicians; there are hardly any physicians who did not in some fashion participate in hereditary health proceedings."[80]

Institutions and organizations that were deemed specifically National Socialist in orientation were disbanded. These included Nazi party institutions involved in racial hygiene and social medicine activities, hygiene departments, the Hygiene Institute of the SS, and the National Socialist Reich Physicians' League. In the Soviet zone, the Reich Medical Association was disbanded, whereas in the Western zones the authorities were content to seize its assets.[81]

Public Health Guidelines in the SBZ and the GDR

The German Democratic Republic concept of a "democratic health care system" that corresponded with Soviet ideas included universal, direct access, free of charge, to all medical institutions, even specialists, and a unified social insurance program in case of illness, disability, and old age. The priority was general health care. Prevention and prophylaxis were the central goals of all medical efforts. In order to achieve this goal, the state would need to assume overall responsibility for the medical care of its population and thus for the system of public health.

From its formation in July 1945, the German Council of Public Health, which would become the German Ministry of Health after 1949, had primary responsibility for the organization of health policy issues. After the dissolution of the Länder, district and municipal physicians retained their health supervisory functions, which were comparable to the functions of the head of a health department in the Federal Republic. However, these district and municipal physicians had little authority to intervene in developing problems, such as in the case of threatened epidemics. However, they did have the authority to issue directives to all public health institutions, hospitals, and even to physicians in private practice. Since the legal and economic planning framework (the two-, five-, and seven-year plans) for the health care system was issued by the Ministry of Health for the entire GDR, there was little opportunity for a regional health policy to develop. The health and social apparatuses of large industries and businesses were also an important feature of the system.[82]

In line with overall political developments, the Socialist Unity Party of Germany (Sozialistische Einheitspartei Deutschlands) began to dominate the health care system. On the level of the central party, the Central Committee and the party apparatus began to assume the dominant role. The Socialist Unity Party initially relied on its cadres to fill important departmental leadership positions within the ministry. Most of these people, who were trained in medicine at German universities, had been social democrats or communists under the Weimar Republic. After the mid-1950s, the Socialist Unity Party began to expand the party's supervisory authority, even establishing its own health division in 1958.

On both the municipal and the industrial levels, the expansion of the state institutions responsible for outpatient health care—the polyclinics, outpatient clinics, and health centers—aimed to dissolve the traditionally dominant pattern of individual, private practice among physicians. The population retained the right to free choice of physicians. Existing private practices were not threatened with closure; however, the barriers to establishing a new private practice were virtually insurmountable. The incentives for physicians to work in state institutions were systematically raised, resulting in a substantial increase in the scope of state outpatient health care institutions in this period.

Physicians' control over the terms of discourse and the dominance of medical thought in all questions of health and disease, however, remained astonishingly intact. Certificates of birth and death, the certification of illness and the ability or inability to work, and certifications for the right to specific jobs and social benefits, including everything from sick pay to day-care spots, continued to remain solely the province of the medical profession. The unbroken belief in the findings of science—a science based on the teachings of scientific socialism—increasingly also influenced political decision making and thus strengthened the academically schooled medical profession. Although their positions on faculties and their professional practice may have been subjected to political pressures, in the end physicians were largely unaffected by political restrictions. In the conduct of their medical duties, even those physicians who occupied university chairs of social medicine were little affected by the content of social hygiene.

"Health Protection" Instead of "Medical Care"

Like Article 161 of the Weimar Republic's constitution, Article 16 of the October 1949 constitution of the German Democratic Republic established the citizen's right to the "preservation of health and ability to work." A "uniform, comprehensive social insurance system" would guarantee this claim.[83] In contrast to the Federal Republic during the 1950s, the GDR's social security offered the entire population full health coverage in case of illness.[84] In the Health Ministry's view, regardless of social standing, "everyone, absolutely everyone . . . possesses—in contrast to before—an unlimited right to the protection of health that is, above all, independent of economic circumstances."[85] The concept of "health protection" that determined health policy in the GDR presupposed a relationship between an individual's social standing and his or her physical state of health. First, social differences shaped the situation of health and illness. Second, illness itself played a part in creating social inequalities. Those who participated in constructing the GDR's explicitly "democratic" health care system sought to create the conditions necessary to provide all citizens with the "right" to "realize all their physical and mental capabilities."[86]

Their rationale drew on Alfred Grotjahn's 1912 reflections on social hygiene, as well as on demands from the German workers' movement during the Weimar Republic.[87] Grotjahn had stressed health policy reforms in his insistence that medicine serve the purpose of social hygiene. In contrast, policy makers in the GDR emphasized the importance of changes in basic social conditions.[88] In formulating health-protection objectives, East German policy makers also drew on the Soviet health care system, itself influenced both by Grotjahn and by the notions of health protection articulated by the

Russian commissar of public health, Nikolai A. Semashko.[89] In absorbing individual traditions deriving from German social hygiene, the GDR chose to emphasize state responsibility, establishing a centralized health system that incorporated new forms of health care for the population, such as polyclinics, outpatient clinics, and health centers.[90]

Underlying the development of health protection in the Socialist Unity Party of East Germany was the belief that health policy was a matter of concern to the entire population and all state institutions, rather than the domain solely of medical and social policy experts and medical science. Health policy thus needed to take all aspects of social life into account.[91] Above all, and in contrast to the case of the Western zones and the Federal Republic, health protection in the SBZ and the GDR did not focus on prevention in the strict sense of the term. Rather, it was founded on the principle of the "unity of prevention, medical care, and rehabilitation."

Health protection was centrally organized. The Ministry of Health issued political guidelines, orders, and instructions for the entire GDR. The result was that there was "little political space for flexible, innovative and context-specific (decentralized) regulatory mechanisms."[92] The concept of health protection was embedded in a wide-ranging and multifaceted political agenda for the promotion of health. These policies were aimed at specific groups of people (mothers, infants, children and youth, families with many children) and at infrastructural institutions (kindergartens, health centers, polyclinics, and housing). Institutions located outside the health system also bore responsibility for health protection. Among the most important such institutions were the medical facilities established by industrial enterprises and the rural medical facilities, neither of which can be analyzed in detail here.

The right to health security stemmed from the interrelationship between the "obligation of the individual towards the whole and of the state towards working people."[93] This right was expressed in the following maxim: "An essential prerequisite for the simple and extended reproduction of the workforce entails securing the conditions for a normal relationship between the depletion of the workforce and its replenishment. At the same time, an absolute reduction of available social and individual work capacity through accidents and illness must be prevented. This necessitates protecting working people, who are the bearers of the workforce, from temporary and long-term damage to health."[94] One of the GDR's most important social hygienists, Kurt Winter, described the political significance of health protection as follows: "Only after we have realized the principle: 'Protecting the health of the working population is a matter of concern to the working population itself'—only then will we have accomplished the democratization of health care."[95]

Conclusion

Within the zones administered by the various occupying authorities, different concepts of medical care developed. These concepts included ideas about the role of physicians within the health care system, about social security, and about outpatient care. Whereas the Federal Republic made the individual responsible for his or her own health, in East Germany the state assumed responsibility. In the West, health policy makers criticized the newly introduced federal structure as a negative reaction to National Socialism's centralism. In the East, health policy makers drew on traditions dating from the Weimar Republic to demand the centralization of the public health system.

Generally speaking, the British occupying authorities envisioned reviving what they deemed positive forces within Germany to facilitate reeducation and democratization. Britain's comparatively large administrative apparatus was to serve as a support, but was not to direct the process of reconstruction from above. For this reason, it is difficult to document the implementation of specific British ideas and agendas within the realm of public health.

As my analysis demonstrates, the policies and perceptions of National Socialism had such a profound influence on the medical sphere that leading German medical officials were unable to conceive of a public health system that would not function as a "sanitation police."[96] The British occupying authorities regretfully took notice of this fact. The revival of social hygiene in West Germany as a whole and Lower Saxony in particular must be interpreted against this backdrop. The concept of social hygiene in the postwar period displayed clear connotations of an authoritarian state. These connotations included sociobiological components that, even when stripped of the vocabulary of racial biology, clearly derived from an earlier era. Alfred Grotjahn's ideas were influential in both German states. However, East and West Germany chose to emphasize different aspects of this tradition in accordance with their different political frameworks.

In reconstructing the public health system in the zone they occupied, the Soviet occupying authorities revived concepts originally formulated by the Social Democratic Party and the Communist Party, some of which had been implemented in the Weimar Republic. The Soviet occupying authorities believed in these concepts. For the Soviet authorities in Germany, the "fit" was not strained: they had, after all been reared in the principles of the "new Soviet medicine," which itself included concepts borrowed from German social hygiene.

The precondition for establishing this system of public health care was the state's assumption of comprehensive responsibility for the protection of health. This required the participation of classical medical institutions such as hospitals, physicians, and health departments. However, and even more important, it necessitated the participation of all socially responsible state and economic institutions and individuals. A central authority was necessary to enact the new system of public health. This realization led to the establishment of the Ministry of Health, the first institution of its kind in German history. The East German public health system thus established a network of local and industrial polyclinics for health protection, comprehensive social insurance, and science founded on concepts of social hygiene. These features differed significantly from the public health system in the Federal Republic.

But the similarities between the East and West German systems of public health become apparent in international comparison. In both East and West Germany, the principle of social insurance was upheld in contrast to a wholly publicly financed system; the free choice of physicians was preserved against a system of primary physician care; and medical training and the organization of medical faculties remained rooted in German traditions. For this reason, physicians, dentists, pharmacists, nurses, orderlies, medical technicians, and paramedics who had trained in the GDR could later be easily hired to positions in the Federal Republic. In fact, a relatively great number of East German physicians "went West." After the fall of the Berlin Wall in 1989, the West German system of public health was established in the east.

Notes

This essay developed in the course of discussions with Udo Schagen during our work heading a research project on the history of public health after 1945. U. Schagen and S. Schleiermacher, "Gesundheitswesen und Sicherung bei Krankheit und im Pflegefall. Einleitung: Rahmenbedingung für die Reorganisation des Gesundheitswesens. Die Sowjetische Besatzungszone und Berlin," Bundesministerium für Arbeit und Sozialordnung, Bundesarchiv, ed., *Geschichte der Sozialpolitik in Deutschland seit 1945*; v 2/1: 1945–1949; *Die Zeit der Besatzungszonen* (Baden-Baden: Nomos Verlag, 2001), 464–528. Documents in Bd. 2/2; *Im Zeichen des Aufbaus des Sozialismus DDR 1949–1961*, ed. Dierk Hoffmann and Michael Schwartz. Bd. 8 (Baden-Baden: Nomos Verlag, 2004), 390–433.

1. National Archives Record Administration, Washington, DC, RG 331, Box 7. German Basic Handbook, ABC of German Administration and Public Services, November 12, 1944; H. E. Sigerist, "From Bismarck to Beveridge," *Bulletin of the History of Medicine* 13 (1943): 365–88.

2. R. A. Leiby, "Public Health in Occupied Germany, 1945–1949" (University Microfilms International, University of Delaware, 1985), 92. T. J. Beatty, "Soziale Sicherheit in Großbritannien," *Arbeitsblatt für die britische Zone* 2 (1949): 338–40, 419–22; H. G. Hockerts, "Deutsche Nachkriegssozialpolitik vor dem Hintergrund

des Beveridge-Plans. Einige Beobachtungen zur Vorbereitung einer vergleichenden Analyse," in *Die Entstehung des Wohlfahrtsstaats in Großbritannien und Deutschland 1850–1950*, ed. W. J. Mommsen, 325–50 (Stuttgart: Klett Cotta Verlag, 1982).

3. V. Hentschel, "Das System der sozialen Sicherung in historischer Sicht 1880–1975," *Archiv für Sozialgeschichte* 18 (1978): 312–13.

4. G. A. Ritter, *Der Sozialstaat. Entstehung und Entwicklung im internationalen Vergleich* (Munich: Oldenbourg Wissenschaftsverlag, 1989), 63–64.

5. F. Tennstedt, "Sozialgeschichte der Sozialversicherung," in *Handbuch der Sozialmedizin*, vol. 3, ed. M. Blohmke (Stuttgart: Enke Verlag, 1976), 403, 408.

6. R. Schuster, ed., *Verfassung des Deutschen Reichs (Weimarer Verfassung) vom 11. August 1919: Deutsche Verfassungen* (Munich: Goldmann Verlag, 1992), 203.

7. L. Preller, *Sozialpolitik in der Weimarer Republik* (Stuttgart: Athenäum/Droste Verlag, 1949), 85.

8. In the following, I refer to F. Tennstedt, *Geschichte der Selbstverwaltung in der Krankenversicherung von der Mitte des 19. Jahrhunderts bis zur Gründung der Bundesrepublik Deutschland* (Bonn: Verlag der Ortskrankenkassen, 1977), 184–91; R. Schwoch, *Ärztliche Standespolitik im Nationalsozialismus. Julius Hadrich und Karl Haedenkamp als Beispiele* (Husum: Matthiesen Verlag, 2001), 164–225.

9. Tennstedt, *Selbstverwaltung*, 196–219.

10. Hentschel, "Das System," 322–23.

11. A. Gütt et al., eds., *Gesetz zur Verhütung erbkranken Nachwuchses vom 14. Juli 1933 mit Auszug aus dem Gesetz gegen gefährliche Gewohnheitsverbrecher und über Maßregeln der Sicherung und Besserung vom 24. Nov. 1933* (Munich: J. F. Lehmann Verlag, 1934), 58, 165–66.

12. Schwoch, "Standespolitik," 220.

13. Tennstedt, "Sozialgeschichte," 388–89.

14. P. Thomsen, *Ärzte auf dem Weg ins „Dritte Reich." Studien zur Arbeitsmarktsituation, zum Selbstverständnis und zur Standespolitik der Ärzteschaft gegenüber der staatlichen Sozialversicherung während der Weimarer Republik* (Husum: Matthiesen Verlag, 1996), 55.

15. Tennstedt, "Sozialgeschichte," 398; E. Wolff, "Mehr als nur materielle Interessen. Die organisierte Ärzteschaft im Ersten Weltkrieg und in der Weimarer Republik 1914–1933," in *Geschichte der deutschen Ärzteschaft. Organisierte Berufs- und Gesundheitspolitik im 19. und 20. Jahrhundert*, ed. Robert Jütte (Cologne: Deutscher Ärzte-Verlag, 1997), 113.

16. E. Hansen et al., *Seit über einem Jahrhundert . . . : Verschüttete Alternativen in der Sozialpolitik. Sozialer Fortschritt, organisierte Dienstleistermacht und nationalsozialistische Machtergreifung: Der Fall der Ambulatorien in den Unterweserstädten und Berlin* (Cologne: Bund-Verlag, 1981).

17. M. H. Kater, "Professionalization and Socialization of Physicians in Wilhemine and Weimar Germany," *Journal of Contemporary History* 20 (1985): 677–701; M. H. Kater, *The Nazi Party: A Social Profile of Members and Leaders, 1919–1945* (Cambridge, MA: Harvard University Press, 1983); M. H. Kater, *Doctors Under Hitler* (Chapel Hill: University of North Carolina Press, 1989).

18. M. Rüther, "Ärztliches Standeswesen im Nationalsozialismus 1933–1945," in *Geschichte der deutschen Ärzteschaft*, ed. R. Jütte (Cologne: Deutscher Ärzte-Verlag, 1997), 143, 147.

19. G. Baader, "Politisch motivierte Emigration deutscher Ärzte," *Berichte zur Wissenschaftsgeschichte* 7 (1984): 72–73; S. Leibfried and F. Tennstedt, *Berufsverbote und Sozialpolitik 1933. Die Auswirkungen der nationalsozialistischen Machtergreifung auf die Krankenkassenverwaltung und die Kassenärzte*, Arbeitspapiere des Forschungsschwerpunktes Reproduktionsrisiken, Soziale Bewegungen und Sozialpolitik (Bremen: Universität Bremen, 1980), 20.

20. Baader, "Emigration," 73.

21. Rüther, "Standeswesen," 192.

22. Health care programs included marital health counseling; medical care for pregnant women and new mothers; care for infants, toddlers, and schoolchildren; tuberculosis treatment; treatment of alcoholics; medical care for the prevention of sexually transmitted diseases; care for the physically disabled; and care for the mentally ill and the criminally mentally ill. C. Sachße, *Mütterlichkeit als Beruf. Sozialarbeit, Sozialreform und Frauenbewegung 1871–1929* (Frankfurt am Main: Suhrkamp Verlag, 1986), 204.

23. M. Mosse and G. Tugendreich, eds., *Krankheit und soziale Lage*, 3rd ed. (Göttingen: Wisomed Verlag, 1981).

24. C. Sachße and F. Tennstedt, *Geschichte der Armenfürsorge in Deutschland*, vol. 2, *Fürsorge und Wohlfahrtspflege 1871–1929* (Berlin and Cologne: Verlag W. Kohlhammer, 1988), 20–21.

25. "Sitzung des Interkommunalen Ausschusses für das Gesundheitswesen am 8 Dezember 1930 in Berlin," *Zeitschrift für Gesundheitsverwaltung und Gesundheitsfürsorge* 2 (1931): 185–91.

26. *Die Eugenik im Dienste der Volkswohlfahrt. Bericht über die Verhandlungen eines zusammengesetzten Ausschusses des Preußischen Landesgesundheitsrats vom 2. Juli 1932*, Veröffentlichungen aus dem Gebiet der Medizinalverwaltung, Bd. XXXVIII, Heft 5 (Berlin: Richard Schoetz Verlag, 1932). Among the most important "hereditary and racial laws" passed beginning in 1933 were the laws and decrees for the promotion of marriage and the granting of marriage loans (June 20, 1933), the Law for the Prevention of Hereditarily Diseased Offspring (July 14, 1933), the Law for the Protection of the Hereditary Health of the German *Volk* (October 18, 1935) as well as the "Euthanasia" program (after 1939).

27. F. Klose, "Die Krise des deutschen öffentlichen Gesundheitswesens," *Ärztliche Mitteilungen* 2 (1948): 287.

28. E. Schütt and N. Wollenweber, eds., *Der Arzt des öffentlichen Gesundheitswesens 1941* (Leipzig: Georg Thieme Verlag, 1941), 1–20, 387–90.

29. The guideline was the "elimination of National Socialism and militarism from the administration, justice, and the economy as well as from all aspects of public life; the reeductation of Germans to democratic ways of life; . . . the prevention of 'fraternization' between occupation soldiers and the German population; the solution of fundamental postwar problems with the help of a German administration and management (the principle of *indirect rule*); . . . the start-up of the economic infrastructure and revitalization of the German peace economy on a reduced level." Germany and Austria in the Post-Surrender Period: Policy Directives for Allied Commanders-in-Chief, FO 371/C1071/24/18/46730, Public Record Office, London (hereafter PRO); quoted in U. Schneider, "Niedersachsen unter britischer Besatzung 1945.

Besatzungsmacht, deutsche Verwaltung und die Probleme der unmittelbaren Nachkriegszeit," *Niedersächsisches Jahrbuch für Landesgeschichte* 54 (1982): 254–55.

30. Die Organisation des Gesundheitswesens in der britischen Zone (probably formulated in 1948), Nds 300 Acc 48/68 III 7, Niedersächsisches Hauptstaatsarchiv (hereafter NHSta).

31. Eröffnungsrede des Direktors der Abteilung öffentliche Gesundheitswesen in der Kontrollkommission vom 25.10.1945, Nds 300 Acc 48/65 III/15a, NHSta.

32. Report by Dr. E. L. Sturdee and Mr. T. Lindsay on Public Health Organization in the British Zone of Germany, based on a tour made by them between April 2 and April 17, 1948, 7, Nds 300 Acc 48/65 III Nr 7, NHSta.

33. Sturdee and Lindsay report, 6f.

34. A. Dorendorf, *Der Zonenbeirat der britisch besetzten Zone. Ein Rückblick auf seine Tätigkeit,* Monographien zur Politik, ed. Forschungsinstitut für Sozial- und Verwaltungswissenschaften der Universität Köln, Abteilung Sozialpolitik, Heft 2 (Göttingen: Schwartz Verlag, 1953), 24, 98.

35. Der Minister für Arbeit, Aufbau und Gesundheit Karl Abel an den Ministerpräsidenten 6.2.1947, Nds 300 Acc 48/65 Nr 7, NHSta.

36. Buurman at the "Konferenz der Zonal Advisers on Public Health and Deutsche Amtsärzte am 25. und 26. Februar 1948," Nds 300 Acc 48/65 III Nr 7, NHSta.

37. Sturdee and Lindsay report, 7.

38. Public Health Organization in the British Zone, 16, Nds 300 Acc 48/65 III, NHSta.

39. Brig. St. Martins Comments on the Report by Sturdee and Lindsay, August 17, 1948, Nds 300 Acc 48/65 III, Nr 7, NHSta.

40. H.-U. Sons, *Gesundheitspolitik während der Besatzungszeit. Das öffentliche Gesundheitswesen in Nordrhein-Westfalen 1945–1949* (Wuppertal: Peter Hammer Verlag, 1983), 53.

41. Sons, *Gesundheitspolitik,* 57–58.

42. Schneider, "Niedersachsen," 276–77.

43. Schneider, "Niedersachsen," 271.

44. Otto Buurman, personal file, Nds 300 Acc 21/80, Nr 5/1, NHSta.

45. Otto Buurman, personal file, Nds 300 Acc 21/80, Nr 5/1, NHSta; H. Kater, *Politiker und Ärzte. 600 Kurzbiographien und Porträts,* 3rd ed. (Hameln: C.W. Niemeyer Verlag, 1968), 69.

46. "In Krakow, the public health officer headed a health department that had a German, a Polish, and intially also a Jewish division; the latter had a Polish-Jewish director. The majority of the Polish medical apparatus continued to work in the cities and in the countryside under the direction and control of the Germans." Comment from Buurman, October 5, 1962, 206 AR 1211/60, 40–42, Zentralstelle Ludwigsburg; quoted in W. Dressen and V. Rieß, "Ausbeutung und Vernichtung. Gesundheitspolitik im Generalgouvernement," in *Medizin und Gesundheitspolitik in der NS-Zeit,* Sondernummer Schriftenreihe der Vierteljahreshefte für Zeitgeschichte, ed. N. Frei (Munich: R. Oldenbourg Verlag, 1991), 160.

47. U. Caumanns and M. G. Esch, "Fleckfieber und Fleckfieberbekämpfung im Warschauer Getto und die Tätigkeit der deutschen Gesundheitsverwaltung 1941/42," in *Geschichte der Gesundheitspolitik in Deutschland. Von der Weimarer Republik bis*

in die Frühgeschichte der „doppelten Staatsgründung," ed. W. Woelk and J. Vögele, 225–62 (Berlin: Duncker & Humblot Verlag, 2002).

48. Franz Ickert, personal file, Nds 300 Acc 21/80 Nr 19, NHSta.

49. Buurman 1.4.1948, Nds 300 Acc 21/80 Nr 10, NHSta.

50. Heinrich Ernst, personal file, A Rep. 001–06, Nr 4682, Landesarchiv Berlin.

51. Gesetz Nr 1, vom 20. September 1945, Amtsblatt des Kontrollrats in Deutschland 1, zweite, korrigierte Auflage, published in Berlin 29.10.1945, 6–8.

52. A. Labisch and F. Tennstedt, Der Weg zum "Gesetz über die Vereinheitlichung des Gesundheitswesens" vom 3. Juli 1934. Entwicklungslinien und -momente des staatlichen und kommunalen Gesundheitswesens, Schriftenreihe der Akademie für öffentliches Gesundheitswesen in Düsseldorf v 13,1 and 13,2 (Düsseldorf: Akademie des öffentlichen Gesunheitswesens, 1985), 313–32.

53. Rudolf Wilsch, "Die öffentliche Gesundheitspflege in Hannover," in 20 Jahre Gesundheitsamt Hannover, ed. Presseamt Hannover (Hannover: Buchdruckwerkstätten, 1955), 22.

54. W. Auerbach, "Gedanken zum Neuaufbau der Niedersächsischen Gesundheitsverwaltung," Mitteilungen des Niedersächsischen Landesgesundheitsrates, vol. 1 (Hannover: Stephansstift Buchdruckerei, 1948), 13.

55. L. Federhen, "Eugenik," in Der Arzt des öffentlichen Gesundheitsdienstes, ed. L. Federhen, 479–98 (Stuttgart: Georg Thieme Verlag, 1950).

56. Draft for Law on Conjugal Health, Beratungsausschuß des deutschen Gesundheitsdienstes vom 5. und 6. Februar 1946 in Bünde, Nds 300 Acc 48/65, III/15b, NHSta.

57. Auerbach, "Gedanken," 14.

58. O. Buurman, Gesundheitspolitik (Stuttgart: Georg Thieme Verlag, 1953), 6.

59. E. Schröder, "Gesundheitspflege als Aufgabe von Gesetzgebung und Verwaltung," Der öffentliche Gesundheitsdienst 12 (1950): 324.

60. Buurman, Gesundheitspolitik, 48.

61. S. Münchow, "Über die Gründung der Akademie für Staatsmedizin in Hamburg," Hamburger Ärzteblatt 21 (1967): 302–5.

62. S. Schleiermacher, "Experte und Lobbyist für Bevölkerungspolitik: Hans Harmsen in der Weimarer Republik, Nationalsozialismus und Bevölkerungspolitik," in Experten und Politik: Wissenschaftliche Politikberatung in geschichtlicher Perspektive, ed. S. Fisch and W. Rudloff, 211–38 (Berlin: Duncker & Humblot Verlag, 2004).

63. H. A. Welsh, "Deutsche Zentralverwaltung für das Gesundheitswesen (DZVG)," in SBZ-Handbuch. Staatliche Verwaltungen, Parteien, gesellschaftliche Organisationen und ihre Führungskräfte in der Sowjetischen Besatzungszone 1945–1949, 2nd ed., ed. M. Broszat and H. Weber (Munich: R. Oldenbourg Verlag, 1993), 244–52, 294–95; W. Zank, "Wirtschaftliche Zentralverwaltungen und Deutsche Wirtschaftskommission," in Broszat and Weber, SBZ-Handbuch, 253–90.

64. Statut der Zentralverwaltung für das Deutsche Gesundheitswesen in der Sowjetischen Okkupationszone. Übergeben durch Oberst Sokolow am 15 September 1945, DQ1 1615, Bl.1–2, Bundesarchiv Berlin/Lichterfelde (hereafter BArch).

65. For more biographical information about Konitzer, see U. Schagen, "Kongruenz der Gesundheitspolitik von Arbeiterparteien, Militäradministration und der Zentralverwaltung für das Gesundheitswesen in der Sowjetischen Besatzungszone," in Woelk and Vögele, Geschichte der Gesundheitspolitik in Deutschland, 379–404.

66. Archiv Biografien des Forschungsschwerpunkts Zeitgeschichte der Medizin, Institut für Geschichte der Medizin, Charité Berlin.

67. Archiv Biografien des Forschungsschwerpunkts Zeitgeschichte der Medizin, Institut für Geschichte der Medizin, Charité Berlin.

68. Mitteilung des Vizepräsidenten Zetkin vom 7. Juni 1946, DQ1 1326, 120, BArch.

69. Welsh, Deutsche Zentralverwaltung, 245, DQ1 243, Bl. 387–92; 244, Bl. 32; 542a, Bl. 134–53, BArch.

70. Archiv Biografien des Forschungsschwerpunktes Zeitgeschichte der Medizin, Institut für Geschichte der Medizin, Charité Berlin.

71. L. Büttner and B. Meyer, *Gesundheitspolitik der revolutionären deutschen Arbeiterbewegung. Vom Bund der Kommunisten bis zum Thälmannschen ZK der KPD*, vol. 25, *Medizin und Gesellschaft* (Berlin: VEB Verlag Volk und Gesundheit, 1984), 82–84; A. Labisch, "Alfred Grotjahn (1869–1931) und das gesundheitspolitische Programm der Mehrheitssozialdemokraten von 1922," *Medizin, Mensch, Gesellschaft* 8 (1983): 194; I. Winter, "Zur Geschichte der Gesundheitspolitik der KPD in der Weimarer Republik (Teil I)," *Zeitschrift für ärztliche Fortbildung* 67 (1973): 455.

72. A.-S. Ernst, *„Die beste Prophylaxe ist der Sozialismus" Ärzte und medizinische Hochschullehrer in der SBZ/DDR* (Münster; New York: Waxmann Verlag GmbH, 1997), 143–206; C. Vollnhals, ed., *Entnazifizierung. Politische Säuberung und Rehabilitierung in den vier Besatzungszonen 1945–1949* (Munich: Deutscher Taschenbuch Verlag, 1991), 43.

73. Gesetz der Landesverwaltung Thüringen über die Reinigung der öffentlichen Verwaltung von Nazi-Elementen vom 23. Juli 1945 in Vollnhals, *Entnazifizierung*, 180–86.

74. DQ 1–1336, BArch. The German Central Administration for Public Health (CGPH) guideline "On the Purging of Nazi Elements from the Independent Medical Professions in the SBZ of 13 November 1945" was designed to prohibit the professional practice of medicine by former members of the SD, the Gestapo, the SS, and individuals who joined the Nazi party prior to January 1933.

75. Gesetz über die Reinigung des Ärzteberufes und des Apothekerberufes von Nazi-Elementen vom 1. Oktober 1945, 242–43, DQ 1–1336, BArch.

76. Ernst, *Prophylaxe*, 177–78.

77. Entwurf zur Ärzteplanung, Aktennotiz vom 18, März 1946, DQ 1–93. Bl. 128, BArch; Tagung der Personalreferenten der Landesgesundheitsämter 21. Dezember 1946, DQ 1–182, Bl. 187, BArch; *Schreiben des Präsidenten des Landes Mecklenburg-Vorpommern an die DZVG 9 October 1945*, DQ 1–95, Bl. 261, BArch; Ernst, *Prophylaxe*, 174; H. Domeinski, "Zur Entnazifizierung der Ärzteschaft im Lande Thüringen," in *Medizin im Faschismus. Symposium über das Schicksal der Medizin in der Zeit des Faschismus in Deutschland 1933–1945*, ed. A. Thom and H. Spaar (Berlin: VEB Verlag Volk und Gesundheit, 1983), 322.

78. G. Moser, *"Im Interesse der Volksgesundheit . . ." Sozialhygiene und öffentliches Gesundheitswesen in der Weimarer Republik und der frühen SBZ/DDR. Ein Beitrag zur Sozialgeschichte des deutschen Gesundheitswesens im 20. Jahrhundert* (Basel: VAS Verlag, 1999), 166–67; Ernst, *Prophylaxe*, 185.

79. Ernst, *Prophylaxe*, 204, 205.

80. C. Meyer-Seitz, *Die Verfolgung von NS-Straftaten in der Sowjetischen Besatzungszone* (Berlin: Berlin Verlag Spitz, 1998), 54.

81. J. W. Bösche, "Die Reichsärztekammer im Lichte von Gesetzgebung und Rechtsprechung der Bundesrepublik Deutschland," *Deutsches Ärzteblatt* 94 (1997): A 1406–10.

82. "Befehl des Obersten Chefs der Sowjetischen Militärverwaltung—Oberkommandierenden der sowjetischen Besatzungstruppen in Deutschland—Nr 234 vom 9.10.1947. Über Maßnahmen zur Steigerung der Arbeitsproduktivität und zur weiteren Verbesserung der materiellen Lage der Arbeiter und Angestellten in der Industrie und im Verkehrswesen," *Das Deutsche Gesundheitswesen* 2 (1947): 684–88; G. Tietze, *Das Wesen des Gesundheits- und Arbeitsschutzes im Kapitalismus und Sozialismus. Die sozialistischen Prinzipien und die Organisation des Gesundheits- und Arbeitsschutzes in den Betrieben der Deutschen Demokratischen Republik* ([East] Berlin: Eigenverlag FDGB Freier Deutscher Gewerkschaftsbund, Bundesvorstand, 1961), 11.

83. D. Hoffmann, *Sozialpolitische Neuordnung in der SBZ/DDR. Der Umbau der Sozialversicherung* (Munich: R. Oldenbourg Verlag, 1996), 85–89.

84. This meant that the costs for all in- and outpatient services were covered without extra payment by those patients. It also meant that no differentiations were made among population groups, as there were in the Federal Republic between civil servants, white-collar workers, and blue-collar workers, or the working and nonworking (pensioners, unemployed). Finally, in the GDR, prevention became an integral part of health protection. Das Zentralsekretariat der Sozialistischen Einheitspartei Deutschlands, *Beschluss über gesundheitspolitische Richtlinien. Berlin, 31. März 1947. Dokumente der Sozialistischen Einheitspartei Deutschlands. Beschlüsse und Erklärungen des Zentralsekretariats und des Parteivorstandes*, Bd.1, 2nd ed. ([East] Berlin: Dietz Verlag, 1951), 171–75.

85. Ministerium für Arbeit und Gesundheitswesen der DDR, Hauptabteilung Gesundheitswesen, ed., *Das demokratische Gesundheitswesen in der Deutschen Demokratischen Republik* (Berlin: Arbeitsgemeinschaft medizinischer Verlage, 1950), 3.

86. K. Winter, *Lehrbuch der Sozialhygiene*, 2nd ed. (Berlin: VEB Verlag Volk und Gesundheit, 1980), 149.

87. D. Tutzke, *Alfred Grotjahn, Biographien hervorragender Naturwissenschaftler, Techniker und Mediziner*, vol. 36 (Leipzig: Teubner Verlag, 1979); K. Renker and K. Winter, "Sozialhygiene und Gesundheitsschutz im Sozialismus am Beispiel der DDR. Zur gesellschaftlichen Bedingtheit der Medizin in der Geschichte," in *Medizin und Gesellschaft. Beihefte zur Zeitschrift für ärztliche Fortbildung*, vol. 10, ed. D. Tutzke, 200–212 (Jena: Gustav Fischer Verlag, 1981).

88. A. Beyer and K. Winter, *Lehrbuch der Sozialhygiene* (Berlin: VEB Verlag Volk und Gesundheit, 1953), 10–11; E. Marcusson, *Sozialhygiene. Grundlagen und Organisation des Gesundheitsschutzes* (Leipzig: VEB Georg Thieme Verlag, 1954), 30–31.

89. I. Winter, "Begründer der Sowjet-Medizin. Zum 100. Geburtstag von N. A. Semaschko," *humanitas* Berlin (East) 14 (1974).

90. Beyer and Winter, *Sozialhygiene*, 62–89.

91. H. Lehmann, *Vorwort zu den gesundheitspolitischen Richtlinien der SED vom 31. 3. 1947* ([East] Berlin: Dietz Verlag, 1947), 1.

92. J.-U. Niehoff and T. Röding, "Steuerung und Regulierung von Prävention in der Deutschen Demokratischen Republik," in *Prävention und Prophylaxe: Theorie und Praxis eines gesundheitspolitischen Grundmotivs in zwei deutschen Staaten*, ed. T. Elkeles, J.-U. Niehoff, R. Rosenbrock, and F. Schneider (Berlin: Edition Sigma, 1991), 163.

93. Beyer and Winter, *Sozialhygiene*, 66.

94. Tietze, *Wesen*, 10.

95. K. Winter, "Die Gestaltung der Fürsorge für Mutter und Kind im neuen demokratischen Gesundheitswesen," *Das deutsches Gesundheitswesen* 4 (1949): 526.

96. For the tradition of "medical police" in Germany in the late eighteenth century, see George Rosen, *A History of Public Health* (New York: MD Publications, 1958), 335–36.

Chapter Eight

British Public Health and the Problem of Local Demographic Structure

GRAHAM MOONEY

"Demography," as a recent critique of the discipline has observed, "offers its wares to a range of agencies."[1] The purpose of this chapter is to focus on demography as a realm of expert knowledge that has applications in the practice of one of these agencies, public health. By demography, we mean the study and analysis of population structure (age, sex, ethnicity, spatial distribution, and so on) and the dynamic components of fertility, marriage and divorce, migration, and mortality. We might assume that public health would be more concerned with the last of these components—mortality—than perhaps with the others, though practitioners working in reproductive and sexual health, and those addressing questions of (for example) refugee health justifiably might beg to differ. This chapter considers not only how, over the twentieth century, knowledge concerning three basic aspects of population—the total number of people, the age structure, and the male/female composition—was used in the evaluation of public health policy at the local level, but also how it shaped the measurement, calculation, and deployment of mortality rates in the practice of public health. The interplay between national policy and local implementation is an enduring theme in the history of public health. By moving between these ends of the spectrum, it is possible to comprehend the variable political meaning of, and sensitivity to, mortality rates as instruments of public health intelligence.[2]

At its most basic, this is a story about the shifting and uncertain role of demographic standardization in the localities. Throughout the twentieth century, central government statisticians provided local public health authorities with methods of demographic standardization to eliminate the distorting effects of a skewed population structure on the level of mortality. These methods changed over the course of the twentieth century, but the imperative that differences in the structure of local populations had to be methodologically controlled did not. As we shall see, by the beginning of the twenty-first century, life expectancy had replaced crude and standardized death rates as the most commonly used summary measure of local mortality. In turn, the structural, aggregate-level difficulties that "age" and "sex" presented to demographers have been partially recast as nonmodifiable, individual-level risk factors. These factors are one feature of a theoretical model of health inequalities that tends to be silent on the implications of local population structures and dynamic demographic change. At the same time, public health activities at the local level are replete with programs that are directed at particular age groups and the sexes.

Much of the spotlight in this chapter will be trained on Liverpool, with the public health reports of the city from years clustering around 1901, 1951, and 2003 (the most recent available at the time of writing) forming the evidential basis of the chapter. It is important to acknowledge here that the uses of demography in public health are shaped by complex interactions between public health and the state that may or may not be immediately evident from a small selection of local administrative documents such as medical officer of health (MOH) annual reports.[3] The selection of Liverpool is partly one of convenience, determined by my personal experience of the public health sector in that city. The city's self-conscious position in the vanguard of public health policy and practice from the mid-nineteenth century to the present also makes it an interesting case study.[4]

Crude Death Rates

At the dawn of the twentieth century, the use of population figures and trends was a key feature of public health discourse. Rare indeed was the occasion when a British local public health annual report did not open with the basic facts of birth and death and population total estimates. There is now a substantial historical narrative about how this came to be the case.[5] The creation of a national, centralized, state-funded department of registration in 1836 has long been identified as a crucial landmark. The General Register Office (GRO) became responsible for administering both the system of vital registration and the decennial census enumerations.[6] The annual reports of the GRO, which contained copious tables of demographic information and interpretation, emerged as an important tool in the campaign for improved public health.[7] In the hands of Dr. William Farr, compiler of abstracts at the GRO, mortality data were manipulated and arranged to act as a "biometer" of the shocking conditions of urban life.[8]

Reference to the question of mortality measurement in the twentieth century cannot ignore developments in the previous century. Various groups of experts—epidemiologists, statisticians, and public health professionals—carried on an intense debate about the validity of demographic methodologies that were endowed with policy implications. A key feature of the arguments about mortality rates—and one that would be instantly recognizable to today's practitioners, who are familiar with mortality target setting—was the use of the crude death rate (CDR, the number of deaths per thousand total population) as a benchmark of healthiness or insalubrity. Clearly, such yardsticks take on a localized meaning only in the presence of a national rate, or a collection of other local rates, to serve as comparisons. Mortality therefore became embedded in a discourse over what was deemed to be "average." During the early nineteenth century this embedding was a key feature in the movement for social statistics more generally, which studied large numbers to establish regularities and, in turn, pinpoint irregularities that could be the focus of reform in education, crime, employment, poor relief, and other areas of social life.[9]

The "formation of sanitary statistics," however, is seen "as the major event of the statistical movement," and the CDR was the centerpiece of the sanitarian's statistical arsenal.[10] As early as 1848, a CDR of above 23 per 1,000 in a locality was sufficient to trigger the creation of a local Board of Health. Farr eventually used a CDR of 17 per 1,000 as the dividing line between healthy and unhealthy districts. During the early twentieth century, local MOHs came to be educated to monitor their own locality's death rate with obsessive zeal: the CDR was the key demographic statistic by which their efforts were judged. Moreover, the competent use of demographic and epidemiologic methods was a way in which the newly professionalized body of medical officers identified themselves as members of the scientific community at the end of the nineteenth century. MOHs duly were advised that although the statistical calculations required for their periodical reports to the local sanitary authority were "simple enough," errors were nevertheless commonplace and it remained "easy . . . to misinterpret the results."[11] Indeed, the cognoscenti preferred the term "crude" death rate as an indication of the measure's rough-and-readiness; alternative terms such as the "general" death rate or the "national" death rate were frowned on, as they were seen to confer a degree of authority on the statistic that was undeserved.[12]

Disagreements about the validity of the CDR did not in fact center on the credibility of death registration itself, which by the mid-1870s was considered reliable and more or less comprehensive. Concerns were more commonly expressed over the distorting effect of hospital and workhouse deaths, which inflated the CDRs of institutionally replete urban communities.[13] The boundary definitions of registration districts also became an issue, because they frequently did not correspond to the administrative boundaries of urban and rural sanitary districts for which local MOHs were responsible.[14] By and large, these difficulties were overcome in the years immediately before World War I by ensuring that deaths in institutions were reallocated to the deceased's place of residence and by allocating deaths in registration districts to other administrative constituencies.[15] More troubling, defects in the estimation of the total population of a locality, and the failure to account for local differences in population composition as broken down into males, females, and age groups, were seen as corrupting the validity of the CDR as a measure of public health progress.

The notion of progress hints at the political sensitivity of death rates. This sensitivity went much deeper than Farr's propagandizing from the GRO. As Philip Kreager has recently noted, it relates to the inseparability of "representation" on the one hand (in this case, the calculated rate of mortality) and "intervention" on the other (that is, public health policy).[16] First, by the beginning of the twentieth century, national legislation required that each MOH send a copy of their annual report to the central government authority for public health, at that time the Local Government Board (LGB). It was not lost on MOHs that the LGB often used these reports as sticks with which to beat local health authorities into sanitary submission. The board achieved this goal largely by a system of medical inspection and surveillance, a form of central government interference that local authorities tended to view with hostility. Although the LGB might commend an MOH's "vigilance" in pointing out defects in the sanitary condition of his district, one commentator warned that it "will probably be condemned" by the MOH's employer, the sanitary authority, "as officiousness and audacity."[17] Although MOHs were unable to avoid including mortality rates in their annual reports, if they valued their jobs it might be unwise for them to comment too forcefully on how these rates might be reduced. The most judicious course of action was to refer "very cautiously . . . to large measures of reform, if they require considerable outlay, or are strongly disapproved of by his [the MOH's] S.A. [sanitary authority]."[18] The precarious nature of the MOH's position with regard to annual reporting relaxed somewhat once the LGB was succeeded by the Ministry of Health in 1919. According to John Welshman, the ministry "interpreted its powers narrowly, and was reluctant to advise MOHs on matters of 'professional opinion.'"[19] Meanwhile, MOHs could always find refuge for ideas that might be controversial locally in professional journals such as *Public Health*, the *Medical Officer*, and the *Journal of State Medicine*.[20]

The second reason that mortality rates were politically sensitive at the local level was because MOHs routinely presented a report to their council's health committee meetings, which in most large towns and cities were held at weekly or biweekly intervals and on a quarterly basis in small towns and rural districts. These reports were rarely printed and commonly were not forwarded to central government. Besides recounting his own activities and those of his staff in their role as environmental police, the MOH would also include weekly totals of deaths by cause, crude death rates, and the incidence of infectious diseases. Weekly reports were the immediate means by which the sanitary authority gauged threats to the health of its local population. In conjunction with information and opinion from a variety of other sources and agencies, it was on these weekly reports, rather than their annual counterparts, that local administrations based the vast majority of their everyday decisions. Furthermore, this information tended to find its way into full town council debates that were recounted verbatim in local newspapers and subjected to intense media scrutiny. The weekly mortality rate was a visceral indication that organized public health was a responsive discipline as much as a preventive one.

Under these circumstances, it is hardly surprising that local MOHs set great store by the accuracy of their demographic measures. Indeed, one of their guidebooks described the procedure for estimating the "weekly population" in order to calculate a CDR using the weekly total of deaths. This method involved dividing the total population by 52.17747, which was the precise number of weeks in the year (as opposed to just 52 weeks).[21] The figure of 52.17747 weeks was based on dividing by 7 the number of days in a year—365.25 (taking into account leap years). If a monthly or quarterly CDR was required, then the MOH was expected to calculate a *daily* population total (using 365.25 as the number of days in a year) and multiply that figure by the number of days in that month or quarter. In the context of this discussion, the methods used matter less than the level of precision that was deemed necessary to attain. Weekly representations of mortality were driven by the political process. MOHs were tailoring demographic calculations to maximize their political impact and underscore their relevance to intervention. The use of such a method, though expedient, overlooked the fact that comparisons of CDRs either between places or over time were influenced by differences in the structure of the populations in question. It also assumed that the original estimate of population was accurate. It is to these issues that we now turn.

The Population Composition Problem

Edward Hope, the MOH for Liverpool, noted in 1901:

> The total population is the foundation upon which all figures relating to births, deaths, and the incidence of disease are based, and if this foundation is inaccurate, all deductions from the figures are worse than useless; but if it is fairly accurate it furnishes undoubtedly the simplest and most popular way in which the results of sanitary measures can be gauged.[22]

One fundamental problem in the calculation of death rates was how the local population was estimated in the absence of an annual census. In estimating a district population of any year other than a census year (which, in England and Wales, was always the first year of a new decade, such as 1901, 1911, and so on), the GRO applied the logarithm of the rate of population growth between the two previous censuses to the most recent census population total. Given that most towns and cities urbanized in fits and starts during the later nineteenth century, such a method was clearly inappropriate. For example, Liverpool's population increased at an average annual rate of 1.81 percent during the 1870s, which slowed in the subsequent decade to 0.63 percent.[23] During the twentieth century, the collapse of Britain's northern industrial economies was reflected in plummeting population figures: between 1951 and 1971, Liverpool's population declined from 784,800 to 610,114. Under these dramatically changing social conditions, arriving at an accurate intercensal population figure was a hazardous undertaking. For the calculation of the mortality rate, the implications of providing a flawed population total are obvious: overestimation of the population at risk leads to an underestimate of the CDR (all other things, such as the quality of death registration, being equal) and vice versa. For a politically sensitive indicator such as the death rate, this imprecision was unacceptable to public health professionals. Historically, the GRO had been known to correct population estimates if a town could provide sufficient corroborating evidence (for example, a local census or the construction of many new houses), although Noel Humphreys, a high-ranking statistician at the GRO in possession of a nice line in irony, had been quick to point out the "curious fact" that it had never received a complaint that a population estimate was too *high*—which, of course, would lower the mortality rate.[24]

In addition to this total population problem, the CDR fails to take into account a district's age and sex composition. This creates a difficulty because death rates differ among age groups and between the sexes. Furthermore, such death rates vary between places and over time depending on the prevailing characteristics of the epidemiological regime. Communities with high proportions of young and old people were more likely to have a steeper CDR if death rates were high in these age groups compared with those among teenagers and young adults. For example, in London in 1901–10, the mortality rate for one- to four-year-olds was 20.4 per 1,000; for five- to fourteen-year-olds it was 2.9 per 1,000; in the thirty-five to forty-four age group it was 9.6; and for fifty-five- to sixty-four-year-olds the rate was 30.4. However, comparisons between the sexes also produce some startling anomalies. In the same decade, the death rate for London men between the ages of twenty and sixty was more than 30 percent than for women.[25] Thus, the argument went, towns and cities might register artificially high rates of mortality simply because they were home to excessive numbers of adult males, children, and senior citizens. These differential age- and sex-specific death rates were driven by the fact that some causes of death strike particular age groups more severely. Many infectious diseases—such as whooping cough and measles—kill disproportionate numbers of young children. Pulmonary tuberculosis is primarily a condition of young adults, whereas older people more commonly succumb to chronic ailments such as heart disease. But such impacts are not fixed in time, since epidemiological landscapes shift, sometimes quite rapidly. For example, 33 percent of all deaths in Liverpool in 1921 occurred in children under five years of age. By 1951, the corresponding figure had fallen sharply to 7 percent, as the combined number of respiratory, digestive, and infectious-disease (including measles, whooping cough, diphtheria, and scarlet fever) deaths in this age group fell from 1,184 to a paltry 38.[26]

There were two possible ways to circumvent the problem of variations in local population structure, both of which are familiar to students of demography and public health today. One solution was to calculate life tables, which produce an estimate of the average length of remaining life at any given age, from zero years up.[27] A life table transforms age-specific mortality rates into the probability of dying, but the amount of data manipulation involved and the detailed statistical knowledge required to create one was laborious, not to mention beyond the technical capacity and material resources of most local public health officials.[28] The author of a popular handbook for MOHs in 1901 expressed knowledge of just four local life tables produced by MOHs in Brighton, Manchester, Oldham, and Glasgow.[29] Indeed, only six national life tables were calculated for England and Wales before the start of the twentieth century, and no more than fifteen have been produced to date.[30] These tables are associated with the decennial census enumerations; interim life tables are calculated in between.[31] It was not until the 1990s that estimates of life expectancy were computed on a consistent basis for local authorities in Great Britain.

An alternative, more practical, course was to standardize the mortality rate. As we have already noted, albeit briefly, notions about healthy and unhealthy places centered on what came to be considered the "average" rate of mortality. The demography of public health in the early twentieth century not only deployed notions of "average" for mortality; it also utilized the concept of "normal" for the populations that were used as the denominator in the mortality equation.[32] Thus, in Edward Willoughby's 1893 *Handbook of Public Health and Demography*, a "normal" population was a "growing" population.[33] (Interestingly enough, no mention of demography had been made in the title of earlier editions, which appeared as *Hygiene: Its Principles as Applied to Public Health*.) The population structure from which standard mortality rates should be calculated was "the *normal* constitution of the population according to age and sex in the country at large."[34] With this in mind, standardization was retrospectively carried out by the GRO in its *Annual Report* for 1901, when it presented age- and sex-"corrected" annual mortality rates for England and Wales from 1838 to 1901. The GRO adopted what is known as the direct method of standardization, whereby the age- and sex-specific death rates of the populations being compared are applied to the numbers in the corresponding age and sex group of the standard population. This calculation provides the number of deaths that would occur (the "expected" deaths) in the standard population, given the death rates in the study populations. The numbers of expected deaths in all the age groups are then added together and divided by the total standard population to produce an age-standardized death rate for the study population. In theory, any population can be used as the standard. In this case, national mortality rates for each year between 1838 and 1900 were applied to the population structure of England and Wales in 1901, thereby controlling for changes in the national population structure over time. The method can also be adopted cross-sectionally to compare different places at the same moment in time. In 1911, at the recommendation of the Society of Medical Officers of Health, the GRO provided standardized mortality rates for county boroughs, urban districts, and rural districts, thus providing local calculations to supplement the national picture.[35]

It is doubtful whether these methodological refinements had any affect on public health practice in subsequent years. This may well reflect an inherent tension between the two types of experts: whereas demographers overcame variations between places to render them comparable, public health practitioners were required to identify and remedy such variations. Despite the problems outlined above, throughout the twentieth century, local public health agencies seemingly continued to accept the annual intercensal estimate of total population that was provided by the registrar-general, and this number was routinely deployed in the calculation of annual mortality rates. Moreover, the *Annual Report* on the health of Liverpool for 1951 finds the MOH, William Frazer, using the term "general" death rate, a worrying slip that doubtless would have enraged those of his predecessors who sought to ensure that the CDR indicated precisely that: crudeness.[36] A more disturbing feature of the report would appear to be Frazer's dependence on the CDR and his unwillingness to use or discuss death rates that were corrected for the age and sex composition of the population.[37] By the early 1940s, however, the GRO itself questioned the method of calculating standardized mortality rates that it had employed since 1901; in part this may explain Frazer's reluctance to use the corrected rates provided by the GRO. (Another potential reason will be mentioned below.)

The source of the GRO's anxiety about the calculation of standardized mortality rates was the selection of an appropriate standard population. This concern may have been prompted by the arrival of Dr. Percy Stocks at the

GRO, which, in the words of Eddy Higgs, heralded an "increasing statistical sophistication."[38] As noted above, the England and Wales population in 1901 was used as the standard in a retrospective analysis stretching back to 1838. This standard continued to be used until World War II, but around this time the GRO began to worry that the choice of the 1901 standard no longer possessed "some regard to the population conditions in which the mortalities are actually experienced." The statistical review of 1941 suggested that "the population of 1901 has for some time ceased to be a satisfactory standard in this respect owing to the great change in proportionate age distribution since that date."[39] Long- and short-range examples were offered to substantiate the claim that use of the 1901 standard distorted the impression of mortality change over time. The first, long-range, comparison used two different standard populations. With the 1901 population standard, national death rates (all causes) per 1,000 population were 16.9 in 1901 and 8.5 in 1939, suggesting a relative mortality decline of 50 percent. Use of the 1939 population as the standard, however, produced rates of 19.6 and 12.1, respectively, resulting in a decline of only 38 percent. It was argued that "in such circumstance it is reasonable to assume that the use of either the 1901 or the 1939 populations alone tends to bias the comparison in opposite directions and that a preferable representation of the decline would be one somewhere between 50 and 38 percent."[40] The second, short-range, comparison considered male mortality in 1938 and 1939. The 1901 standardized rate for 1939 was 0.6 percent lower than that of 1938. Substituting the 1901 standard population with that of the mean population for 1938 and 1939 produced a contradictory result: an increase in male mortality of 1.6 percent between the two years (the actual rates were not provided in the commentary). "In this case," argued the registrar-general, "neither of the experiences has any direct relation with the conditions of 1901 and the second measure will clearly be preferred as the more realistic index of the change."[41]

The upshot of the GRO's discomfort was the discontinuation of the 1901-based standardized mortality rate for localities. In its place at the national level came the comparative mortality index (CMI), a single number by which a national death rate (either crude or cause specific) was multiplied to make it comparable to previous years. At the first time of calculation, the index was the ratio of deaths for the year in question (1941) to deaths in 1938, reached by applying the age- and sex-specific death rates of 1941 and 1938, respectively to a "common" population. The proportion in each age and sex group in this common population was in fact the mean of the age and sex groups of the two years in question.[42] Being the year immediately preceding the outbreak of war, 1938 was an obvious choice for the new "base," but it was also the year of lowest mortality ever recorded, "and will thus be stringent rather than otherwise in its influence on the measurement of any subsequent mortality improvement."[43] For reasons that were not elaborated on, the use of the CMI was discontinued by the medical statisticians in 1958, at which point the standardized mortality ratio replaced it.[44] This ratio expresses the number of deaths registered in the year of experience as a percentage of those that would have been expected in that year had the age- and sex- specific mortalities of a standard period operated on the age and sex composition of the population of the year of experience. The standard population chosen towards the end of the 1950s was the national average of the three-year period 1950–52.

Of course, the method used to measure mortality has repercussions for policy debate at the national level, but as we have seen, arguably the political implications of demographic methods are more keenly felt at the local scale. As a consequence, the GRO sought an alternative way to control for local variations in the age and sex structure that could be applied to subnational areas. Thus, the area comparability factor (ACF), an indirect method of standardization, was introduced in 1934 to correct local CDRs.[45] Here, death rates for the sexes were calculated in the "smallest number . . . of age groups consistent with reasonable accuracy in the resulting factor."[46] The age groups used were under 5, 5 to 34, 35 to 54, 55 to 64, 65 to 74, 75 to 84, and over 85. Already the small number of deaths in late childhood and early adulthood meant that ages five to thirty-four had to be combined. Each of these age- and sex-specific death rates was then divided by the sum of the death rate for all ages, yielding a series of weighting factors for each group. The number in the local population of each age and sex group was multiplied by the relevant weighting factor and the products summed. The ACF was arrived at by dividing the total population of the local area by this result. Use of the ACF was suspended between 1940 and 1947 due to disruption in the age and sex profiles of localities caused by enlistment into and discharge from the armed forces and migration within the country during wartime.[47] With minor methodological refinements, the ACF continued to be tabulated for health areas and local authorities after the reorganization of the National Health Service in 1974.[48] However, it should be noted that coincident with the introduction of computerization at the GRO, standardized mortality ratios by cause and area—that is, regions, conurbations, urban and rural aggregates, and hospital regions—were produced from 1963.

The very use of the terms *comparative mortality index* and *area comparability factor* (as opposed to, say, "correction factor," "standardization factor," or "adjustment factor") is fascinating in itself, seemingly an indication of the continuing desire to make reliable comparisons among localities. Eddy Higgs has argued that during the interwar years,

> [t]he work undertaken by the GRO in this period also showed a growing emphasis on national trends as opposed to local conditions. . . . [T]he central spatial variables used to investigate mortality in this period were not specific place or

locality but settlement type (county borough, small town, rural, etc) and, above all, region. . . . Environment was now seen in terms of general causal factors operating across whole regions, rather than the local space over which political action needed to be mobilised.[49]

This loss of the "local" was in large part due to the reining in of the GRO's independence following its administrative subordination to the Ministry of Health in 1919. In short, the GRO was to provide the Ministry of Health (and other ministries for that matter) with statistical services. Analysis and interpretation of the GRO's data was to be carried out separately, in this case by medical statisticians in the Ministry of Health. Policy implications of the statistical evidence also were to be handled by the ministry without interference from the GRO.[50] It is perhaps for these reasons that annual trends in local mortality based on the ACF went without remark, and observations on the detailed geography of mortality were relegated to the *Decennial Supplement*.[51]

Until the production of local life expectancies in the mid-1990s, the GRO developed three different methods to render local mortality rates reliably comparable from a demographic perspective: the standardized mortality rate, the area comparability factor, and the standardized mortality ratio. In attempting to fulfill a basic requirement that had been identified by public health professionals and epidemiologists in the nineteenth century, demographic standardization and indexing methods facilitated the correction of local mortality rates. Regardless of their relative merits, these demographic indicators represent the central statistical authority's ongoing search for the most efficient and effective way to negate the uniqueness of local population structures. Each indicator gives the appearance of a nongeography of population. Since the CDR was inherently unreliable, this served public health purposes in the sense that neither the "progress" nor the "regression" of a place could be claimed on the basis of flawed evidence, a particularly important consideration given the long-standing tradition of mortality tables that ranked districts according to their CDR.

However, reductionist measures of demographic standardization conceal as much as they reveal. Paradoxically, the concealed population structures are of central concern to public health practitioners. Taking Liverpool in 1951 as an example, the table in which the ACF (labeled the "comparability factor") appeared is shown in figure 8.1. Reading along the row for the CDR per 1,000 population, Liverpool's CDR registered at 13.60, coming third in the urban sample behind Bradford (15.37) and Manchester (13.82). We can see from the vertical axis of the accompanying chart (figure 8.2) that the transformation of these death rates by use of the ACF results in a noticeable shift in the rank order, whereby Liverpool's adjusted death rate swaps places with Bradford's to become the worst in the urban sample by quite a margin. This demotion of Liverpool may provide a supplemental reason that

TABLE SHOWING POPULATION, BIRTH RATES, DEATH RATES,
RATES OF 12 LARGE TOWNS IN ZYMOTIC DEATH RATES, INFANT
AND MATERIAL MORTALITY ENGLAND AND WALES FOR 1951.

	Birmingham	Bradford	Bristol	Cardiff	Kingston-upon-Hill
Registrar Generals' estimated population for 1951:—					
(a) civil	—	—	—	—	—
(b) total	1,110,900	289,800	442,700	243,500	298,100
Comparability factor—					
(a) births	0·96	1·01	0·99	0·97	1·00
(b) deaths	1·12	0·97	0·97	1·06	1·14
Crude birth rate per 1,000 population ...	16·52	16·46	15·52	17·77	19·00
Birth rate as adjusted by factor	15·86	16·62	15·37	17·24	19·00
Crude death rate per 1,000 population ...	11·43	15·37	12·70	13·06	12·03
Death rate as adjusted by factor ...	12·80	14·91	12·32	13·85	13·71
Infantile mortality rate per 1,000 live births	29·69	43·6	20·37	32	46
Neonatal mortality rate per 1,000 live births	19·2	22·2	13·39	18·95	24
Stillbirth rate per 1,000 total births ...	22·2	23·9	22·06	28·51	23·1
Maternal mortality rate per 1,000 total births from—					
(a) Sepsis	0·26	0.41	0·14	—	—
(b) Other Causes	0·48	0.82	0·85	1·57	1·38
Total	0·74	1.23	0·99	1·57	1·38
Tuberculosis rates per 100,000 total population—					
(a) Primary notifications—					
Respiratory	106·5	79	135·1	145	107·0
Non-Respiratory	12·8	20	15·8	23	14·4
(b) Deaths—					
Respiratory	34·4	29·67	33·9	43·1	31·2
Non-Respiratory	3·2	6·55	3·2	4·9	2·3
Death Rates per 1,000 Population from—					
Cancer (all forms)	1·78	2·27	1·997	2·.5	1·90
Typhoid & Para;typhoid Fever ...	—	0·00	0·002	—	—
Meningococcal Infections	0·00	0·00	—	0·004	0·01
Scarlet Fever	0·00	0·00	0·002	—	—
Whooping Cough	0·01	0·10	0·005	0·02	0·03
Diphtheria	0·00	0·003	—	—	—
Influenza	0·26	0·32	0·416	0·28	0·18
Measles	0·01	0·017		0·008	0·00
Acute Poliomyelitis and Encephalitis	0·00	0·007	0·009	—	—
Acute Infectious Encephalitis ...	0·00	0·014	—	—	0·00
Smallpox	0·00	0·00	—	—	—
Diarrhoea (under 2 years) ...	0·03	0·055	0·009	0·01	0·07

† 1 death

Figure 8.1. Demographic indicators, Liverpool, 1951. From W. Frazer, *Report on the Health of the City of Liverpool for the Year 1951* (Liverpool: n.d.), facing p. 2. Courtesy of Liverpool Record Office, Liverpool Libraries.

Leeds	Leicester	Liverpool	Manchester	Newcastle-upon-Tyne	Notingham	Sheffield
—	—	—	—	—	—	—
503,030	284,700	784,800	699,900	291,700	306,600	510,000
0·96	0·98	0·96	0·95	0·97	0·96	0·99
1·07	1·01	1·19	1·11	1·09	1·19	1·07
16·0	16·2	19·9	17·77	16·46	19·9	14·18
15·4	15·9	18·1	16·88	15·97	18·1	14·01
13·5	12·4	13·6	13·82	13·38	13·6	13·01
14·5	12·5	16·2	15·34	14·58	16·2	13·92
31	25·2	35·1	35·29	34·56	32·6	30·55
17·5	15·625	20·3	20·18	20·82	20·5	19·08
23·5	22·28	24·8	25·01	24·57	22·7	2·23
0·12	0·000	0·125	0·39	—	0·19	0·135
0·49	0·848	0·500	1·10	0·203	0·37	0·270
0·61	0·848	0·625	1·49	0·203	0·56	0·405
94·6	121	195	101	160·3	160	134·5
20·7	13	20	15	24·34	4·9	14·7
33·0	35	52	45	37·71	27·7	29·4
3·18	2·5	5	6	4·80	3·6	4·9
1·96	2·00	1·98	1·98	2·005	1·9	2·009
—	0·00	—	—	0·000	—	—
0·01	0·007	0·01	0·01	0·010	0·01	0·002
—	0·00	0·00	—	0·000	—	—
0·008	0·007	0·02	0·02	0·020	0·02	0·006
—	0·0035	—	—	0·007	—	—
0·29	0·41	0·66	0·66	0·329	0·32	0·237
0·006	0·007	0·00	0·00	0·003	0·00	0·008
—	0·0035	0·01	0·01	0·007	†0·00	0·008
—	0·00	0·00	0·00	0·007	—	0·002
—	0·00	—	—	0·000	—	—
0·14	0·018	0·04	0·04	0·017	0·01	0·018

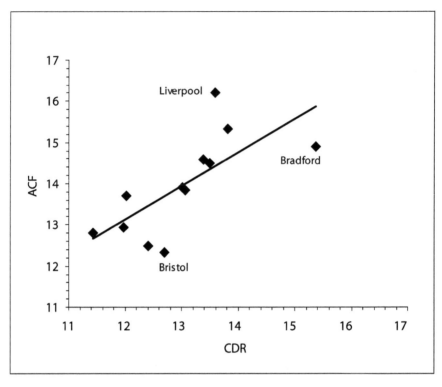

Figure 8.2. Mortality in twelve English and Welsh large towns: crude death rate (CDR) and CDR adjusted with area comparability factor (ACF), 1951. From W. Frazer, *Report on the Health of the City of Liverpool for the Year 1951* (Liverpool: n.d.), facing p. 2. Courtesy of Liverpool Record Office, Liverpool Libraries.

MOH William Frazer was so reluctant to use the comparability factor. But what explains this shuffling of the urban order? The probable answer is that Liverpool had a much younger population than Bradford. In 1951, 26 percent of Liverpool's population was under fifteen years of age, and 9 percent was over sixty-five. The figures for Bradford were 21 and 12 percent, respectively. When the effect of a youthful population was ironed out, Liverpool's mortality rate rose. The key point here is that although in 1951 a youthful urban population tended toward lower overall mortality, this may not necessarily have been the case thirty years previously, when, as discussed earlier, Liverpool's childhood mortality rates were much higher.

Although mortality standardization was desirable for comparative purposes, it simultaneously downplayed the impact of demographic developments that were otherwise crucial to the practice of public health, such as population aging and outmigration. A limitation of abstract demographic

The Main Determinants of Health

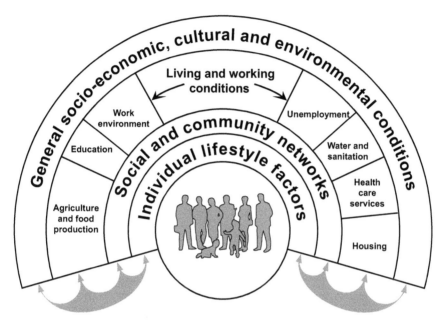

Figure 8.3. Model of factors influencing health. From G. Dahlgren and M. White-head, *Policies and Strategies to Promote Social Equity in Health* (Stockholm: Institute for Futures Studies, 1991). Courtesy of the Institute for Futures Studies, 11.

methodologies that are "given to mathematical tractability" is that their neutrality "renders them invalid as detailed guides to practical action with respect to any particular social context or local environment."[52] It may not, then, be exaggerating Frazer's position in the mid-twentieth century to say that in this case at least, public health practitioners were not buying the "wares" demographers had to offer.

Health Inequality and the Problem of Population Structure

In recent years, public health has witnessed two important developments that have impinged heavily on practice at the local level. The first is the reassertion of the health inequalities agenda that came about with the election of a Labour government in May 1997.[53] The second is the lifestyle agenda that has been set, in part, by the predominance of risk factor epidemiology. The pairing of these developments, I will argue, has complicated the nongeography of population structure that emerged earlier in the twentieth century.

These twin agendas are well reflected by the multilayered model of factors influencing health elaborated by Gören Dahlgren and Margaret Whitehead in the early 1990s (figure 8.3).[54] This model has been widely adopted and formed the conceptual basis of the UK Independent Inquiry into Inequalities in Health chaired by Sir Donald Acheson (the Acheson Report).[55] This inquiry was commissioned in July 1997 by the newly elected Labour government as part of a stated mission to tackle health inequalities.[56] The inquiry was conducted by a team drawn from sociology, epidemiology, and public health, including Margaret Whitehead. Although the inquiry put the issue of health inequalities on the political agenda in a way the previous Conservative government had declined to do, reception of the Acheson Report was somewhat mixed, with criticism concentrating primarily, though not solely, on the diffuse focus of the report's recommendations.[57] Evaluations of its long-term impact are ongoing.[58] The Acheson Report summarized the Dahlgren-Whitehead model as follows:

> We have adopted a socioeconomic model of health and its inequalities. This is in line with the weight of scientific evidence. Figure 1 [reproduced here in figure 8.3] shows the main determinants of health as layers of influence, one over another. At the centre are individuals, endowed with age, sex and constitutional factors which undoubtedly influence their health potential, but which are fixed. Surrounding the individuals are layers of influence that, in theory, could be modified. The innermost layer represents the personal behaviour and way of life adopted by individuals, containing factors such as smoking habits and physical activity, with the potential to promote or damage health. But individuals do not exist in a vacuum: they interact with friends, relatives and their immediate community, and come under the social and community influences represented in the next layer. Mutual support within a community can sustain the health of its members in otherwise unfavourable conditions. The wider influences on a person's ability to maintain health (shown in the third layer) include their living and working conditions, food supplies and access to essential goods and services. Overall there are the economic, cultural and environmental conditions prevalent in society as a whole, represented in the outermost layer.[59]

Thus age and sex are categorized alongside genetics as innate individual-level characteristics that exist in a health model as nonmodifiable risk factors, visually underscored by the depiction of a group of silhouetted individuals at the center of the diagram. When recommending future policy developments in relation to social and health services and public health interventions, the Acheson Report used age- and sex-based categorizations of population characteristics, such as "mothers," "children," "young people," "adults of working age," and "older people." ("Ethnicity" and "gender" were also used).

Significantly, a version of the Dahlgren-Whitehead model is reproduced in the 2003 report of the Central Liverpool Primary Care Trust (CLPCT). In miniature form, the figure of the model is the signature logo of the document. An excerpt from the introduction to this report outlines the pairing of the inequalities and the lifestyles agendas rather well:

> Health inequalities are primarily the product of differences in living conditions. Different social groups may face different barriers to accessing facilities such as sports centres and hospitals. These may be located in places that are hard to reach without a car, or may not be open at suitable hours for those who are employed or have caring responsibilities. Levels of well-being and life expectancy are closely associated with the availability of local services such as transport and health services.
>
> Changing unhealthy lifestyles is key to improving quality of life and preventing disease development. The key risk factors for developing a number of diseases, such as heart disease, stroke and lung cancer, are lifestyle factors, for example smoking, alcohol, and substance misuse, diet and exercise. Yet we know that changing behaviour is difficult, particularly if individuals, families and communities are living in deprived areas.[60]

Both structural inequalities—the provision of health services and transport, and living and working conditions—and the individual behaviors that lead to health inequalities reside in localities. It is among the second, third, and fourth layers of the model that local health agencies such as the CLPCT operate most naturally, modifying personal behaviors, influencing the health-related aspects of local communities, and intervening to improve work and living conditions. In following the Dahlgren-Whitehead model, the CLPCT sees age and sex as "fixed factors" that "determine their [individual's] health to a certain extent" but over which health agencies have little control.[61] As a result, a chapter on "age, sex and heredity factors" places age and sex alongside unmodifiable—for the present at least—genetic risk factors. However, when the age and sex profiles of the individuals that form the core of the model are aggregated, the inevitable result—local population composition—mysteriously dissipates, perhaps to the outer layer of the model, though this is not made explicit. One must assume that local demographic structures become part of "the economic, cultural and environmental conditions prevalent in society as a whole."[62] Otherwise, how else can the model explain that young, single men and women in central Liverpool are a section of the population that requires particular forms of health provision "to maximise health gains and reduce health inequalities"?[63]

Although public health is historically wedded to the conceptual and empirical significance of "population health,"[64] it seems curious that the most commonly used model of health determinants can sidestep, if only in a theoretical sense, the issue of how local population structures affect health outcomes. If population structures, particularly "age" and "sex," are to be relocated as significant components of health inequalities that are shaped by the makeup of places, then more consideration should be given to situating them less in the core layer of fixed variables or even in the outer layer of economic, cultural, and environmental factors affecting health, and more prominently and explicitly in the three inner layers.

Conclusion

Although disjunction between the production and use of demographic information in a wide variety of settings has recently attracted scholarly interest, published research into the relationship between demography and local public health in twentieth-century Britain is still rare.[65] (Paradoxically, the nineteenth century is comparatively well served.) It seems safe to say, however, that basic demographic criteria such death rates and life expectancies remain the most conventional yardsticks by which public health is evaluated. It is remarkable how little this particular landscape has changed since the beginning of the twentieth century (though national sample surveys of health status are now performed). In Liverpool and elsewhere, life expectancies produced by the Office for National Statistics have gradually replaced the crude—or, for that matter, standardized—death rate as the key summary health measure. Although it would appear that this shift came about only in the latter part of the twentieth century as life-expectancy calculations were made and released by the central government on a consistent basis, the tendency toward a reductionist approach has a deep history. This is hardly surprising and perfectly understandable, given that year-by-year local health surveys, which may provide alternative criteria to mortality benchmarks, are expensive to administer; given that public health is managed in a target-setting culture;[66] and given that however blunt the instrument of life expectancy, it continues to illustrate stark and basic inequalities. In 2000–2002, for example, males born in Central Liverpool could expect to live 71.4 years, compared to 74.7 years in South Liverpool; the respective figures for females were 77.1 years and 79.2 years.[67]

This chapter has emphasized, albeit briefly, ways in which the geography of population structure has played on the minds of government statisticians and public health practitioners alike in the twentieth century. These concerns can be traced back to the very beginnings of state public health in the middle of the nineteenth century, when crude mortality rates for local areas began to be used as indicators of sanitary progress. The early twentieth century witnessed the first methodologically successful wide-scale attempts at reducing the distorting impact of local population structures on the measurement of mortality via standardization. Additional refinements included the area comparability factor and the short-lived comparative mortality index. Now that local-level estimates can easily be calculated for localities, life expectancy is widely used as the "gold standard," though it is deployed alongside standardized mortality ratios that continue to be important for describing and analyzing patterns of specific causes of death. In the context of managerialist, target-setting approaches to health improvement, these summary standardized indices of mortality remain as important to public health practitioners at the beginning of the twenty-first century as the CDR was at the beginning of the twentieth century. Detailed archival research needs to be conducted in order to understand fully the political fate of the weekly mortality rate in the localities. I would speculate that more than one force was at work. With the decline of infectious diseases the CDR probably lost much of its power to motivate administrators. The well-documented difficulties in redefining the role of the public health profession after the reorganization of the health service in 1974 may also have played its part.[68]

If methodological complexities in age and sex standardization for mortality analyses are any indication, it would appear that demographers largely have come to terms with their struggle to exercise professional control over the local. But whereas demographers endeavor to iron out the distortions caused by topographies of age and sex composition, public health practice seeks to uncover, map, and intervene to reduce the detriments to health brought about, in part, by these varying topographies; it is now replete with programs that focus specifically or exclusively on children, young adults, senior citizens, and women. As always, the size and significance (in health terms) of these demographic groups varies from place to place, though this does not seem to be explicitly acknowledged in the dominant model of health inequalities. It is important to think critically about interactions between the production of statistics and their use as public health intelligence. By considering the instrumentality of mortality rates at the local level, this chapter has demonstrated the possibility of seeing beyond the veneer of objectivity that demographic analysis purports to convey.

Notes

I would like to thank Harry Marks and the editors of this volume for their many helpful comments and suggestions on earlier versions of this chapter.

1. S. Szreter, H. Sholkamy, and A. Dharmalingam, "Contextualizing Categories: Towards a Critical Reflexive Demography," in *Categories and Contexts: Anthropological and Historical Studies in Critical Demography*, ed. S. Szreter, H. Sholkamy and A. Dharmalingam (Oxford: Oxford University Press, 2004), 11.

2. Gerry Kearns uses the term *sanitary intelligence* for the mid-nineteenth century to describe "all those means whereby information was gathered and analyzed, and conclusions published." See G. Kearns, "Town Hall and Whitehall: Sanitary Intelligence in Liverpool, 1840–63," in *Body and City: Histories of Urban Public Health*, ed. S. Sheard and H. Power, 89–108 (Aldershot: Ashgate, 2000).

3. A. Hardy, *Health and Medicine in Britain since 1860* (Basingstoke: Palgrave, 2001); H. Jones, *Health and Society in Twentieth-Century Britain* (Harlow: Longman, 1994); J. Lewis, *What Price Community Medicine? The Philosophy, Practice, and Politics of Public Health since 1919* (Brighton: Wheatsheaf Books, 1986); J. Welshman, *Municipal Medicine: Public Health in Twentieth-Century Britain* (Oxford: Lang, 2000).

4. J. Ashton and H. Seymour, *The New Public Health: The Liverpool Experience* (Milton Keynes: Open University Press, 1988), 184.

5. E. Higgs, *Life, Death, and Statistics: Civil Registration, Censuses, and the Work of the General Register Office, 1836–1952* (Hatfield: Local Population Studies, 2004).

6. J. Eyler, *Victorian Social Medicine: The Ideas and Methods of William Farr* (Baltimore: Johns Hopkins University Press, 1979).

7. S. Szreter, "The Importance of Social Intervention in Britain's Mortality Decline c. 1850–1914: A Re-Interpretation of the Role of Public Health," *Social History of Medicine* 1 (1988): 1–37.

8. Eyler, *Victorian Social Medicine*, Chapter 4.

9. S. E. Igo, *The Averaged American: Surveys, Citizens and the Making of a Mass Public* (London: Harvard University Press, 2007).

10. K. Metz, "Paupers and Numbers: The Statistical Argument for Social Reform in Britain During the Period of Industrialization," in *The Probabilistic Revolution*, vol. 1, *Ideas in History*, ed. L. Krüger, L. J. Daston, and M. Heidelberger (Cambridge, MA: MIT Press, 1990), 345; W. Rothstein, *Public Health and the Risk Factor: A History of an Uneven Medical Revolution* (Rochester, NY: University of Rochester Press, 2003), 22–49; T. M. Porter, *The Rise of Statistical Thinking, 1820–1900* (Princeton, NJ: Princeton University Press, 1986), 23–39.

11. T. W. Hime, *The Practical Guide to the Public Health Acts. A Vade Mecum for Officers of Health and Inspectors of Nuisances*, 2nd ed. (London: Baillière, Tindall and Cox, 1901), 520.

12. G. Mooney, "Professionalisation in Public Health and the Measurement of Sanitary Progress in Nineteenth Century England and Wales," *Social History of Medicine* 10 (1997): 53–78.

13. G. Mooney, B. Luckin, and A. Tanner, "Patient Pathways: Solving the Problem of Institutional Mortality in London During the Later Nineteenth Century," *Social History of Medicine* 12 (1999): 227–69.

14. F. Lewes, "The GRO and the Provinces in the Nineteenth Century," *Social History of Medicine* 4 (1991): 492–93.

15. E. Higgs, "The Statistical Big Bang of 1911: Ideology, Technological Innovation, and the Production of Medical Statistics," *Social History of Medicine* 9 (1996): 421–25.

16. P. Kreager, "Objectifying Demographic Identities," in *Categories and Contexts*, ed. S. Szreter, H. Sholkamy, and A. Dharmalingam, 33–56 (Oxford: Oxford University Press, 2004).

17. Hime, *The Practical Guide*, 413.

18. Hime, *The Practical Guide*, 413.

19. Welshman, *Municipal Medicine*, 256.

20. Welshman, *Municipal Medicine*, 114.

21. Hime, *The Practical Guide*, 528–33.

22. E. Hope, *Report on the Health of Liverpool During 1901* (Liverpool, 1902), 3.

23. Rates calculated from census returns. Population totals: 581,203 (1871); 686,303 (1881); 729,743 (1891). Liverpool here comprises the registration districts of Liverpool, West Derby, and Toxteth Park.

24. N. Humphreys, "The Value of Death-Rates as a Test of Sanitary Condition," *Journal of the Royal Statistical Society* 37 (1874): 461. Noel Humphreys (1837–1923) entered the GRO in 1856 where he was employed for the next fifty years, becoming chief clerk in 1898. See "Obituary. Noel Algernon Humphreys," *Journal of the Royal Statistical Society* 86 (1923): 277. According to Simon Szreter, Humphreys "had considerable status and influence . . . especially . . . during his last fifteen years when his authority was probably on a par with both Ogle and Tatham, Farr's successors." S. R. S. Szreter, *Fertility, Class and Gender in Britain, 1860–1940* (Cambridge: Cambridge University Press, 1996), 79.

25. Registrar-General for England and Wales, *Decennial Supplement, Part III, Registration Summary Tables, 1901–10* (London: HMSO, 1914).

26. W. Frazer, *Report on the Health of the City of Liverpool for the Year 1951* (Liverpool, n.d.).

27. Kreager, "Objectifying Demographic Identities," 36–37.

28. Mooney, "Professionalisation in Public Health," 56; H. Wolfenden, "On the Methods of Comparing the Mortalities of Two Or More Communities, and the Standardization of Death-Rates," *Journal of the Royal Statistical Society* 86 (1923): 399–411.

29. Hime, *The Practical Guide*, Appendix, 179. See also J. M. Eyler, *Sir Arthur Newsholme and State Medicine, 1885–1935* (Cambridge: Cambridge University Press, 1997), 38.

30. R. Woods, *The Demography of Victorian England and Wales* (Cambridge: Cambridge University Press, 2000).

31. Great Britain Office for National Statistics, *English Life Tables no. 15, 1990–1992* (London: HMSO, 1997).

32. For discussion of "normal" and "average" in a broader context, see I. Hacking, *The Taming of Chance* (Cambridge: Cambridge University Press, 1990), 160–88.

33. E. Willoughby, *Handbook of Public Health and Demography* (London and New York: Macmillan, 1893), 410.

34. Willoughby, *Handbook*, 411–12 (emphasis added).

35. Mooney, "Professionalisation in Public Health," 60–61.

36. William Mowll Frazer (1888–1958) was Liverpool's MOH from 1931 to 1953 and was appointed professor of hygiene at the University of Liverpool in 1933. "Obituary. Prof. W. M. Frazer," *The Times*, September 9, 1958, 11. He is best known to historians of public health for his *Duncan of Liverpool. An Account of the Work of Dr. W. H. Duncan Medical Officer of Health of Liverpool, 1847–63* (London: Hamish Hamilton, 1947) and *A History of English Public Health, 1834–1939* (London: Baillière, Tindall and Cox, 1950).

37. Frazer, *Report on the Health of the City of Liverpool for the Year 1951*.

38. Higgs, *Life, Death, and Statistics*, 208. In 1921 Stocks was recruited by Karl Pearson to the Galton Laboratory at University College London. He was a regular

contributor to the journals *Biometrika* and the *Annals of Eugenics*, publishing papers on various aspects of epidemiology. He was appointed chief medical statistician at the GRO in 1933, a post that he held until his retirement in 1950. Doll has noted that Stocks "wrote extensively, but often anonymously" in the GRO's *Annual Reports*. R. Doll, "Stocks, Percy (1889–1974)," in *Oxford Dictionary of National Biography* (Oxford: Oxford University Press, 2004).

39. Registrar-General for England and Wales, *Statistical Review of England and Wales for the Year 1941 (New Annual Series no. 21) Tables. Part I. Medical* (London: HMSO, 1945), 320.

40. Registrar-General for England and Wales, *Statistical Review for 1941*, 320.

41. Registrar-General for England and Wales, *Statistical Review for 1941*, 320.

42. The clearest mathematical representation appeared in the 1942 *Statistical Review*.

$$CMI = \Sigma\, m(r + r^1)/2 \; / \; \Sigma\, m^1(r + r^1)/2$$

where m is the death rate in a particular age group; r is the ratio of the population at those ages to the total population at all ages in the year for which the CMI is required; and where m^1 and r^1 are the corresponding values in the base year (1938).

43. Registrar-General for England and Wales, *Statistical Review for 1941*, 321.

44. Registrar-General for England and Wales, *Statistical Review of England and Wales for the Year 1958. Part III. Commentary* (London: HMSO, 1960), 56–58.

45. Higgs, *Life, Death, and Statistics*, 208.

46. Registrar-General for England and Wales, *Statistical Review of England and Wales for the Year 1954. Part III. Commentary* (London: HMSO, 1957), 57.

47. Registrar-General for England and Wales, *Statistical Review of England and Wales for the Two Years 1948–1949. Text, Medical* (London: HMSO, 1953), 17. See also M. P. Newton and J. R. Jeffery, *Internal Migration: Some Aspects of Population Movements within England and Wales* (London: HMSO, 1951).

48. Great Britain Office of Population Censuses and Surveys, *Vital Statistics for Administrative and Health Areas of England and Wales, 1980, Series VS no. 7* (London: HMSO, 1982). On the 1974 government changes, see C. Webster, *The National Health Service: A Political History*, 2nd ed. (Oxford: Oxford University Press, 2002), 107–11.

49. Higgs, *Life, Death, and Statistics*, 199–200.

50. See Higgs, *Life, Death, and Statistics*, 188–201 for a discussion of the relationship between the GRO and the Ministry of Health.

51. See, for example, Registrar-General for England and Wales, *Decennial Supplement for England and Wales, 1951, Area Mortality* (London: HMSO, 1958).

52. Szreter, Sholkamy, and Dharmalingam, "Contextualizing Categories," 11–12. See also N. E. Riley and J. McCarthy, *Demography in the Age of the Postmodern* (Cambridge: Cambridge University Press, 2003), 11–12.

53. N. Krieger, "Historical Roots of Social Epidemiology: Socioeconomic Gradients in Health and Contextual Analysis," *International Journal of Epidemiology* 30 (2001): 899–900. S. Macintyre, "Before and After the Black Report: Four Fallacies," in *Poor Health: Social Inequality Before and After the Black Report*, ed. V. Berridge and S. Blume, 198–219 (London: Frank Cass, 2003).

54. M. Whitehead, "The Concepts and Principles of Equity and Health," *International Journal of Health Services* 22 (1992): 429–46.

55. D. Acheson, *Independent Inquiry into Inequalities in Health Report* (London: The Stationery Office, 1998), http://www.archive.official-documents.co.uk/document/doh/ih/ih.htm (accessed July 19, 2007).

56. M. Exworthy, "The 'Second Black Report'? The Acheson Report as Another Opportunity to Tackle Health Inequalities," in *Poor Health: Social Inequality Before and After the Black Report*, ed. V. Berridge and S. Blume, 175–97 (London: Frank Cass, 2003); M. Exworthy and M. Powell, "Variations on a Theme: New Labour, Health Inequalities and Policy Failure," in *Analysing Health Policy*, ed. A. Hann, 45–62 (Aldershot: Ashgate, 2000).

57. R. Illsley, "Reducing Health Inequalities: Britain's Latest Attempt," *Health Affairs*, May–June 1999, 45–46; A. Williams, "Commentary on the Acheson Report," *Health Economics* 8 (1997): 297–99; S. Birch, "The 39 Steps: The Mystery of Health Inequalities in the UK," *Health Economics* 8 (1997): 301–8; G. Davey Smith, J. N. Morris, and M. Shaw, "The Independent Inquiry into Inequalities in Health Is Welcome, But Its Recommendations Are Too Cautious and Vague," *British Medical Journal* 317 (1998): 1465–66.

58. D. Black, J. N. Morris, C. Smith, and P. Townsend, "Better Benefits for Health: Plan to Implement the Central Recommendation of the Acheson Report," *British Medical Journal* 318 (1999): 724–27; M. Exworthy, L. Berney, and M. Powell, "'How Great Expectations in Westminster May Be Dashed Locally': The Local Implementation of National Policy on Health Inequalities," *Policy & Politics* 30 (2002): 79–96.

59. Acheson, *Independent Inquiry*, Introduction.

60. Central Liverpool Primary Care Trust, *Public Health Annual Report 2003. Life in Central Liverpool: Reviving the Health of Our Population* (Liverpool: Central Liverpool Primary Care Trust, n.d.), 6.

61. Central Liverpool Primary Care Trust, *Public Health Annual Report 2003*, 6.

62. Acheson, *Independent Inquiry*, Introduction.

63. Central Liverpool Primary Care Trust, *Public Health Annual Report 2003*, 9.

64. S. Szreter, "The Population Health Approach in Historical Perspective," *American Journal of Public Health* 93 (2003): 421–31.

65. See contributions to Szreter, Sholkamy, and Dharmalingam, eds. *Categories and Contexts*. The links between demography and public health in the Weimar Republic are explored in G. Moser and J. Fleischhacker, "People's Health and Nation's Body: The Modernisation of Statistics, Demography and Social Hygiene in the Weimar Republic," in *The Politics of the Healthy Life: An International Perspective*, ed. E. Rodríguez-Ocaña, 151–79 (Sheffield: European Association for the History of Medicine and Health, 2002).

66. M. Whitehead, "Editorial: Setting Targets—Still Reaching for the Sky?" *Health Education Journal* 59 (2000): 119.

67. Central Liverpool Primary Care Trust, *Public Health Annual Report 2003*, 18.

68. Lewis, *What Price Community Medicine*, 125–64; Webster, *The National Health Service*, 124–26; Welshman, *Municipal Medicine*, 34 and 38.

Part Four

Navigating between
International and Local

Chapter Nine

A Matter of "Reach"

Fact-Finding in Public Health in the Wake of World War I

Susan Gross Solomon

The finding and measurement of social facts are critical components of statecraft. These activities, James Scott tells us, help policy makers to make their society "legible," to read it, and then to shape it.[1] Fact-finding "away from home" has a different raison d'être: it allows those who craft policies at home to situate their nation in a larger world that they have designated as relevant, and it provides them with baselines against which they may judge that world—and themselves.

The decade after World War I saw exponential growth in travel by public health experts to European countries to find the facts about systems of health care delivery other than their own. Sponsored by international health agencies, national health care administrations, or private philanthropies with transnational aspirations, foreign fact-finding was driven by an acknowledgement that the experiences of countries in fighting disease and promoting wellness might have relevance beyond their borders.

Elsewhere, I have examined the reception by domestic patrons of fact-finding conducted abroad.[2] This chapter engages public health fact-finding at a much earlier stage in the process—before experts extracted "lessons" from their inquiries. It focuses on the decisions that experts (and their patrons) make when they set out to find the facts about public health in "foreign parts." Which aspects of foreign public health systems and practices are important to know? Which countries must be studied? Which might be ignored? Can a single fact-finding template be designed to apply to a range of countries, or do countries have to be studied individually? Can a brief site visit yield reliable knowledge, or is long immersion required? How reliable is the information from fact-finders' networks? The answers to these questions shaped fact-finding agendas and procedures in the field.

Approaches to fact-finding vary significantly from patron to patron, expert to expert, and nation to nation. The variation reflects differing assumptions about what is knowable across borders and how to know it. But behind epistemology and methodology lie deeper issues. The decision to apply abroad fact-finding approaches developed at home inevitably brings into play political judgments about which countries are like "us" and which are not, which differences among countries are salient and which are not.

This chapter compares two approaches to public health fact-finding used in the 1920s—one American, the other Soviet. The American approach relied on instruments of fact-finding; the Soviet approach depended on persons. In both cases, the design of the information retrieval reflected the patron's assessment of the degree of variation among European countries. American information gathering was premised on the relative homogeneity of European countries; the Soviet approach was calibrated to take account of important variations from country to country.

In the 1920s, committed as they were to advancing public health "the world over," American philanthropies such as the Rockefeller Foundation and the Milbank Memorial Fund commissioned studies of public health facilities and training in an array of countries. In conducting these studies, fact-finders used templates developed in—or for—America. Typically, the fact-finding template was deployed on a site visit by a foundation officer or a commissioned expert. The modal "fact-finder" had a background in public health or medicine and international experience; there were no country specialists. The purpose of the exercise was to assess the "fit" of a given country with programs offered by, or policy initiatives advocated by, the sponsoring agency. The templates were prized for their ability to yield standardized results. In the name of standardization, those who designed the templates tended to relegate the political and social context of health systems to the category of "background information."

In the same decade, in the effort to overcome the isolation of Russian public health and medical research that followed the Bolshevik seizure of power in 1917,[3] the Russian Commissariat of Public Health (Narkomzdrav RSFSR) honed an approach to foreign fact-finding that stationed "representatives" of the commissariat's newly created Bureau of Foreign Information in a variety of countries.[4] The representatives were charged with retrieving information on foreign health-care systems and with disseminating abroad information on the new Soviet public health. The bureau's modal "representative" had some experience in public health research or practice, good political credentials (Communist party membership or sympathy with the Soviet government), and facility in the language of the host country. From their foreign perches, representatives developed informal networks of health specialists on whom they relied for fact-finding and dissemination. Over time, the "send-and-receive" functions became looped, allowing representatives not only to find the facts about their host countries, but also to shape those facts.

Neither approach to fact-finding was totally new. The American embrace of standardized surveys and questionnaires built on over three decades of experience in the use of surveys and on the fascination with positivist methods of gathering and processing information.[5] What *was* novel was the application of quantitative methods to the "art of giving."[6] The Soviet dependence on representatives embedded in foreign countries drew on the time-honored practice of sending epidemiologists (military and civilian) into the field to monitor the outbreak of disease.[7] What *was* novel was the explicit looping of the sending and receiving of information.

The fact-finding that is at the center of this chapter catches these two nations at a distinct moment in their histories. In the wake of World War I, with the emphasis in the paradigm of American foreign policy shifting from "isolationism" to a "missionary" focus,[8] the United States was, as Daniel Rogers writes, "particularly open to foreign models and ideas."[9] In the 1920s, in the aftermath of a violent revolution and civil war, Russia was facing not only the challenge of creating a new domestic political order but also the task of breaking down the international isolation in which the country found itself. Russia's effort to reclaim its place in the international arena was accompanied by a real curiosity about the outside world and sensitivity to its variations. In 1920s Russia, the "West" was not the undifferentiated category it would become and remain for a long time.[10]

The "reach" of an approach to fact-finding, which is built into its design, is revealed by how it accommodates the unexpected. The elasticity of the American fact-finding templates was challenged by the call to include Russia among the European nations surveyed. The elasticity of the Russian send-and-receive loop was tested by the visit of the Russian commissar of public health to European countries in which the bureau's representatives were stationed. The adaptability of fact-finding approaches to the unexpected lays bare not only their "reach," but the assumptions underlying their creation.

One Size Fits All:
American Philanthropies and Fact-Finding Abroad

In Progressive-era America, private philanthropies committed to improving public health at home and abroad began increasingly to look to the continent of Europe—whether to alleviate postwar social and economic ills; to spread American-style training in medicine and public health; or to see how countries addressed problems of health care, funding, and administration that were also besetting America.[11] Whatever the impulse, gripped by the promise of "scientific philanthropy," the foundations insisted that launching programs for public health and medicine required knowing the "local." But was that "local" to be known from the inside or from the outside?

For much of the 1920s and early 1930s, in the belief that wielding a single tool in a range of different venues would produce replicable and reliable knowledge, experts commissioned by American foundations deployed abroad templates refined at home. In the late 1920s, for a variety of reasons, American experts (and their patrons) expanded the range of countries they studied to include Bolshevik Russia. Could the existing templates be used for Russia, with its commitment to free, universally accessible, high-quality medicine? If not, did American experts modify the template, set it aside, or stretch the case to fit the template?

Discussions in the American philanthropies about whether the standardized fact-finding instruments could be applied to Russia turned on the issue of Europe's boundaries. Was Russia part of Europe or outside its frame? Did the sociopolitical changes that the Bolshevik revolution introduced disqualify Russia from inclusion in Europe?

The present-day reader might identify in those discussions a question relevant to all foreign fact-finding: how important is the fit between the socioeconomic setting in which a fact-finding instrument is developed and the setting in which it is applied? The assumption by American foundation officers in the 1920s that the countries of Europe surveyed were largely "like" America made the problem of "fit" appear specific to Russia.

If It's Tuesday, It Must Be Belgium: The Rockefeller Philanthropies

In deciding which countries would be included in their coveted international programs, the Rockefeller philanthropies set great store by the "survey of local conditions." Introduced in 1916 in Latin America by the Rockefeller Foundation's International Health Board,[12] over the course of the 1920s the survey became the instrument of fact-finding on which the foundation's Division of Medical Education (DME) based its determinations in Europe. Abraham Flexner conducted a landmark survey of medical education in the United States and Canada for the Carnegie Foundation for the Advancement of Teaching in 1910.[13] But the DME surveys went well beyond Flexner's study, both in the range of data collected and in their reach to Europe.

Applied by talented foundation officers in Belgium and Poland (1920); Germany and Austria (1922); Holland, London, Bulgaria, Romania, Switzerland, and Constantinople (1923); Denmark, Hungary, Scotland, and

Spain (1924); the Baltics, Italy, France, Ireland, and Norway (1925); England and Wales (1926); Iceland and Russia (1927); Sweden (1929); Finland and Greece (1930); and Portugal (1931), the surveys yielded a storehouse of comparative data on European medical education and training.[14]

The DME's surveys followed a standard format. The opening section provided substantial background on a country's location, natural resources, form of government, and history. The "background" included data on public health agencies and medical practice, prevalent diseases, the ratio of doctors to population, conditions of medical licensing, and regulations regarding foreign physicians. Primary, secondary, and university education were also described.

The main section of the survey covered the academic and administrative organization of the country's medical schools. In keeping with the (American) model of medical education favored by the foundation, the survey paid particular attention to the role of laboratory-based teaching, the strength of clinical faculties, the integration of biomedical research, and teaching.[15] The final section contained specific recommendations for the Division of Medical Education. Additional materials, including previous "surveys" by the foundation, were included in an appendix.

The architecture of the DME surveys is worth notice. The background section had no links to the main section on the content of medical education. The survey acknowledged the existence of the "local," or sociopolitical surround, but hived it off, treating it as colorful background. Equally important, the use of categories developed in America meant that medical education in the countries surveyed was compared with the (American) model. How would the fact-finding instruments be applied to settings for which they had not been designed? What were the limits to the transportability of the instruments?

Tailoring the Case to the Template

The decision to survey a country signaled the interest of the Rockefeller philanthropies in extending their programs to that country. The issue of whether to open to Russia was hotly debated within the foundation for four years.[16] In 1927, the foundation sent Alan Gregg, the associate director of DME, on a three-week site visit to Russia, armed with a mandate to "look after the distribution of literature and to investigate possible fellowships."[17] How useful would the survey template prove in a case for which it had not been designed?

As it did routinely for officers conducting site visits abroad, the foundation's Information Service prepared a briefing book for Gregg. The Russia briefing book was a pastiche of information gathered from first-hand observers such as Horsley Gantt, the American physiologist working with Pavlov in Leningrad; English-language texts on Russia; and material on Soviet public health supplied by Alexander Rubakin, the representative of the Russian Commissariat of Public Health in Paris.

The first half of the briefing book provided background on Russia's history, political system, economic conditions, social agenda and problems, topography, and educational system, and the foreign contacts of its scientists and cultural diplomats. Unlike the DME "surveys of local conditions," the briefing book connected background and medical education. Using Rubakin's information on the Bolshevik project for public health, the author of the briefing book identified two distinctive features of the Soviet medical curriculum—the inclusion of hygiene (experimental, labor, school, social) in the courses compulsory for students in their last two years of medical training and the strong preventive emphasis in public health.[18]

Having digested the briefing book, Alan Gregg left on December 5, 1927. Gregg (1890–1957) had considerable foreign experience. After serving with the Harvard Medical Unit in France during World War I, he spent three years in Brazil with the foundation's International Health Board, working on hookworm. The Brazil sojourn sensitized Gregg to the importance of culture for the understanding of disease.[19] Would Gregg see Russian medical education through the prism of the briefing book, which stressed Russian particularity? Or would he rely on the DME survey template, which treated medical education as a generic product, unaffected by its sociocultural surround?

In Russia, Gregg enjoyed high-level access: very early in his visit, he had an audience with Nikolai A. Semashko, the Russian commissar of public health; with the head of that commissariat's Bureau of Foreign Information; and with the physician in charge of medical education at the Russian Commissariat of Education. But his mandate from the DME encouraged Gregg to focus on terrain familiar to him as an expert on comparative medical education—laboratories, clinical teaching, curricula, the professoriate, the student body, and financial support for medical training.

In the course of eight days in Moscow, he inspected (and interviewed physicians at) a staggering number of scientific and medical institutions—the Institute of Experimental Biology, the Institute for Venereal Diseases, the Institute for Social Hygiene, and the Institute of Biochemistry, as well as clinics and laboratories of the Moscow universities—many of which impressed him favorably. In nine days in Leningrad, Gregg visited some of that city's best-known institutions—including the Institute of Botany, the Institute of Pharmacology, the Obstetrical Clinic, the Military-Medical Academy, the Lesgaft Institute of Natural Sciences, the Institute of Epidemiology and Bacteriology, and the Institute of Hygiene.[20] The highlight of his Leningrad sojourn was his meeting with the Nobel laureate Ivan Pavlov.

As Gregg's travel diary reveals, within days of his arrival, he moved away from the link between Russian context and core writ large in the briefing book. Focusing on the details of Soviet medical education, Gregg reduced the unfamiliar Russian context to "background." He decoupled medical training from Soviet ideology and political practice. His contacts with colleagues led him to distinguish those for whom politics was a full-time occupation from those in medical administration "who had to work with and around politics."[21]

To be sure, Gregg encountered some of what the briefing book had identified as distinctive features of Soviet medical education—for example, the prominence of prevention in Soviet medical training and health care. But from the field, Gregg described the curriculum as "saturated with hygiene and preventive medicine," and noted Soviet colleagues' complaints that the focus on hygiene was "robbing the clinical courses."[22] Gregg's view of medical education, which was shaped by the Rockefeller endorsement of the separation of medical and public health teaching,[23] predisposed him to privilege the Soviet critics of prevention, as opposed to those who championed the Bolshevik project.[24]

Handwritten notes reveal that Gregg planned his Russian report to be a "searching analysis nine years after the inauguration of Communism."[25] The report, dated 1927 but written in Paris in May of 1928,[26] ended by being a hundred-page account of medical education, accompanied by a further hundred pages of appendices, some from Soviet sources. Ironically, as with many of the country studies, much of the material in the report had appeared in the briefing book. The two-hundred-page report was preceded by a mere seven pages (!) of general thoughts on Russia—clear evidence of Gregg's reluctance to come to grips with the "surround" of Soviet medical training and care.

Gregg assessed Soviet medical training using both American yardsticks (which led him to approve the delegation of administrative positions to the communists, which freed scientists to work "as they liked") and metrics unique to Russia (which prompted him to suggest that strict political control may have been less harmful to universities in Russia than elsewhere, because it "prevents the slide into anarchy.")[27] What Gregg did not do was to measure Soviet medical education by the goals of its architects. He tagged as "residues" the focus on prevention and on public health instruction, features that the briefing book had presented—neutrally—as distinctive to the Soviet system. By depicting these features as holdovers from early Bolshevik enthusiasm, Gregg was able to dismiss them and fit Soviet medical education to the DME template. He reported being impressed by how much—not how little—Soviet medical education resembled its largely state-controlled counterparts in western Europe. That resemblance cleared the way for Gregg to urge the inclusion of Russia in the Rockefeller's fellowship program for medical education.[28]

"The Method of Sampling": The Milbank Memorial Fund

In 1928, the trustees of the Milbank Memorial Fund[29] commissioned the leading British health statesman, Sir Arthur Newsholme, to conduct a large cross-national study of the relationship between the "private and official" practice of medicine in the "chief" countries of Europe.[30] As part of an escalating discussion in America over the costs and quality of health care delivery,[31] in 1923, the Milbank Memorial Fund had launched a series of "health demonstrations" in New York City and New York State aimed at making health care delivery more efficient and economical. The fund's "demonstrations" drew protests from physicians in New York.[32] In the hope that evidence from abroad might prompt Americans to rethink the fraught relationship between public and private medicine that was impeding the reform of American medical care, John A. Kingsbury, executive secretary of the Milbank Memorial Fund, persuaded Albert Milbank to ask Newsholme to conduct a large cross-national study.

Unlike the "fact demonstration," which was the heart of the New York pilot projects,[33] the Milbank mandate to Newsholme called for *fact-finding*. In late 1929 and early 1930, Newsholme traveled for four months by car across Europe with a secretary-interpreter. He interviewed health officials, observed facilities, and collected statistical reports on a single issue—the relationship of private and "official" (that is, public) medicine.[34] The results of the fact-finding appeared as *International Studies on the Relationship between the Private and Official Practice of Medicine,* a three-volume "structured-focused" study of the relation between private and public medicine in eighteen European countries: the Netherlands, Denmark, Sweden, Norway, Germany, Austria, and Switzerland (volume I); Belgium, France, Italy, Yugoslavia, Hungary, Poland, and Czechoslovakia (volume II); and England, Scotland, Wales, and Ireland (volume III).[35] In his cross-national inquiry, Newsholme applied a template based on British administrative categories (sickness insurance, hospitals, midwifery, infant and child welfare, school medical work, the prevention of tuberculosis, and the prevention of venereal disease).[36] The findings of the eighteen-country study were summarized in a fourth volume, *Medicine and the State.*[37]

Russia was not among the countries surveyed. As Newsholme put it, he "scarcely thought that Russian experience was likely to give important guidance as to the direction and character of advances and reforms needed in American or English communities."[38] But in July of 1932, with the American Committee on the Costs of Medical Care set to deliver its Final Report amid internal opposition to provisions for national health insurance, Kingsbury persuaded Newsholme to include the Soviet Union among the cases potentially instructive for America.

In September of 1932, Newsholme, accompanied by Kingsbury, embarked on a month-long, 8,500-mile journey through Russia to see "how the Soviets handle their public health problem."[39] The team's findings, detailed in their travel diary, were framed and reframed several times before appearing as *Red Medicine*, a book published by Doubleday in 1933.[40]

The fact-finders tapped by the Milbank—John Adams Kingsbury (1876–1956) and Sir Arthur Newsholme (1857–1943)—were part of the American public health establishment. Kingsbury had been executive secretary of the Milbank Memorial Fund since 1921, a post he would retain until 1935. Between 1914 and 1918, he had been commissioner of public charities in New York City; during World War I, he had served as assistant director of general relief with the American Red Cross in France.[41] As principal medical officer of the Local Government Board from 1908 to 1919, Arthur Newsholme had effectively been head of the English public health service. Knighted in 1917, he retired from the British civil service in 1919. At the invitation of Dr. William Welch, the first dean of The Johns Hopkins University School of Medicine, he taught at the newly created Johns Hopkins School of Hygiene and Public Health for two years and then lectured and wrote extensively on public health.[42]

Setting the Template Aside

Kingsbury and Newsholme's original plan was to make the study of Russia into Volume IV of Newsholme's series International Studies. This would have meant focusing on the factor privileged in Newsholme's volumes—the relationship of private and "official" medicine.

Even before they left for Russia, the pair had decided—at Kingsbury's suggestion—to study Soviet public health as a single case with unique features.[43] That decision prompted a dual shift from Newsholme's template: the Russian study would examine more facets of public health, and it would provide more country-specific background than Newsholme's surveys of public health in other European countries.

Kingsbury instructed an assistant to retrieve the best material (in English and German) on public health in tsarist Russia and the Soviet Union—its administration, its leaders, and its operation in the republics as well as in the center. The materials were compiled by General Viktor Yakhontoff, the former assistant secretary of war under Alexander Kerensky.[44] At this stage, Kingsbury and Newsholme projected an eighteen-chapter book: a substantial introductory chapter (on the country, its population, its government, and its vital statistics, and sociomedical background) would be followed by chapters on the provision of services, the measures to combat diseases, work-related injuries, and aspects of social deviance (alcoholism, prostitution).

Kingsbury and Newsholme's Russian itinerary was tailored to their aspirations. The fact-finders visited a staggering array of medical facilities in the course of one month: the Central Tuberculosis Institute and the Institute for Skin and Venereal Diseases in Moscow, the Institute for the Protection of Motherhood and Childhood in Leningrad, a large university clinic in Kazan, the Hospital for Bone Tuberculosis in Rostov, a state sanitorium in Yalta, the Roentgen Institute in Kiev, a day preventorium for children in Kiev, and the Institute of Hygiene and Pathology of Labor in Kharkov—to name but a few.[45] Site visits were interspersed with interviews with "medical leaders and officials," including Dr. M. F. Vladimirskii, the Soviet commissar of public health. While in the field, the fact-finders took detailed notes and wrote drafts of some chapters. After leaving Russia, they divided the work between them; the book was written and rewritten at least twice.

The decision to treat the Russian case in the round allowed the fact-finders to include detailed descriptions of facilities they visited, many of which impressed the pair with the commitment of health care workers and administrators to comprehensive health care, both preventive and curative. Equally important, the fact-finders' choice to conduct a context-rich case study made it possible to include a considerable amount of nonmedical material. The authors explained, "We have thought it wise to give a somewhat detailed account of social and economic life in Russia in order that its medicine of today may be seen in its natural setting."[46] But how much of an account? And what should be included? Newsholme favored including more material. Kingsbury was for less, writing to Newsholme, "I agree with you that an account of the medical problem alone is a 'baby unclad,' and I agree that the general national position and history is essential to an understanding of the specialist problem. . . . Nevertheless, I do think it is slightly out of proportion."[47]

The amount of nonmedical material included was less the issue than the nature of that material. The authors provided a substantial discussion of the sociopolitical surround of the health care system and drew links between that surround and the government's commitment to treating the health of an individual as a social concern. The authors diverged over how much weight to give the gap between ideology and reality. Newsholme did not shy away from exposing Russia's "warts." Thus, after praising the fact that Soviet employers (the state or a cooperative) bore the cost of social insurance, Newsholme listed the "deprived persons" excluded from these benefits—"former landlords, Bourgeoisie, nobles, Tsarist officials, Merchants, kulaks, and Tsarist army officers"—and noted that insurance benefits had yet to be extended to peasants.[48] Kingsbury, who favored "comparing Russians with themselves,"[49] feared that the "warts" would mar the picture. To Newsholme he wrote, "The criticism I have . . . is that you lay a good deal of stress on warts which are not on the face at least of our "subject." . . . [W]e are concerned primarily with the medical problems and . . . cannot give adequate discussion of 'class hatred,' 'class government' 'preference to the workers,' 'cruelty to the kulaks' unless we really enter into quite a detailed discussion of 'communism' 'revolution' and the class struggle generally. . . . I wonder if it is necessary to go into the discussion of such questions quite as fully as you do."[50]

The fact-finders compromised (not always seamlessly): they brought out both the "warts" and the innovations of the Soviet system. The compromise did not wash with their patron, Albert Milbank. In May 1933, after reading a draft of *Red Medicine,* he commented that the frequent references to medicine and the state sounded to him like "propaganda." Most disconcerting was the authors' deference to British socialist and reformer Sidney Webb, who read and commented on every chapter. "Despite Sidney Webb's reputation among the intelligentsia and despite the fact that he was in part a collaborator, I am questioning whether you have not brought out too clearly his views. He is recognized generally both in England and in this country as a rather extreme Socialist. . . . [Y]ou are opening yourselves to the criticism that the book is not so much the product of an American and an Englishman interested in the health movement, as the product of men who . . . became enamored of Sidney Webb's interpretation of the whole Russian movement."[51]

In its published form, *Red Medicine* went beyond a context-rich description of the Soviet system to compare Soviet and American health care. The binary comparison was prompted by the final report of the American Committee on the Costs of Health Care, which recommended voluntary, rather than compulsory health insurance, as Kingsbury had hoped.[52] Each of the authors wrote a comparative chapter. In his, Newsholme measured the Soviet system against the ten "maladjustments" in American health care cited in the committee's final report. The comparison showed that Soviet health care suffered less from the maladjustments of the American system than did the United States! Invoking the template used in *International Studies,* Newsholme concluded that the Soviet system "has the great merit that the direct payment of fees has ceased and with it . . . the burning problem of the relation between the private and public practice of medicine, which in capitalist countries is always with us."[53]

Kingsbury's comparison, which appeared in "Concluding Observations," positioned Russia as an outlier, an exception among nations. The chapter focused on Russia's political, social, and economic system, which the author characterized as "the most gigantic experiment in the deliberate public organization of social and economic life in the history of the world." Kingsbury's brief discussion of the "socialization of medicine," defined as the provision of medical care out of communal funds, underlined the distinctive position of Russia. "The position of the U.S.S.R. . . . is very special. In some essential particulars it has surpassed all other countries in its socialization of medicine." Kingsbury doubted that the Soviet model could be replicated. "Other countries . . . may well envy Soviet Russia's elaborately centralized government . . . [, which] has been able to brush aside all complexities and to initiate a nearly universal national medical system on unified lines, untrammeled by such complications as exist in western Europe and America. . . . [A]lmost certainly progress in western countries toward the goal of a national medical service will not follow the exact procedure."[54]

The years following the publication of *Red Medicine* saw increasing discussion in America of compulsory health insurance, which drew shrill protests from the American Medical Association (AMA). In that context, as I have shown elsewhere, the authors' decision to add a binary comparison to the context-rich study doomed the project. Though *Red Medicine* was published to considerable acclaim, in 1935 Albert Milbank summarily fired Kingsbury from his position at the Milbank Memorial Fund.[55]

The call to include Russia in foreign fact-finding challenged the approaches honed by the Rockefeller philanthropies and the Milbank Memorial Fund. The responses to the challenge varied. To accommodate the case of Russia, the Rockefeller fact-finders shelved the sociopolitical background of Soviet health care, whereas the Milbank fact-finders replaced their standardized template with a detailed study that included aspects of the Russian sociopolitical surround that they considered indispensable to understanding the country's public health system. In neither case did the original fact-finding instrument prove elastic enough to accommodate the Russian case without fundamental change.

The Send and Receive Loop: Narkomzdrav's Biuro Zagranichnoi Informatsii

In 1920, with the civil war still raging in Russia, the Russian commissar of public health, Nikolai Semashko, signed a decree creating a new Department of Foreign Information under the Russian Commissariat of Public Health (Narkomzdrav RSFSR).[56] Opened on February 7, 1921, the department, renamed in 1924 the Bureau of Foreign Information (Biuro Zagranichnoi Informatsii, or BZI), was responsible for a two-way flow of information: the gathering of information on health and medicine abroad and the dissemination outside Russia of material on Soviet health and medicine.

BZI was the first Bolshevik governmental agency to engage in information collection and dissemination abroad. The factors prodding the commissariat to create the bureau were plain.[57] Researchers in Russian public health and medicine (like their counterparts in science) were desperate to offset the effects of the international isolation of Russia that followed World War I and the Bolshevik revolution. To ensure the vitality of Russian science, they needed access to foreign research, colleagues, and medical equipment, and the capacity to publicize their own work abroad. Further, spokesmen for Russian public health and medicine were eager to position themselves internationally. In 1918, the Russian Commissariat of Public Health introduced a new approach to public health, which guaranteed universal and free access to medical care and called for the integration of preventive and curative medicine in physician training and patient treatment. To publicize the new approach effectively, spokesmen needed sufficient familiarity with foreign health care to reassure themselves that their blueprint had "gotten it right."

BZI did not operate by remote control. It relied on a group of physicians whom it stationed as "representatives" (*predstaviteli*) in Germany, France, the United States, England, Italy, and Switzerland.[58] Over time, the representatives developed networks that shaped their fact-finding and information dissemination. With usage, the send-and-receive functions between Moscow and its representatives became looped. For example, in 1923, BZI charged representatives to "find facts" on curiosity about Russian medicine in their respective countries. This material was to be included in a chapter on Western interest in Russian science in a forthcoming book marking the fifth anniversary of Soviet public health slated for distribution abroad. The book was published without the chapter in question.[59] How tightly were the send-and-receive information functions looped? How easily did the system accommodate new information?

There is almost no scholarly research on Russian gathering of foreign information or dissemination of information abroad in the 1920s. The fascination with Soviet espionage on the one hand[60] and Soviet foreign propaganda on the other[61] left little room for reflection on how the fledgling Bolshevik regime, like other European states of the day, used openly available foreign information to shape their agendas at home and their image abroad.[62] Publicly available information was BZI's stock in trade. The lion's share of the materials that BZI representatives collected for Moscow—journal articles, published reports, book reviews—was in the public domain, though effectively inaccessible to Russian health researchers: during the early 1920s, Russia lacked the hard currency to renew journal subscriptions, buy books, and send its scientists to conferences. Likewise, most of the material that BZI disseminated—articles, government reports, statistical compilations—had been published in Russia, but was unavailable to the outside world because Russia had yet to exploit channels to publicize abroad the work of its scientists and because the materials were written in Russian. Of course, we cannot preclude the possibility that some of BZI's representatives had "second" jobs, covertly sending and receiving information not in the public domain.[63] The local police occasionally monitored the activities of

BZI's representatives.[64] But that monitoring paled in comparison to the surveillance of Russia's political representatives and the representatives of the Ministry of Foreign Trade.

Analysis of the content of BZI's send-and-receive information loops illuminates how spokesmen for Soviet health care understood the outside world in the 1920s, as they worked to make and remake their social order. Which facets of their system did they see as marketable abroad? Looking at BZI's send-and-receive loops of information as an *iterative* process, as we do here, draws attention to the capacity of the system to cope with new information.

Terms of Reference

The mandate of BZI, as set forth in a document of November 1922, specified three functions:

1. "Politico-Organizational and Official" (that is, "cultural diplomacy"): conducting relations with state, social, medical, and other organizations in Western Europe and America; exchanging information on the principles of health care in Russia; arranging for the participation of NKZ in sanitary conventions and agreements; and strengthening contacts with visiting physicians.

2. "Scientific-Medical" (that is, "scientific exchange"): organizing Russian participation in international conferences; disseminating published information on health care in the RSFSR; exchanging scientific literature and information about new discoveries in medical science.

3. "Intermediary Function" (that is, "middleman"): facilitating acquisition of medico-surgical and laboratory equipment and instruments.[65]

Two points command attention. First, unlike an earlier version,[66] the November mandate treated scientific-medical exchange as distinct from cultural diplomacy. Second, Narkomzdrav was "selling" two different products: Soviet medical research and Soviet socialized health care, which was an integral part of the Bolshevik project. Could the two be sold simultaneously? How did Moscow decide which of these two products to emphasize in a given locale?

For over a half decade, the bureau and its representatives performed all three mandated tasks, with skeletal staff and no local structure to speak of.[67] As the 1920s wore on, BZI's cultural diplomacy was curtailed, as foreign policy making became centralized in the Commissariat of Foreign Affairs, and foreign cultural relations were claimed by the All-Union Society for Cultural Ties Abroad (VOKS).[68] BZI's "middleman" function shrank as the Commissariat of Foreign Trade increasingly controlled acquisition of foreign medical equipment, supplies, and pharmaceuticals. BZI's scientific exchange function eroded, as institutions like the Russian Academy of Science began to deal directly with foreign counterparts. In late 1927, the bureau—renamed the All-Union Bureau of Foreign Sanitary Information (OBZSI)—was directed to cease cultural diplomacy and to collect and disseminate only sanitary data. In the 1928–29 budget, allocations for BZI's foreign representations were slashed. Only the American representation retained its political function, because there were no diplomatic ties between Russia and the United States. The representations were slated to close by autumn of 1928,[69] though some representatives remained in place until the turn of 1929.

On the Ground

Moscow and its "men on the ground" conducted an iterative dialogue. The representatives functioned as "clipping services," sending notices of local conferences and publications. They dispatched "reports"—fact-finding documents of ten to twenty pages (occasionally with budgets), covering periods from three months to five years—which described the local scene, touted accomplishments, and negotiated targets for the next period. Representatives also peppered Moscow with brief letters and telegrams on urgent matters—visas, travel itineraries, and modalities for equipment or pharmaceutical purchases. From Moscow, in telegrams, letters, or cryptic notes, came requests for fact-finding, suggestions for disseminating Russian material—and the occasional rebuke for instructions misunderstood.

BZI had distinctive ties to each of its representatives. As the comparison of Germany and France suggests, those ties were a function of political relations between Russia and the host countries, personal relations between Semashko and the representatives, and the character of the local networks the representatives constructed.

Berlin, Lindenstrasse 25

The German representation opened in Berlin in August of 1921, just six months after the creation of BZI. By that point, Germany and Russia were already taking the steps that would culminate in the Treaty of Rapallo of April 1922.[70] The German representation had de jure status: with the consent of the German government, it was located in what the historian Karl Schloegel has termed the "archipelago" of the Russian embassy.[71]

BZI's German representative was Iakov Rafailovich Gol'denberg (born in 1876 in Warsaw), who was posted to Berlin in 1921 as representative of the Russian Commissariat of Public Health and of the Comintern.[72] Gol'denberg had strong political credentials. A committed communist from the early twentieth century, he joined the Polish party (SDKPiL) in 1902. In France during World War I, he joined the French Communist party in 1917. Arrested that year for spreading "Bolshevik propaganda" among Russian soldiers, he was deported from France in 1921 and posted to Germany, where he continued his involvement (illegally) with the French Communist party.[73]

Gol'denberg was the dean of BZI's foreign representatives.[74] He acted as the conduit between Moscow and BZI's representatives in Paris and New York, particularly before the Paris representation was opened formally in 1925. He exerted quality control: in 1924, when his Paris counterpart was setting up a bilingual medical journal, Gol'denberg set out the conditions.[75] Gol'denberg's authority derived from his long-standing, close ties to Semashko.[76]

In August 1928, when the representation in Berlin was being liquidated and merged with the Red Cross office, in a "secret" letter, the Russian ambassador to Germany urged Semashko to appoint as Gol'denberg's successor someone who, like Gol'denberg, was a socially oriented physician, knew Soviet sanitary activity, and spoke German. The designated replacement was purely a political operative, whose training would prevent him from doing informational work.[77] Gol'denberg remained in Berlin until mid-January 1929; two months later, he was appointed a member of the administration of the State Medical Publishing House in Moscow.[78]

During his tenure in Berlin, Gol'denberg emphasized the role of "propaganda" in securing foreign recognition of Soviet achievements in medicine and public health.[79] He saw Germany as fertile soil for Soviet ideas: the widespread destruction that followed the war had raised German interest in how the USSR addressed maternal and infant care, sanitary enlightenment, collective nutrition, housing, and social insurance.[80] Himself a specialist in social medicine,[81] Gol'denberg gave talks and wrote articles on Soviet public health for German publications[82] in the belief that "doing propaganda for social medicine [i.e., "public health"] was the best way to market socialist ideas."[83] For his Moscow patrons, Gol'denberg retrieved information on German public health and social medicine.[84]

There were important links between prominent German and Russian medical researchers,[85] but Gol'denberg was never accepted by the elite of German medical science. His best connections in the German medical world were in fringe specialties such as sexology and eugenics.[86]

Knowing Narkomzdrav's interest in connecting to German scientific circles,[87] Gol'denberg published articles in German journals on bilateral scientific cooperation.[88] But in a candid report, he admitted difficulty getting a hearing for Soviet scientific medicine.[89] In 1924, he tried unsuccessfully to found a bilingual joint medical journal, *Folia Medica*.[90] In October 1925, he managed to launch the bilingual *German-Russian Medical Journal* (*Deutsch-Russische Medizinische Zeitschrift/ Russko-Nemetskii Meditsinskii Zhurnal*) with Semashko and Dr. Friedrich Kraus, head of the II Medical Clinic, Charité, as coeditors. The journal, which lasted through 1928, carried articles by Soviet physicians in German and by German physicians in Russian. Despite its title, the journal devoted far more attention to public health than to biomedicine. Even articles on public health were hard to commission, Gol'denberg admitted; many researchers preferred to get their articles into a journal with a "name."[91]

Paris, 7 avenue Président Wilson

In 1925, just a year after French recognition of Soviet Russia, BZI opened its Paris representation.[92] In fact, BZI's representative, A. N. Rubakin, had been working since 1922 under the guidance of Gol'denberg.[93] Located on avenue Président Wilson, the Paris representation did not have de jure status. The French government refused Rubakin's requests to move the representation inside the embassy. A reference (by Semashko) in 1927 to the representation as being "under the aegis of the Embassy" angered the French government. Rubakin was informed that the representation could present itself only as a scientific center.[94] Such diplomatic niceties were lost on the outside world: a Rockefeller Foundation document identified Rubakin as "a Russian physician connected with the Embassy of the URSS in Paris."[95]

Alexander Nikolaevich Rubakin (born 1889 in St. Petersburg) had a life in parts. Arrested in 1906 for publishing revolutionary literature, he escaped to France, where he studied medicine from 1916 to 1919 and served as physician in the French army in 1918–19. In 1921, he escaped deportation thanks to his French wife, who was a schoolteacher.[96] In 1923, he became a Soviet citizen.[97] In March 1925, the political attaché at the Russian embassy commended Rubakin to Semashko as "a good man to appoint in some way or other"; six months later, Rubakin was appointed BZI's representative in Paris.[98] In July 1927, Rubakin secured an official Soviet passport.[99] Rubakin had a literary side: through his sojourn in France, his poetry was published in French journals (under the pseudonym "Junior") and in the Russian émigré press.

In mid-August 1928, with the liquidation of the French representation looming, Rubakin cast about for a place. He wrote to the Rockefeller Foundation officer Daniel O'Brien that he wanted to return to work in bacteriology.[100] He expected a position in the USSR, but nothing permanent materialized. In the summer of 1929, he began a two-year stint in Geneva as an expert for the Hygiene Section of the Secretariat of the League of Nations Health Committee.[101] During this period, he published articles in France on Soviet public health.[102] He spent 1932–33 as a fellow of the Rockefeller Foundation's International Health Division in America, where he wrote a book on Soviet public health.[103] In Paris between 1933 and 1941, he taught hygiene in a French high school and read lectures at the Worker's University, which was under the aegis of the French Communist party. In 1941, Rubakin was interned first in Le Vernet in France and then in Camp Djelfa in Algeria, where he remained for two years. John A. Kingsbury, who had met Rubakin in America, offered to sponsor his entry to the United States.[104] Nothing came of the offer. Liberated in 1943, Rubakin returned to Moscow where two years later, he began working as a professor of hygiene at I Moscow Medical Institute.[105]

As the bureau's "man" in Paris, Rubakin was involved in one way or another in all medical and scientific traffic between France and Russia.[106] Over time, Rubakin's quarterly reports or "Bulletins" expanded to cover activity in such far-flung places as French North Africa.[107] Rubakin's contacts in France were in biomedical circles. As he put it in March 1925, "Opening contacts with the doctors was not necessary for me; I had them already."[108] In August 1924, even before his official appointment, Rubakin launched two Russian-French medical journals: *Revue Franco-Russe de Médecine et de biologie* and *Novosti frantsuzskoi meditsiny i biologii*.[109] In the preface to the first issue (1924) of the *Revue*, the editor explained, "Germany alone opened her doors to Russia and . . . tried to establish a monopoly on the importation of scientific ideas. But the Russian genius . . . so eager to know everything, could not content itself . . . to receive at the hands of the Germans ideas about the scientific tendencies of French science."[110] To Semashko, Rubakin insisted that the journals would "do propaganda for Soviet Russia and will get bilateral relations going."[111]

The journals were mirror opposites. *Novosti frantsuzskoi meditsiny*, with its articles and reviews from French medical journals, targeted Russian readers. The journal attracted French luminaries of the National Committee for Defense against Tuberculosis such as Fernand Bezançon, Albert Calmette, Léon Bernard, and Robert Debré, though critics of the Bolshevik regime tried to dissuade French physicians from contributing.[112] The *Revue Franco-Russe*, with its abstracts by Russian scientists on medicine and biology, news of Russian science, and reports on the structure of Soviet medical care, targeted French readers. A planned section on Narkomzdrav and a sanitary chronicle did not materialize. But between the wars, the three major French public health journals carried only a handful of articles on Soviet public health, several of which were written by Rubakin himself.[113] Gol'denberg warned Rubakin that the *Revue Franco-Russe* must present the full range of Soviet activity—scientific, clinical, laboratory, and social medicine; otherwise it would be "no good."[114] But the strong biomedical focus corresponded to the portrait of French medical life that emerges from Rubakin's reports: the French doctor was bourgeois in his attitudes; his social concern was stirred only by the problem of tuberculosis.[115]

Creating the Loop: The Commissar Writes for Foreign Readers

In 1924, the Commissariat of Public Health began its outreach to Europe. Over an eighteen-month period, articles by Semashko appeared in the German and French press. A comparison of Semashko's German and French publications shows the commissar crafting his presentations with his representatives' readings in mind.

In 1925, in its section on public health, the German medical journal *Deutsche medizinische Wochenschrift,* ran fourteen short pieces by Semashko that showcased Soviet strength in areas of interest to Germans.[116] He led with a piece on the centralization of Soviet health care. A report to BZI on health care in Germany revealed the decentralization of German health care.[117] His pieces on epidemic control depicted the Soviets behaving responsibly: no doubt the memory of the 1922 League of Nations conference in Warsaw, which had extended the policy of cordon sanitaire to most of European Russia, was still fresh.[118] Building on Gol'denberg's information, in his discussion of Soviet work on social diseases (tuberculosis, venereal disease) Semashko highlighted Narkomzdrav's social approach to health. But he glossed over the Soviet state's commitment to the social insurance of workers, cost-free hospitals and outpatient units—perhaps because Germany's law on social insurance dated from 1883. Writing on maternal and infant care, Semashko did not mention the 1920 Soviet decree on free abortions; he knew that, except for women physicians and some socialist physicians, most German doctors opposed paragraph 218, which called for free abortion.[119]

Semashko's articles were not confined to public health. The final piece dealt with the contribution of medical science to medical care. Appended was a list of Russia's premier institutes, headed by biomedical units. All the "soft" fields—psychiatry and orthopedics, social hygiene, maternal and infancy, venereal disease—were lumped together as "practical units." Personally Semashko was committed to social hygiene. He taught the subject at I Moscow Medical Institute and wrote a brief text. He instructed BZI's representatives to send all foreign material on social hygiene to him.[120] But as commissar, Semashko saw his German publications as an opportunity to make the case for Russian medical science.

In roughly the same period, Semashko published in France a long-two part article entitled "Hygiene in Soviet Russia."[121] The article appeared not in the mainline medical press, but in the new *Revue Franco-Russe de Médecine et de biologie*, with its illustrious editorial board led by the serologist A. M. Besredka. Semashko opened the two-part article with an extensive discussion of the structure and functions of the Russian Commissariat of Public Health. With its strong organizational cast, the article was an outlier in the issue. Indeed, though Semashko's portrait appeared at the front page of the issue, his was not the lead article.

At the end of the first piece, Semashko reverted to type with a list of institutions under Narkomzdrav. The list was headed by institutes devoted to research.

As an aside, Semashko mentioned that in Russia hygiene and medicine were under one umbrella. Rubakin may well have told him that some reformers in France wanted closer links between medicine and hygiene in the education of doctors, but were wary of state intervention.[122] In detailing the role of the Soviet state in combating epidemics, the commissar noted that nurses were going into factories as well as dwellings; this reflected a degree of cooperation between the ministries of health and labor that Semashko's French counterparts might well have envied.[123]

Semashko's emphasis on Soviet medicine in France and social medicine in Germany reflected an acceptance of variation in BZI's outposts. That acceptance was writ large in BZI's 1925–26 plan, formulated in mid-1925, for the representations.[124] The plan for Germany targeted extended ties to public health circles; the plan for France called for more links to biomedical circles. In effect, the plan was an exercise in the "art of the possible" rather than a call for new directions.

The send-and-receive loops between Moscow and its Berlin and Paris outposts depended on the nature of Gol'denberg's and Rubakin's local networks. Would the German and French representatives' "read" of their local situations survive direct contact between Moscow and the "field"? The commissar's site visit to Berlin and Paris (1925) would test the German and French loops.

Moscow Calling: Semashko Visits Berlin and Paris

In October 1925, Semashko embarked on a trip to Berlin and Paris.[125] In both capitals, BZI's representatives acted as "handlers," introducing the commissar to the "right" audiences. Was Semashko's itinerary limited by the send-and-receive loops shaped by BZI's representatives? Or he did he venture "outside the box"? What impact did Semashko's first-hand reconnoitering have on the send-and-receive loops?

Germany: Creating Two Tracks

In Gol'denberg's view, Semashko's visit, which provided the first opportunity for German government ministers to meet the Soviet minister face to face, was the high point of BZI's outreach in Germany. Gol'denberg took pains to introduce the commissar to "official and social circles."[126] At a festive evening at the Soviet embassy, Semashko met informally with political and scientific leaders.[127] But for Gol'denberg, the centerpiece of the visit was the press conference that Semashko gave at the embassy on November 4, which was reported in the general and the medical press.[128] The press conference format allowed Semashko to get his message out: the USSR was instituting sanitary measures to deal with the social diseases (tuberculosis and syphilis), "milieu" diseases (exacerbated by poverty, cultural backwardness, and cramped living conditions), and infectious diseases (malaria) that confronted the country.

Semashko's visit was not simply an exercise in cultural diplomacy. The commissar met with "faculty groups and societies."[129] Sources suggest that Semashko was steered to groups sympathetic to Soviet Russia. On November 5, he addressed the Association of Socialist Doctors, a group founded in 1913.[130] Speaking to an audience that included representatives of medical science, members of parliaments, and spokesmen for medical unions, the commissar contrasted the socialist approach of Russian health care to bourgeois approaches. He acknowledged Germany as the fount of social medicine but added, "We are the best students." Answering critics who charged that Russian socialist health care was an exercise in theory, Semashko detailed the practice of Soviet health care, its organization, and its principal policies.[131] He gave a short address at a reception hosted by the Society of the Friends of New Russia, a group that included prominent figures in German arts and sciences favorably disposed to Russia. Here Semashko underscored the commissariat's belief that health care involved raising the sociocultural level of the population, not only curing disease: hence Narkomzdrav's extensive hygiene education programs. Catering to his audience, Semashko hailed the ties between Russian and German medical science.[132]

During the visit, German journals ran articles by Semashko on the Soviet health system. In *Das Neue Russland*, Semasko presented the system's core principles—its centralized organization, its commitment to prevention and cure, and its provision of insured care to the population.[133] The issue of *Der sozialistischer Arzt* that carried Semashko's address to the Association of Socialist Physicians reprinted the text of a 1924 Russian regulation on the entitlement to abortion and a notice for Semashko's recently issued book, which collected his *Deutsche Medizinische Wochenschriftt* articles of the previous year.[134] The flagship issue of the *German-Russian Medical Journal* featured an article in which Semashko explained the role of prophylaxis in Russia in a country rife with "milieu" (that is, "socioeconomic context") diseases.[135] Even the mainline German medical journal *Münchener medizinische Wochenschrift* carried a piece on Semashko's work.[136]

During his stay, Semashko managed what Gol'denberg had failed to do—namely, to open contact with German medical scientists. Friedrich Kraus, who coedited the *German-Russian Medical Journal* with Semashko, invited the commissar to give a talk to the II Medical Clinic of Charité.[137] To this audience, Semashko spoke of the tasks and achievements of the Soviet sanitary system.[138]

The way had been prepared for Semashko's opening to German medical scientists. In September 1925, during the celebrations of the two hundredth anniversary of the Russian Academy of Sciences in Leningrad, Friedrich Schmidt-Ott, head of the Notgemeinschaft der deutschen Wissenschaft, discussed with a high-level Russian delegation the possibility of joint scientific endeavors. (The delegation included Nikolai Gorbunov, head of the Department of Scientific Institutions of the Council of People's Commissars; Sergei Oldenburg, permanent secretary of the Academy of Sciences; and Anatoli Lunacharskii, the commissar of education.)[139] On October 1, 1925, Schmidt-Ott and Nikolai Gorbunov met in Berlin to discuss specific joint ventures.[140] That same month, the flagship issue of the *German-Russian Medical Journal* appeared.[141] Coedited by Semashko and Kraus, the journal had a stellar editorial board: Ludwig Aschoff (pathology), Alexei I. Abrikosov (pathology), Ludolph Brauer (internal medicine), Nikolai Burdenko (surgery), Adalbert Czerny (pediatrics), Georgii F. Lang (pathology), Otto Lubarsch (pathology), Fred Neufeld (epidemiology), Dmitri D. Pletnev (bacteriology), Lev A. Tarasevich (immunology), Hermann Thoms (pharmacy), and Grigorii I. Rossolimo (neuropsychiatry). The masthead signaled that the Russians saw themselves as suitable partners for German medical researchers.

After Semashko's visit, German-Russian cooperation in medical science grew exponentially. Medical researchers began regularly attending conferences across borders.[142] In 1926, a joint research expedition to Buriat Mongolia to study endemic syphilis went into the field.[143] Cooperation reached its peak in June 1927 with the celebration in Berlin of the Week of Soviet Science, organized by the Society for the Study of East Europe to showcase the achievements of Soviet science. Semashko headed the Russian delegation.[144]

Did the outreach to German medical researchers begun during Semashko's 1925 visit loosen the send-and-receive loop Gol'denberg had fashioned? In 1926 and the first half of 1927, Gol'denberg expanded information retrieval and dissemination in fields of public health such as occupational health[145] and intensified interaction in some fringe fields of medicine such as sexology.[146] He filled requests from Moscow for material on German research in medical science,[147] but there is no evidence that he animated or initiated contact with German medical researchers.

Consider the German-Russian syphilis expedition to Buriat Mongolia, which Gol'denberg listed among his achievements.[148] He attended a meeting of German venereologists interested in going to Russia and Russian spokesmen for science, but the negotiations that put the venture in place were carried out government to government.[149] He secured visas for two prominent German researchers who made the trip and forwarded to Moscow a copy of the report presented by the lead German researcher.[150]

Or consider Gol'denberg's pet project—the bilingual medical journal. The German medical scientists on the masthead were not part of Gol'denberg's network: Friedrich Kraus issued the invitations to join.[151] In a 1925 memorandum on the operation of the journal, Gol'denberg appeared as the translator of texts.[152] In summer 1928, when he tried to renegotiate the financing and prolong the life of the German-Russian journal, he drew criticism from Ludwig Aschoff and Oskar Vogt (with anti-Semitic overtones).[153] Lacking high-level scientific credentials, Gol'denberg was never accepted by the German scientific elite. In January 1929, Schmidt-Ott wrote Semashko to ask him to oppose all further actions by Gol'denberg regarding the journal.[154]

After Semashko's visit, a two-track connection between Berlin and Moscow emerged—one track for public health and social medicine, the other for medical science. The 1922 mandate of BZI to market both proved unworkable. In good part, the reason lay in the very strength of the networks—Gol'denberg's network in public health and the network of German medical science. But the vitality of those networks was a function of the broader landscape of German-Russian contacts, whose number and variation was encouraged by the German government as proof of Germany's *Sonderverhältnis* (special relation) with Russia.[155]

France: Switching Tracks

Semashko's visit to Paris had its own resonance. For French government ministers, meeting Semashko face to face was not necessarily a "happening." With French recognition of Soviet Russia just over a year old, Rubakin still considered relations ginger.[156] Further, because Russian monarchists were everywhere in Paris in the mid-1920s, Rubakin could not guarantee Semashko protected settings. What Rubakin could draw on were his excellent relations with the French medical elite, which largely revolved around the two French-Russian medical journals.[157]

Semashko's French visit had two high points. On October 26, 1925, "with the whole French professoriate in attendance" (Rubakin's description) Semashko delivered a talk entitled "Some Observations about Soviet Hygiene" to the medical faculty of the University of Paris.[158] The talk was sponsored by the Association for the Development of Medical Relations between France and Allied or Friendly Countries (A.D.R.M.), a broad-based association founded in 1920 to facilitate the stay in Paris of foreign doctors and medical students.[159] Sponsorship was likely arranged through Dr. M. Hartmann, president of the association's bureau, who had attended the Academy of Sciences celebration in Leningrad. The A.D.R.M minutes reveal that some members thought Hartmann should have denied Semashko a platform.[160] Rubakin reported only that Semashko's talk was controversial.

To counter the "lies and calumny" that were circulating, the editors of *Revue Franco-Russe* decided to reprint the full text of Semashko's talk. Semashko opened with the declaration that the fundamental principle of Soviet health care was the centralization of all services—not a topic Rubakin had reported as of interest in French medical circles. Despite Rubakin's information that the typical French physician was not socially conscious, Semashko referred to the social aspects of Soviet health care (the commitment to eliminate social diseases, to make the workplace healthy, to provide universal access to care, and so on). The commissar even mentioned the Soviet legalization of abortion of 1920; he almost certainly knew that in 1920 France had passed a law maintaining the criminal status of abortion and making incitement to abortion punishable by imprisonment.[161]

At the end of the talk, Semashko regained safe ground. He stressed the need to preserve the great Russian scientific institutions; in a clear crowd-pleaser, Semashko noted that many leading Soviet medical scientists had studied with the great French medical researchers.

Semashko's decision to lead with the organization of Soviet health care may have been prompted by a letter sent to the Soviet ambassador in France in December 1924 by Dr. Hervé, a member of the French Communist party and a physician with the Union of the Unitary Trade Unions of the Seine. Hervé reported that French physicians were uninterested in social issues, but were intrigued by the social organization of health care; familiarity with the Soviet approach to practical problems might persuade French physicians of the superiority of the Soviet system. Hervé appended nine pages of questions (on medical practice, social insurance, and level of hygiene) in Russia, which he urged the commissariat to distribute there and then transmit to the French Communist party for distribution among French physicians. In response, BZI instructed Rubakin to send Hervé Semashko's brochure on Soviet health care.[162] That BZI engaged with Hervé suggests its indifference to whether French physicians came to Soviet public health through socialist ideas or through the organization of health care.

Two weeks after Semashko's talk to the medical faculty, Rubakin hosted an informal dinner in his apartment with "many Frenchmen in attendance" to introduce Semashko to the head of the Rockefeller Foundation's Paris office, Selskar Gunn. In a short conversation, Semashko expressed the hope that Gunn would make a trip to Russia.[163] Rubakin had likely explained to Semashko that Rockefeller assistance was contingent on an officer's making a site visit, which required a formal invitation from the country concerned. A few days later, Rubakin paid a follow-up visit to Alan Gregg in the foundation's Paris office to urge the Rockefeller's Division of Medical Education to extend its fellowship program to Russian physicians.[164] Although securing foreign fellowships for young Russian scientists was not part of BZI's mandate, as BZI's "man" in Paris with the right contacts, Rubakin was well suited to the diplomatic follow-through. Rubakin, never modest, wrote "Our diplomats came to Paris without any personal contacts. They succeeded thanks to the representation of NKZ."[165]

In the first half year after Semashko's visit, the traffic in materials between Moscow and Paris changed. Before October 1925, Rubakin had focused on biomedicine, relying on networks in medical science that he had structured around the two bilingual journals.[166] After Semashko left, Rubakin continued, whenever possible, to advance French-Soviet connections in medical science.[167] However, Moscow now began to press for information on French sanitary education, school hygiene, industrial hygiene, social insurance, and sanitary technology and to urge the dissemination in France of Soviet materials on many of the same issues.[168] In his report of early 1927, under the heading "contacts with large circles of physicians" (that is, "public health practitioners" as opposed to the medical science elite), Rubakin explained that interest in social hygiene had increased in France.[169] When the BZI was recast as the All-Union Bureau of Foreign Sanitary Information (OBZSI) in mid-1927, the shift in the send-and-receive loop toward public health and social medicine intensified.[170]

Rubakin ceded his focus on biomedicine with reluctance. In a revealing note to BZI in March 1926, Rubakin reported that he was sending the full text of a talk on Bacille-Calmette-Guerin (BCG), the vaccine that protected against tuberculosis, delivered by Calmette to the Medical Academy. "I still think," he wrote plaintively, "that in addition to information on social medicine . . . it is important to send material on sensational discoveries in medicine."[171]

In 1926, when *Revue de Medicine et de biologie* ceased publication, the structural support for Rubakin's medical network disappeared. In early 1928, Rubakin wrote to inform Moscow that he was trying to organize a nucleus of French physicians interested in Soviet public health: members would present reports to one another on sanitary education, syphilis, tuberculosis, and abortion, and films would be shown. Rubakin would function as a resource person, not as a member of the nucleus. A handwritten note on the document quashed the idea: "Unfortunately we have no money for this."[172]

Rubakin's idea of creating a new network (without him) of public health physicians is intriguing. In 1928, he wrote to the Rockefeller Foundation of his desire to return to bacteriology! But Rubakin was casting about for ways to make himself indispensable to Moscow. When the idea to create a public health network failed, Rubakin began to write articles on public health in French periodicals. Simultaneously, he ramped up his work in cultural diplomacy, positioning himself as an intermediary between the Rockefeller Foundation and Moscow.[173] In late January 1928, Rubakin informed Moscow that Alan Gregg had written that all correspondence between Rockefeller and Moscow about fellowships should go "through us."[174] Rubakin's functions ended in August 1928, but he retained "interest" in the Rockefeller file. In early January 1929, OBZSI in Moscow received an outraged letter from the Red Cross representative who had replaced Rubakin in Paris: without consultation, Rubakin had designated a young Russian physician as a Rockefeller fellow in medical education. How was it possible, the Red Cross representative sputtered, for Rubakin to insist that everything went "through him," when the list of Russian Rockefeller nominees was to be established in Moscow by the Commissariats of Health and Education?! The Red Cross representative suggested the Rockefeller Foundation be informed that Rubakin was no longer working for the Soviets.[175] In 1929, Rubakin moved to Geneva as a consulting expert for the Health Commission of the League of Nations.

Events in Germany and France underscore the role of networks in the BZI send-and-receive system. In Germany, when Moscow's interests in medical science intensified, Gol'denberg's public health network was sidelined. In France, when Moscow shifted its interests to public health, Rubakin's network, weakened by the closing of the journals, was unable to adapt; nor could he raise the resources to create a new network. The story told here points up the personalistic character of the representatives' networks. Despite his friendship with Semashko, Gol'denberg's position was weakened by the antipathy to him of German medical researchers. Rubakin's vulnerability was increased by the resentment of his attempt to monopolize the Rockefeller contact. Ultimately, the durability of the networks was limited by the absence of structural supports.

But the landscape in which the networks were embedded also mattered. In Germany, a splay of contacts was encouraged, which made it possible to close Gol'denberg's network down without imperiling German-Russian scientific relations. In France, there was neither the time nor inclination to develop multiple lines of contact in medicine and science. The landscape (reinforced by Rubakin's insistence that all lines go "through us") encouraged a single track of contacts. When Moscow's interest shifted away from biomedicine, Rubakin's network proved useless.

Afterthoughts

Fact-finding instruments are judged by many yardsticks. Of primary importance is their ability to generate data useful to their patrons. The templates that the American philanthropies used generated an enormous body of standardized information on systems of public health and medical training that is still of interest today. In Russia, the send-and-receive loop yielded for Narkomzdrav information about local interests, cadres, and capacities that was very helpful in the commissariat's crafting of relations with foreign medical and public health researchers.

Fact-finding instruments are also judged by their "reach," or capacity to accommodate cases or data for which they were not intended. The American templates worked well for a large range of cases, but they could not accommodate the case of Russia, in which the socioeconomic surround of health differed strikingly from that of America. The data had to be bent or the frame set aside. The BZI's send-and-receive loop was designed to have a broad reach. It did succeed in engaging as information providers and disseminators reference groups with preexisting ties to Russia. But Semashko's visit revealed the limits of the loop: as a self-reinforcing instrument, it was not able to draw in new professional reference groups that were outside of the loop, uncommitted to one or the other of the products Moscow had on offer.

With hindsight, it is clear that the both the American and Russian approaches to fact-finding described above were artifacts of a particular moment in time. The American fact-finding was premised on a particular approach to "knowing the local." Enchanted by the promise of standardization, American knowing occurred from the outside in—that is, through the application of templates developed in or for the United States. The political surround of a health system was treated as "background"—a view that in itself was anything but apolitical! It may have been possible to maintain this position because the countries surveyed up to 1927 seemed more or less "like" America—though how it was possible in the wake of World War I to maintain that Germany was "like us" would be interesting to explore. During the mid-1930s, as Lion Murard tells us in his chapter, there was a shift. American foundations sounded the call to know the "local" (that is, the"foreign") from inside. Whether this shift was affected by the lessons of the Russian engagement remains to be seen.

BZI fact-finding was based on the assumption that the scientific "lay of the land" could be reliably known through the immersion in foreign parts of a single fact-finder, whose work required building up relations with the "right" (that is, well-placed and, if possible, sympathetic) interlocutors on the ground. In fashioning these networks, the fact-finders worked around existing institutions in the host country, creating groupings of informants that were rarely structurally based. The networks and the send-and-receive loops they spawned varied perforce with place. By the onset of the 1930s, the heterogeneity in relations with the outside world that marked BZI's work was a thing of the past. In its place came the planned information-gathering and tightly managed dissemination of the facts that were so much a part of the post–World War II trope about Russia's relations with the outside world.

Notes

1. J. C. Scott, *Seeing Like a State: How Certain Schemes to Improve Mankind Have Failed* (New Haven: Yale University Press, 1998).

2. S. G. Solomon, "Fact Finding and Policy Making: The Rockefeller Foundation's Division of Medical Education and the 'Russian Matter,' 1925–1927," *Journal of Policy History* 14 (2002): 384–417.

3. E. Crawford, "Internationalism in Science as a Casualty of World War I," *Social Science Information* 27 (1988): 163–201; B. Schroeder-Gudehus, *Les scientifiques et la paix: La communauté scientifique internationale au cours des années 20* (Montreal: Presse de l'Universite de Montréal, 1978).

4. All commissariats (ministries) existed only at the republican level until the USSR was formed in 1923. The first constitution (1924) allocated jusrisdiction over some areas of policy to commissariats at the federal or All-Union level (e.g., defense and foreign policy), but most areas of domestic policy remained in the hands of republican commissariats only. Hence for the period covered by this essay, the most important agency in the health field was the Russian Commissariat of Public Health. At the same time spokesmen for that Commissariat and their interlocutors in government and research institutions routinely referred to Soviet public health.

5. See the essays in M. Bulmer et al., eds., *The Social Survey in Historical Perspective, 1880–1940* (Cambridge: Cambridge University Press, 1991); G. Harp, *Positivist Republic: Auguste Comte and the Reconstruction of American Liberalism, 1865–1920* (University Park: Pennsylvania State University Press, 1995).

6. J. Smith, *The Idea Brokers: Think Tanks and the Rise of the New Policy Elite* (New York: Free Press, 1991), 41.

7. See the essays in N. Rupke, ed., *Medical Geography in Historical Perspective* (London: Wellcome Trust Centre of the History of Medicine at UCL, 2000).

8. W. R. Mead, *Special Providence: American Foreign Policy and How It Changed the World* (New York: Knopf, 2001).

9. D. Rogers, *Atlantic Crossings: Social Politics in a Progressive Age* (Cambridge, MA: Harvard University Press, 1998), 4; L. Murard, "Atlantic Crossings in the Measurement of Health: From American Appraisal Forms to the League of Nations Health Indices, 1915–1955," in *Medicine, the Mass Market and the Mass Media in the 20th Century*, ed. V. Berridge and K. Loughlin, 19–54 (London: Routledge, 2005).

10. In 1990, Russian scholars began again to write of an undifferentiated "West" in relation to Russia. *Rossiia i Zapad: Formirovanie vneshnopoliticheskikh stereotipov v soznanii rossiiskogo obshchestva pervoi poloviny XX veka* (Moscow: Russian Academy of Sciences, 1998).

11. C. Lawrence, *Rockefeller Money, the Laboratory, and Medicine in Edinburgh, 1919–1930: New Science in an Old Country* (Rochester, NY: University of Rochester Press, 2005); J. Sealander, *Private Wealth and Public Life* (Baltimore: Johns Hopkins University Press, 1997); E. Condliffe Lagemann, *The Politics of Knowledge: The Carnegie Corporation, Philanthropy, and Public Policy* (Middletown, CT: Wesleyan University Press, 1989).

12. M. Cueto, "Visions of Science and Development: The Rockefeller Foundation's Latin American Surveys of the 1920s," in *Missionaries of Science: The Rockefeller Foundation and Latin America*, ed. M. Cueto, 1–22 (Bloomington: Indiana University Press, 1994).

13. A. Flexner, *Medical Education in the United States and Canada: A Report to the Carnegie Foundation for the Advancement of Teaching* (New York: Carnegie Foundation for the Advancement of Teaching, 1910).

14. W. Schneider, "The Men Who Followed Flexner: Richard Pearce, Alan Gregg, and the Rockefeller Foundation Medical Divisions, 1919–1951," in *Rockefeller Philanthropy and Modern Biomedicine*, ed. W. Schneider (Bloomington: Indiana University Press, 2002), 18.

15. For the model, see R. Fosdick, *The Story of the Rockefeller Foundation*, 93–123 (New York: Harper & Bros., 1952).

16. S. G. Solomon and N. Krementsov, "Giving and Taking Across National Borders: The Rockefeller Foundation in Russia, 1921–1927," *Minerva* 39 (2001): 265–98.

17. George E. Vincent diary, interview with Richard Pearce, May 1, 1925, RG 12.1, Rockefeller Archive Center, Tarrytown, NY (hereafter RAC).

18. Medical Education in Russia, vol. 2, 71, 785 A Rus, RAC. For the Bolshevik innovations in medical training, see S. G. Solomon, "Social Hygiene in Soviet Medical Schools, 1922–1930," *Journal of the History of Medicine and Allied Sciences* 45 (1990): 153–221.

19. W. Penfield, *The Difficult Art of Giving* (Boston: Little Brown, 1967), 158.

20. Medical Education in Russia, vol. 1, A. Gregg's travel diary, 785 A Rus, RAC.

21. Gregg diary, December 6, 1927, 12.1, RAC.

22. Gregg diary, December 6, 1927.

23. See E. Fee, "Designing Schools for Health in the United States," in *A History of Education in Public Health*, ed. E. Fee and R. Acheson, 155–94 (Oxford: Oxford University Press, 1991); J. Farley, *To Cast Out Disease: A History of the International Health Division of the Rockefeller Foundation, 1913–1951* (Oxford: Oxford University Press, 2004); S. G. Solomon, "Through a Glass Darkly: The Rockefeller Foundation's International Health Board and Soviet Public Health," *Studies in History and Philosophy of Biomedical Science* 31 (2000): 409–18.

24. Gregg made a similar criticism of Jacques Parisot's emphasis on prevention. I am grateful to Lion Murard for this point.

25. A. Gregg, "Russian Report," Rockefeller Foundation 1927–1929, Gregg papers, Box 25, National Library of Medicine Archives, Washington, DC.

26. A. Gregg, "Report on Medical Education in Russia," *Medical Education in Russia*, vol. 1 (1927), 1, 785 A Rus, RAC.

27. Gregg, "Report on Medical Education," 21, 22.

28. Gregg, "Report on Medical Education," 48.

29. The Milbank Memorial Fund, created in 1905 by Elizabeth Milbank Anderson, was dedicated to the "improvement in the general level of public health and public welfare through the translation into practical usefulness of knowledge sustained by scientific research and through the demonstration of principles confirmed by experience." C. Kiser, *The Milbank Memorial Fund* (New York: Milbank Memorial Fund, 1975).

30. J. Eyler, *Sir Arthur Newsholme and State Medicine, 1885–1935* (Cambridge: Cambridge University Press, 1997), 359.

31. For the discussions, see B. Hoffman, *The Wages of Sickness: The Politics of Health Insurance in Progressive America* (Chapel Hill: University of North Carolina Press, 2001).

32. "The New York State Health Demonstrations in Syracuse and in Cattaraugus County," *Milbank Memorial Fund Quarterly Bulletin* 4 (1926): 49–66. For the protests, see Eyler, *Sir Arthur Newsholme and State Medicine*, 359; J. Kingsbury, foreword to *International Studies in the Relation between the Private and Official Practice of Medicine, with Special Reference to the Prevention of Disease*, by A. Newsholme (London: Allen & Unwin, 1931).

33. L. Farrand, "The Philosophy of Health Demonstrations," *American Journal of Public Health* 17 (1927, supplement): 3–4.

34. Eyler, *Sir Arthur Newsholme and State Medicine*, 360.

35. Newsholme, *International Studies in the Relation between the Private and Official Practice of Medicine*. For "structured, focused" research, see A. George, "Case Studies and Theory Development: The Method of Structured Focused Comparison," in *Diplomacy: New Approaches in History, Theory, and Policy*, ed. Paul Gordon Lauren, 27–42 (New York: Free Press, 1979).

36. Eyler, *Sir Arthur Newsholme and State Medicine*, 360–61.

37. A. Newsholme, *Medicine and the State, The Relation between the Practice and Official Practice of Medicine, With Special Reference to Public Health* (London: Allen & Unwin, 1932).

38. A. Newsholme and J. Kingsbury, *Red Medicine: Socialized Health Care in Soviet Russia* (New York: Doubleday, 1933), 2.

39. J. Kingsbury to A. Newsholme, June 23, 1932, Kingsbury Papers, Part II, Box 76 (hereafter II/76), Library of Congress, Manuscript Division, Washington, DC (hereafter JAK, LC).

40. See S. G. Solomon, "The Intermediary as Strategist: John A. Kingsbury, Soviet Socialized Medicine, and 1930s America," (unpublished manuscript).

41. See the biographical notes in JAK, LC, I; A. Viseltear, "Compulsory Health Insurance and the Definition of Public Health," in *Compulsory Health Insurance: The Continuing American Debate*, ed. R. Numbers, 25–55 (Westport, CT: Greenwood Press, 1982).

42. Eyler, *Sir Arthur Newsholme and State Medicine*.

43. C. Ragin, "Turning the Tables: How Case-Oriented Research Challenges Variable-Oriented Research," *Comparative Social Research* 16 (1997): 67–72.

44. V. Freeburg to V. Yakhontoff, July 15, 1932, JAK, II/75, LC.

45. Newsholme and Kingsbury, *Red Medicine*, 29–57.

46. Newsholme and Kingsbury, *Red Medicine*, 5.

47. J. Kingsbury to A. Newsholme, January 23, 1933, JAK, II/76, LC.

48. Newsholme and Kingsbury, *Red Medicine*, 189.

49. Newsholme and Kingsbury, *Red Medicine*, 189.

50. J. Kingsbury to A. Newsholme, January 26, 1933, JAK, II/76, LC.

51. A. Milbank to J. Kingsbury, May 9, 1933, JAK, II/75, LC.

52. Committee on the Costs of Medical Care, *Medical Care for the American People: The Final Report* (Chicago: University of Chicago Press, 1932).

53. Newsholme and Kingsbury, *Red Medicine*, 276–77.

54. Newsholme and Kingsbury, *Red Medicine*, 294, 295, and 309.

55. For the dismissal, see Solomon, "The Intermediary as Strategist."

56. *Rasporiazhenie No. 208*, March 14, 1920, Gosudarstvennyi arkhiv Rossiiskoi Federatsii, Moscow f. A 482, op. 42, d. 2506, l. 4 (hereafter GARF).

57. "Kharakter raboty predstavitel'stv Narkomzdravov," undated, unsigned memorandum, GARF f. A 482, op. 35, d. 253, l. 33–34 ob. Likely date is 1927; probable author was Ia. R. Gol'denberg.

58. N. Semashko to B. Biderman and E. Zigfrid, dated 1922 (month and day illegible), GARF f. A 482, op. 41, d. 18, l. 134. The French, German, and American representations were independent; in Switzerland and Italy, BZI functions were carried out by the Red Cross representatives. Memo, October 1922, GARF f. A 482, op. 35, d. 2, l. 3.

59. I. Kalina to Ia. R. Gol'denberg et al., May 14, 1923, GARF f. A 482, op. 35, d. 58, l. 244. The volume was *Piat' Let Sovetskoi Meditsiny 1918–1923* (Moscow: Narodnyi Kommissariat Zdravookhraneniia, 1923).

60. See D. J. Dallin, *Soviet Espionage* (New Haven: Yale University Press, 1955).

61. F. C. Barghoorn, *Soviet Foreign Propaganda* (Princeton, NJ: Princeton University Press, 1964); F. C. Barghoorn, *The Soviet Cultural Offensive* (Princeton, NJ: Princeton University Press, 1960).

62. E. S. Rosenberg, *Spreading the American Dream: American Economic and Cultural Expansion, 1890–1945* (New York: Hill and Wang, 1942); A. Dubosclard, "Diplomatie culturelle et propaganda aux États-Unis pendant le premier vingtième siècle," *Revue d'historie moderne et contemporaine 48* (2001): 102–19.

63. In autobiographical notes prepared for submission to the Party Control Commission of the Central Committee on May 12, 1944, shortly after he was repatriated to Russia, BZI's representative in France, A. N. Rubakin, reported that while he was working in Geneva from 1929 to 1932 for the Health Organization of the League of Nations, he "informed" on the activities of the League at the request of Valerian Dovgalevskii, the Soviet political representative to France, and of Aleksandr Arosev, the Soviet Ambassador to Prague. Rossiiskii gosudarstvennyi arkhiv sotsial'no-politicheskoi istorii, Moscow (hereafter RGASPI), Archives of the Communist International, f. 495, op. 270, d. 1371, l. 12. Given the addressee of the autobiographical notes and his eagerness to be treated as a member of the Russian Communist Party, Rubakin may have exaggerated his covert activity much as he did other aspects of his career abroad.

64. For example, the apartment of the German representative in Berlin was searched in April of 1922. Protests from the Russian Political Representative to the German Foreign Office followed. See R 83884 (IV Russland Rechtswesen 8: Recht der Extraterritorialen) June 21, 1922, Auswärtiges Amt, Politisches Archiv, Berlin

(hereafter AA Pol Arch). Low level, intermittent surveillance continued, but no further incidents occurred. For the surveillance of the French representative, which was also low level, see May 22, 1926, F/7/13496, Archives Nationales, Paris.

65. "Proekt polozheniia ob otdele zagranichnoi informatsii Narkomzdrava," November 11, 1922, GARF f. A 482, op. 1, d. 528.

66. The previous version was drawn up in October: GARF f. A 482, op. 35, d. 2, l. 3–5.

67. In 1921, BZI had a head, a deputy head, an administrator, and a typist, but no translator: Memo, GARF f. A 482, op. 35, d. 2, l. 5. Each foreign representation had a head, a secretary, and a typist: Memo, GARF f. A 482, op. 41, d. 1b, l. 134.

68. V. Knoll, "Das Volkskommissariat für auswärtige Angelegenheiten im Prozess aussenpolitischer Entscheidungsfindung in den zwanziger und dreissiger Jahren," in *Zwischen Tradition und Revolution: Determinanten und Strukturen sowjetischer Aussenpolitik, 1917–1941*, ed. L. Thomas and V. Knoll, 73–156 (Stuttgart: Steiner, 2000); M. David-Fox, "From Illusory 'Society' to Intellectual 'Public': VOKS, International Travel, and Party-Intelligentsia Relations in the Interwar Period," *Contemporary European History* 11 (2002): 7–32.

69. "Proekt sokrashcheniia smety predstavitel'stv OBZSI do kontsa biudzhetnogo goda," GARF f. A 482, op. 35, d. 253, l. 8. "V Obshchesoiuznoe Biuro Zagranichnoi Sanitarnoi Informatsii," GARF f. A 482, op. 35, d. 253, l. 15–16.

70. P. Weindling, "German Overtures to Russia, 1919–1925: Between Racial Expansion and National Co-existence," in *Doing Medicine Together: Germany and Russia between the Wars*, ed. S. G. Solomon (Toronto: University of Toronto Press, 2006).

71. "Dokladnaia zapiska o deiatel'nosti predstavitel'stva Narkomzdrava v Berline" (undated, likely 1923), GARF f. A 482, op. 35, d. 48, l. 6, 3–4. In November 1925, the representation moved from Lindenstrasse 25 to Unter den Linden 68a. Ia. R. Gol'denberg to BZI, November 21, 1925, GARF f. A 482, op. 35, d. 128, l. 7. This move brought the representation into the Russian Embassy complex. K. Schloegel, *Berlin Ostbahnhof Europas* (Berlin: Seidler, 1998), 117–18.

72. Memo, August 11, 1921, GARF f. A 482, op. 41, d. 16, l. 49; B. Souvarine to N. Semashko, August 4, 1921, GARF f. A 482, op. 41, d. 16, l. 51.

73. "Lichnyi listok No. 1," signed by Ia. R. Gol'denberg, November 2, 1924, GARF f. A 482, op. 41, d. 769, l. 3.

74. "Dokladnaia zapiska," GARF f. A 482, op. 35, d. 48, l. 9.

75. B. Biderman to Ia. R. Gol'denberg, March 3, 1923, GARF f. A 482, op. 35, d. 57, l. 87; Ia. R. Gol'denberg to Moscow, March 22, 1923, GARF f. A 482, op. 35, d. 57, l. 199. For Gol'denberg's "quality control," see Ia. R. Gol'denberg to Editorial Board, July 16, 1924, GARF f. A 482, op. 35, d. 87, l. 9–10.

76. So deep were the ties that when Gol'denberg was accused of malfeasance, Semashko wrote to defend him, citing their long acquaintance and Gol'denberg's exemplary record of service to the Party. N. Semashko to L. Kaganovich, October 1923, GARF f. A 482, op. 41, d. 769, l. 16.

77. N. Krestinskii to N. Semashko, August 16, 1928, GARF f. A 482, op. 41, d. 769. l. 25–28. The letter was stamped "Sekretnyi organ administrativnogo upravleniia NKZdrava RSFSR."

78. Memo, GARF f. A 482, op. 35, d. 261, l. 62; Order, GARF f. A 482, op. 41, d. 769, l. 31.

79. "Dopolnenie k otchetu o deiatel'nosti predstavitel'stva Narkomzdrava v Germanii," July 29, 1924, GARF f. A 482, op. 35, d. 80, l. 111.

80. "Dokladnaia zapiska" (undated, but internal indications suggest late 1922 or early 1923), GARF f. A 482, op. 35, d. 48, l. 6. For German interest in social medicine, see "Obshchii obzor deiatel'nosti predstavitel'stva NKZ za 5-tu letnii period," GARF f. A 482, op. 35, d. 162, l. 29.

81. "Lichnyi Listok No. 1," signed by Ia. R. Gol'denberg, November 2, 1924, GARF f. A 482, op. 41, d. 769. l. 1–3.

82. J. Gol'denberg, "Das Problem der Gesundung der Arbeit in Russland," *Das Neue Russland* 1, no. 3/4 (1924): 22–25; J. Gol'denberg, "Das Sexualleben des Kindes und die soziale Umgebung," *Die neue Generation*, 1926, no. 5, 137–39. For Gol'denberg's talk to the Society of Friends of the New Russia, see GARF f. A 482, op. 35, d. 85, l. 263–264.

83. "Dopolnenie," GARF f. A 482, op. 35, d. 80, l. 113.

84. To illustrate, in just a ten-day period in May 1925, Gol'denberg (or his assistant Binger) sent to Moscow minutes of a meeting of the Berlin Society of Social Health Care and a draft of the German Act on the Protection of Mothers and Children. See GARF f. A 482, op. 35, d. 126, l. 247; GARF f. A 482, op. 35, d. 127, l. 504.

85. See the essays in Solomon, *Doing Medicine Together*.

86. Ia. R. Gol'denberg to BZI, February 7, 1923, GARF f. A 482, op. 35, d. 57, l. 62; M. Hirsch to Ia. R. Gol'denberg, February 27, 1923, GARF f. A 482, op. 35, d. 57, l. 96–98.

87. E. Biderman to Ia. R. Gol'denberg, April 13, 1923, GARF f. A 482, op. 35, d. 57, l. 192.

88. J. Gol'denberg, "Wege und Ausblick der Zusammenarbeit Deutschlands und Sowjetrusslands auf dem Gebiete der Gesundheitspflege," *Osteuropa* 2 (1926/1927): 474–81; J. Gol'denberg, "Zusammenarbeit der deutschen und sowjetischen Medizin," *Deutsch-Russische Medizinsche Zeitschrift* 4 (1928): 562–64.

89. "Deiatel'nost predstavitel'stva Narkomzdrava v Germanii s dekabria 1923 po iiul' 1924," GARF f. A 482, op. 35, d. 702, ch. 2, l. 269.

90. "Protokol soveshchaniia komissii po peresmotru dogovora ob izdanii v Germanii zhurnala Folia Medica," GARF f. A 482, op. 35. d. 85, l. 276.

91. "Otchet predstavitel'stva Narkomzdrava za 1925–1926g.," undated, GARF f. A 482, op. 35, d. 162, l. 46. For the agreement establishing the journal, see "Russische Zeitschrift," GARF f. A 482, op. 35, d. 125, l. 347–348. For the difficulties in getting articles, see "Dokladnaia zapiska Narkomu N. A. Semashko o propagandistko-informatsionnoi rabote pr-va NKZ v Germanii," GARF f. A 482, op. 35, d. 702, ch. 1, l. 185.

92. A. Hogenhuis-Seliverstoff, *Les relations franco-soviétiques*, 1917–1924 (Paris: Publications de la Sorbonne, 1981).

93. Letters from A. N. Rubakin to Ia. R. Gol'denberg, dated from March 22 to 31, 1923, GARF f. A 482, op. 35, d. 57, l. 199–201.

94. A. N. Rubakin, "Kratkii otchet o deiatel'nosti predstavitel'stva Narkomzdrava Narkomzdrava [sic] vo Frantsii," January 1927, GARF f. A 482, op. 35, d. 162, l. 15–17.

95. S. Gunn to F. F. Russell, November 13, 1925, Record Group 5, Series 1.2, Box 238, Folder 3052, RAC.

96. A. N. Rubakin to Kalina, March 20, 1925, GARF f. A 482, op. 35, d. 131, l. 146.

97. A. N. Rubakin, Avtobiografii, No. 1 (undated), Manuscript Division, Russian State Library (hereafter MD/RSL) f. 358 (Rubakin), 494.1.

98. Letter, B. Volin to N. Semashko, March 23, 1925, GARF f. A 482, op. 35, d. 131, l. 145; Soviet Embassy to Ministry of Foreign Affairs, September 7, 1925, Z6482, Archives du Ministère des Affaires Etrangères, Paris (hereafter AMAE); A. N. Rubakin to I. Kalina, March 20, 1925, GARF f. A 482, op. 35, d. 131, l. 146.

99. Letter from A. N. Rubakin to his father, July 15, 1927, MD/RSL f. 358 (Rubakin), 268.42, l. 31.

100. D. O'Brien diaries, August 17, 1928, RG 12.1, RAC. In his memoirs, Rubakin claimed to have run a bacteriological laboratory in Paris; no confirmation was found. "Vospominaniia Errio vosstanovlenie sviazei mezhdu SSSR i Frantsii," MD/RSL f. 358 (N. A. Rubakin), 496.11.

101. S. Munier to L. Rajchman, December 30, 1930, R 5911, 8a/ 12358, League of Nations Archives, Geneva.

102. A. Roubakine, "Avortement, problème sociale, et sa solution dans l'Union des Républiques socialistes soviétiques," *Annales de Médecine Légale* 9 (1929): 153–68; A. Roubakine, "La réforme de l'enseignement de la médecine dans L'Union des républiques socialistes soviétiques," *Revue d'hygiène et de médecine sociales*, March–April 1931, 69–80.

103. R. A. Lambert diaries, October 28, 1932, RG 12.1, RAC; A. N. Rubakin to J. A. Kingsbury, November 22, 1933, JAK, II/18, LC. Rubakin's book was published as A. N. Roubakine, *La protection de la santé publique dans l'URSS, principes et résultats* (Paris: Bureau d'éditions, 1933).

104. For Rubakin's memoirs of his years in France, see A. N. Rubakin, *Frantsuzskie zapisi, 1939–1943* (Moscow: Sovetskii pisatel,' 1947). For Kingsbury's offer, see H. H. Ripley to Department of State, September 15, 1942, JAK, II/18, LC.

105. For Rubakin's liberation, see A. N. Rubakin to J. A. Kingsbury, May 25, 1945, JAK, II/18, LC. I Moscow Medical Institute was formed in 1930 from the medical faculty of the Imperial Moscow University, which dates back to 1758.

106. For French-Russian contact in this period, see S. Coeuré, *La grande lueur á l'Est: Les Français et l'Union soviétique 1917–1929* (Paris: Seuill, 1999).

107. "Biulleten' predstavitel'stva Narkomzdrava RSFSR vo Frantsii, no. 5, aprel'–maia 1927 g.," GARF f. A 482, op. 35, d. 209, l. 98–105.

108. "Kratkii otchet o deiatel'nosti predstavitel'stva Narkomzdrava Narkomzdrava [sic] vo Frantsii," GARF f. A 482, op. 35, d. 162, l. 1.

109. A. N. Rubakin to N. A. Semashko, April 1925 (day not indicated), GARF f. A 482, op. 35, d. 431, l. 137–140.

110. "Préface de la Rédaction," *Revue franco-russe de médecine et de biologie* 1 (1924): 2–3.

111. A. N. Rubakin to N. A. Semashko, April 20, 1925, GARF f. A 482, op. 35, d. 131, l. 137–140.

112. "Kratkii otchet o deiatel'nosti predstavitel'stva Narkomzdrava Narkomzdrava [sic] vo Franstsii," January 1927, GARF f. A 482, op. 35, d. 162, ch. 1, l. 120. For the campaign against the journal, see member of the editorial board to Ia. R. Gol'denberg, October 28, 1924, GARF f. A 482, op. 35, d. 87, l. 236–237.

113. Editorial board of *Revue franco-russe* to editors of *Vrachebnaia gazeta*, August 1924, GARF f. A 482, op. 35, d. 87, l. 17–19, 110–112; L. Murard and P. Zylberman,

"French Social Medicine on the Map of International Public Health in the 1930s," in *The Politics of the Healthy Life: An International Perspective*, ed. E. Rodriguez Ocaña, 197–218 (Sheffield: European Association for the History of Medicine and Health Publications, 2002).

114. Letter, Ia. R. Gol'denberg to editorial board of *Revue franco-russe*, June 26, 1924, GARF f. A 482, op. 35, d. 87, l. 9–10.

115. "Kratkii otchet o deiatel'nosti predstavitel'stva Narkomzdrava Narkomzdrava [sic] vo Franstsii," January 1927, GARF f. A 482, op. 35, d. 162, ch. 1, l. 118, 121.

116. N. Semaschko, "Das Gesundheitswesen in Sowjetrussland," *Deutsche medizinische Wochenschrift*, 1925, no. 4: 117–19; no. 7: 213–14; no. 8: 243–44; no. 11: 344–45; no. 17: 545–46; no. 18: 581–82; no. 22: 722–23; no. 27: 923–24; no. 32: 1090–92; no. 37: 1251–53; no. 46: 1587–88; no. 51: 1807–9.

117. A report on health care in Germany, one of the series of country reports prepared for BZI in 1921, stressed decentralization. See GARF f. A 482, op. 35, d. 131, l. 40–42.

118. P. Weindling, *Epidemics and Genocide in Eastern Europe, 1890–1945* (Oxford: Oxford University Press, 2000), 168–71.

119. For German attitudes to Soviet policy on abortion, see S. G. Solomon, "The Soviet Legalization of Abortion in German Medical Discourse: A Study of the Use of Selective Perceptions in Cross-Cultural Scientific Relations," *Social Studies of Science* 22 (1992): 455–87.

120. N. A. Semashko, *Nauka o zdorov'e obshchestva* (Moscow, 1921). For Semashko's directive to the representatives, see GARF f. A 482, op. 35, d. 58, l. 357.

121. N. A. Semachko, "L'hygiène en Russie soviétique," *Revue franco-russe de médecine et de biologie* 2 (1924): 10–16. N. A. Semachko, "L'hygiène en Russie soviétique II," *Revue franco-russe de médecine et de biologie* 2 (1925): 9–15.

122. For Rubakin's written analysis of the relation between French doctors and the state, see "Raskol sredi frantsuzskikh sindikatov vrachei" (undated, likely late 1925), GARF f. A 482, op. 35, d. 131, l. 38, 48–49.

123. Semachko, "L'hygiène en Russie soviétique II."

124. "Plan rabot na 1925–1926 gody," GARF f. A 482, op. 35, d. 207, l. 65–69.

125. The visit was arranged in September 1925, when German scientists and science administrators attended the celebration of the two hundredth anniversary of the founding of the Russian Academy of Sciences in Leningrad. Karl-Heinz Karbe, "N. A. Semaschko und die deutsch-sowjetischen Wissenschaftsbeziehungen auf dem Gebiet des Gesundheitswesen," *Das Deutsche Gesundheitswesen* 22 (1967): 2072–77.

126. "Otchet predstavitel'stva Narkomzdrava za 1925–1926g.," GARF f. A 482, op. 35, d. 162, l. 47.

127. L. Brauer to N. A. Semashko, January 5, 1926, GARF f. A 482, op. 35, d. 129, l. 263–263 ob.

128. See "Das Gesundheitswesen in Russland," *Berliner Tageblatt*, November 5, 1925, 2. Coverage of the press conference was limited to one paragraph.

129. "Otchet predstavitel'stva Narkomzdrava za 1925–1926g.," GARF f. A 482, op. 35, d. 162, l. 47.

130. For the links between the association and Soviet health, see Christine Böttcher, *Das Bild der sowjetischen Medizin in der ärztlichen Publizistik und Wissenschaftspolitik der Weimarer Republik* (Pfaffenweiler: Centaurus, 1998), 233–62.

131. N. Semaschko, "Sozialistische Gesichtspunkte im Gesundheitswesen Russlands," *Der Sozialistische Arzt* 1, no. 4 (1925): 1–8. For the blue-ribbon audience, see "Semaschkovortrag," *Der Sozialistische Arzt* 1, no. 4 (1925): 53.

132. N. Semaschko, "Ansprache bei dem Empfang der Ärzte und Gelehrten in der 'Gesellschaft der Freunde des neuen Russland,'" *Das Neue Russland* 3, no. 9/10 (1925): 13–14.

133. N. Semaschko, "Sowjetmedizin und Volkshygiene," *Das Neue Russland* 3, no. 9/10 (1925): 12–13.

134. "Rundschreiben des Volkskommissariats für Gesundheitswesen Nr. 221 vom 3. November 1924," *Der Sozialistischer Arzt* 1, no. 4 (1925): 42–43; for the book review, see ibid., 55.

135. N. Semaschko, "Die prophylaktische Richtung in der Sowjetmedizin," *Deutsch-Russische Medizinische Zeitschrift* 1 (1925): 14–16.

136. "Der Volkskommissar für Gesundheitswesen Professor Dr. Semaschko und sein Werk," *Münchener Medizinische Wochenschrift* 72, no. 37 (1925): 2123–24.

137. F. Kraus to E. Bumm, president of the Reichsgesundheitsamt, October 31, 1925, R86, Nr 17, vol. 8, Bundesarchiv Koblenz (hereafter BAK). The talk was given some time before November 4.

138. N. Semaschko, "Das Gesundheitswesen in Russland," 2.

139. "Eine Verständigung zwischen der russischen und deutschen Wissenschaft," R9215, Nr 396, 137–8, Bundesarchiv Berlin (hereafter BAB). See Marina Sorokina, "Partners of Choice/*Faute de /Mieux*? Russians and Germans at the 200th anniversary of the Academy of Sciences, 1925," in *Doing Medicine Together*, ed. Solomon, 61–102.

140. "Unterhaltung zwischen Excellenz Schmidt-Ott und Herrn Gorbunoff," R9215, Nr 396, 131–36, BAB.

141. The first issue appeared on October 28, 1925: GARF f. A 482, op. 35, d. 128, l. 6.

142. Gol'denberg sent a list of programs for upcoming conferences that Soviet researchers might attend. Ia. R. Gol'denberg to BZI, March 1926, GARF f. A 482, op. 35, d. 129, l. 79–80.

143. See S. G. Solomon, "Das Reisetagebuch als Quelle für die Analyse binationaler medizinischer Unternehmungen," in *Lues, Lamas, Leninisten: Tagebuch einer Reise durch Russland in die Burjatische Republik im Sommer 1926*, ed. J. Richter, 1–42 (Pfaffenweiler: Centaurus, 1995).

144. L. Brussilowskii to F. Schmidt-Ott, June 25, 1927, Schmidt-Ott, Nr 47, Rep 92, 130–32, Geheimes Staatsarchiv, Stiftung Preussischer Kulturbesitz (Berlin-Dahlem) (hereafter Geheimes Staatsarchiv); F. Schmidt-Ott to Ia. R. Gol'denberg, June 30, 1925, Schmidt-Ott, Nr 47, Rep 92, 138–140, Geheimes Staatsarchiv; F. Schmidt-Ott, "Die Russische Forscherwoche in Berlin" (undated), Schmidt-Ott, Nr 47, Rep 92, 153–56, Geheimes Staatsarchiv.

145. See Memo, Ia. R. Gol'denberg to BZI, March 31, 1926, GARF f. A 482, op. 35, d. 129, l. 69; Letter, L. Teleky to Narkomzdrav, December 5, 1925, GARF f. A 482, op. 35, d. 124, l. 14.

146. Gol'denberg sent to Moscow a review of G. Batkis's book on sexology: GARF f. A 482, op. 35, d. 129, l. 303–304. He also transmitted correspondence from Magnus Hirschfeld to Semashko. M. Hirschfeld to Ia. R. Gol'denberg, January 29, 1926, GARF f. A 482, op. 35, d. 129, l. 229–230.

147. See Memo, BZI to Dr. Goldenberg, April 12, 1926, GARF f. A 482, op. 35, d. 129, l. 50.

148. "Otchet predstavitel'stva Narkomzdrava za 1925–1926," GARF f. A 482, op. 35, d. 162, l. 48.

149. F. Schmidt-Ott to U. Brockdorf Rantzau, March 18, 1926, 09. 02. Nr. 417, BAP.

150. See Memo, Ia. R. Gol'denberg to BZI, April 23, 1926, GARF f. A 482, op. 35, d. 129, l. 48; "Reziume doklada Prof. Karla Vilmannsa/Geidelberg na Kongresse v Kassele," GARF f. A 482, op. 35, d. 129. l. 306–308.

151. F. Kraus to Ia. R. Gol'denberg, August 12, 1922, GARF f. A 482, op. 35, d. 125, l. 358.

152. See GARF f. A 482, op. 35, d. 125, l. 346–348.

153. F. Schmidt-Ott to O. Vogt, July 20, 1928, R73, 224, BAK; F. Schmidt-Ott to N. A. Semashko, July 24, 1928, R73, Nr 224, BAK; "Aktennotiz," undated, signed by Siegesmund, R 73, Nr 224, BAK. For the anti-Semitic comment, see O. Vogt to L. Aschoff, May 31, 1928, Ordner 58, Nachlass Vogt (Dusseldorf).

154. F. Schmidt-Ott to N. A. Semashko, January 15, 1929, R73, Nr 224, BAK.

155. For the ideology behind the *Sonderverhältnis* and its impact on German-Russian relations, see S. G. Solomon, introduction to *Doing Medicine Together*, 8–9.

156. "Kratkii otchet o deiatel'nosti predstavitel'stva Narkomzdrava Narkomzdrava [sic] vo Frantsii," January 1927, GARF f. A 482, op. 35, d. 162, l. 1.

157. A. N. Rubakin to N. A. Semashko, April (date obscured), 1925, GARF f. A 482, op. 35, d. 131, l. 136–139.

158. N. A. Semashko, "Quelques apercus de l'Hygiene sovietique," *Revue Franco-Russe de médicine et de biologie* 2 (1926): 1–13.

159. Association pour le Développement des Relations Médicales entre la France et les Pays Alliés ou Amis (A.D.R.M.), *Compte-Rendu de L'Assemblée Générale Annuelle* 17 *Novembre* 1924 (Auxerre: Tridon, 1925), 18.

160. *Compte-Rendu de L'Assemblée Générale Annuelle*, 19; "Kratkii otchet o deiatel'nosti predstavitel'stva Narkomzdrava Narkomzdrava [sic] vo Frantsii," GARF f. A 482, op. 35, d. 162, l. 3–4.

161. B. M. Knoppers et al., "Abortion Law in Francophone Countries," *American Journal of Comparative Law* 38, no. 4 (1990): 384.

162. "Exposé des motifs," GARF f. A 482, op. 35, d. 131, l. 151–153; "La vie pratique courante," GARF f. A 482, op. 35. d. 131, l. 154–162. For the reply from Moscow, see I. Kalina to E. Zigfrid, March 21, 1925, GARF f. A 482, op. 35, d. 131, l. 147.

163. S. Gunn to F. F. Russell, November 13, 1925, Record Group 5, Series 1.2, Box 238, Folder 3052, RAC.

164. A. Gregg diary, November 23, 1925, RG 12.1, RAC.

165. "Kratkii otchet o deiatel'nosti predstavitel'stva Narkomzdrava Narkomzdrava [sic] vo Frantsii," January 1927, GARF f. A 482, op. 35, d. 162, l. 118.

166. "Kratkii otchet o deiatel'nosti predstavitel'stva Narkomzdrava Narkomzdrava [sic] vo Frantsii," GARF f. A 482, op. 35, d. 162, l. 120.

167. BZI to A. N. Rubakin, January 26, 1926, GARF f. A 482, op. 35, d. 132, l. 159. The letter records Rubakin's contact with Besredka in Paris.

168. See Rubakin's requests to BZI, GARF f. A 482, op. 35, d. 132, l. 131, 134, 136, 163, 216. Rubakin often did the fact-finding himself, because France had no

central institution that collected data on many topics of interest to Moscow. "Kratkii otchet o deiatel'nosti predstavitel'stva Narkomzdrava Narkomzdrava [sic] vo Frant-sii," GARF f. 482, op. 35, d. 162, l. 10.

169. "Kratkii otchet o deiatel'nosti predstavitel'stva Narkomzdrava Narkomzdrava [sic] vo Frantsii," GARF f. 482, op. 35, d. 162, l. 4.

170. See the orders for material to Rubakin from OBZSI, March 11, 1928, GARF f. A 482, op. 35, d. 262, l. 24.

171. A. N. Rubakin to BZI, March 1, 1926, GARF f. A 482, op, 35, d. 132, l. 149–151. Calmette delivered his talk on February 18, 1926. For discussion of the attitude toward Calmette's discoveries in Russia, see M. Z. David, "Social Welfare or Wasteful Excess? The Legacy of Soviet Tuberculosis Control Programs in Post-Soviet Russia," in *What Is Soviet Now? Identities, Legacies, Memories*, ed. T. Lahusen and P. H. Solomon, Jr., 214–33 (Berlin: LIT Verlag, 2008).

172. A. N. Rubakin to Moscow, February 3, 1928, GARF f. A 482, op. 35, d. 262, l. 36–36 ob.

173. "Kratkii otchet o deiatel'nosti predstavitel'stva Narodnogo Kommissariata Zdravookhraneniia vo Frantsii s 1-go oktabriia 1927 g. po 1-oe ianvariia 1928 g.," GARF f. A 482, op. 35, d. 262, l. 12–14 ob.

174. A. N. Rubakin to OBZSI, January 27, 1928, GARF f. A 482, op. 35, d. 262, l. 47 ob.

175. Gelfand to T. Asatkina, January 10, 1929, GARF f. A 482, op. 35, d. 263, l. 11.

Chapter Ten

A Transatlantic Dispute

The Etiology of Malaria and the Redesign of the Mediterranean Landscape

Patrick Zylberman

On the threshold of the 1930s, malariology was already "a house divided."[1] In Europe, some researchers saw malaria as a "social disease" determined by socioeconomic factors (housing, food, poverty, working conditions). Others, particularly in America, believed it to be a "local disease" contingent on insect and human geography in the affected area.[2] Debates over etiology were reflected in the solutions championed. For partisans of basic health care, the treatment of patients and their dwellings was the priority; for partisans of public health campaigns, the key lay in the struggle against that most important feature of the malarial locale, the mosquitoes.[3] American malariology was profoundly different from social malariology of a European ilk. During the construction of the Panama Canal (1906–13), William Crawford Gorgas, a U.S. Army medical officer, put the struggle against mosquitoes at the center of his strategy. Although its cost was prohibitive and its method never duplicated, the campaign became the wellspring of malaria-eradication efforts in the American South run by the Communicable Disease Center (1946–52), and of programs in Sardinia (1947–51), Italy (1947), and Greece (1946–49) run by national governments with the help of the United Nations Relief and Rehabilitation Administration (UNRRA) and the Rockefeller Foundation. The eradication program conducted under the aegis of the World Health Organization (1956–69) was likewise based on U.S. principles.[4] At the time, the apparent victory over *Anopheles gambiae* in Brazil (1939–40) and in Egypt (1943–45), along with the amazing effectiveness of DDT, reinforced the blind faith of hygienists and of the general public in technological remedies.[5]

The two approaches differed profoundly in their social and institutional structures. Social malariology relied on centralization. After all, socioeconomic improvements are matters of public policy; the Malaria Commission of the League of Nations had a lasting tendency to impose on localities general programs worked out in Geneva. By contrast, if the advocates of the "local disease" paradigm are to be believed, the fight against mosquitoes left the door open to self-centered strategies and to specific programs more attuned to local features. It is small wonder that the participation and engagement of the populations concerned became an issue. As popular participation combined with a sense of place (marshes, mosquitoes, the village) to shape local epidemiology, local culture, and local policy, a bitter controversy developed over matters of locality in the war against malaria.

How did this local culture of malaria develop? How did malaria as a local object of research and policy develop? To what extent did the controversy within malariology promote the differentiation of the "big" concept of the locale itself into "smaller," more technical, intellectual tools for mapping the locality? Analysis of the disagreement in the early 1930s between European and American experts in the Health Organization of the League of Nations can help to answer these questions.

At the outset of the debate, malaria was closely connected to agriculture.[6] In his 1929 history of the retreat of the disease in the United States, M. A. Barber wrote: "[I]t is plain how closely the prevalence of malaria was associated with pioneer life and its decrease with the agricultural development of the country."[7] Malaria was thus strongly associated with underdevelopment—with "barbarism," as Ronald Ross put it[8]—for reasons that were both demographic (its impact on infant/juvenile mortality and population density) and economic (its impact on agricultural productivity).[9] The two models of malaria mentioned above—the "social" and the "local"—constituted weaker and stronger versions of the general relationship between malaria and agriculture.[10]

In this chapter, I consider the genealogy of each of the two models. Next, I explore the confrontation between the Malaria Commission of the League of Nations and the California doctor Lewis Hackett, one of the chief protagonists of U.S. malariology. Geneva was the primary political-scientific theater in which the argument evolved. To be sure, the confrontation has been the subject of a literature that has grown rapidly in the past two decades. But scholarly attention has been selective. Both Gordon Harrison and Hughes Evans, who were among the first to put the confrontation on the agenda, seem to have missed the opportunity to study Hackett's report on the Malaria Commission's June 1928 meeting in Geneva, which was to be the key event of the dispute.[11] John Farley rightly points out that by the mid-1920s the social medicine approach "came face to face" with the antimosquito strategy, and that "the place [of confrontation] was Italy."[12] But Farley's fascination with Hackett biased his understanding of the political implications of the struggle against malaria. In their comprehensive survey of Rockefeller Foundation activity in fascist Italy, Gianfranco Donelli and Enrica Serinaldi offer a much more stimulating portrait of Hackett.[13] Yet quite understandably they show more interest in the complicated relations between the American and the indigenous authorities than in the international debate about malaria strategy.

In this chapter, the scientific underpinnings of the discussion will be of less interest than the depictions of the locale, the pictures that supported those underpinnings. Like most sanitary work, antimalaria campaigns were not only about plasmodium or mosquitoes, but also about rural landscapes, lifestyles, and people's practical knowledge. Whether socioeconomic or ecological, the point of view always conveyed specific images of locality. And divergent descriptions of these particulars spawned different concepts of milieu and local environment. Moving beyond the abatement of the disease and the control or eradication of the insects, I examine how health campaigns staked out the redesign of the villages and the reform of rural life.

Malaria, Scourge of Rural Development

In the interwar period, the socioeconomic model (that is, the "malaria and civilization" model) was prevalent among hygienists and historians of the disease. As early as 1884, Alphonse Laveran wrote that malaria "almost always gave way to man and civilization."[14] To support this thesis, proponents referred to the debate among historians over the impact of malaria on the fate of ancient Greece and Rome.

The philologist and historian W. H. S. Jones is a case in point. Jones claimed that malaria was the necessary, but not the only, cause of the decline of classical civilization.[15] Inspired by Ronald Ross, the winner of the Nobel prize for medicine in 1902 and to whom he dedicated his *Malaria and Greek History* (1909), Jones belonged to that end-of-century generation obsessed with decadence, which believed that the fall of the ancient world was the result of the tragic death of its elites through social strife, incessant war, and religious persecution.[16] Civilization and malaria were at odds. By infecting almost all individuals and "attacking every fresh generation as it is born, [endemic disease] gives the nation which is its victim no chance to recuperate."[17] With the best eliminated by death or emigration, the outcome of generalized malarial infection in ancient societies was the weakness that comes of physical and moral decay and—even worse—national decline.

The writings of Angelo Celli—a professor of hygiene at the University of Rome (from 1887 on), a member of the Italian parliament (1892), and a promoter of a "total" onslaught against malaria (the fight against the parasite and the mosquito coupled with action against the concomitant socioeconomic causes of the disease)—also underscored the tension between malaria and civilization.[18] But in Celli's work, there was no trace of the supposed "inverse natural selection" featured in Jones's writing.[19] According to Celli, malaria, an "eminently biological phenomenon" that caused depopulation even more than debilitation, had been and remained the main obstacle to the agricultural colonization of the Roman countryside. He associated the oscillations in the disease over the centuries with different periods in the peninsula's civilization (prehistoric, Roman empire, Middle Ages, and so on) as defined by their archaeological remnants. Construction of villas, he wrote, reflected periods of prosperity associated with less virulent waves of malaria. In the words of a present-day author, Celli ascribed a "cycle of fluctuations of virulence of *Plasmodium falciparum* malaria in the Roman Campagna throughout history" to a mass of questionable evidence. However, Celli's ideas were accepted by malariologists such as Alberto Missiroli and, as late as the 1980s, by historians such as Yves-Marie Bercé, a fact that present-day historiography has glossed over.[20]

Considered valid for many years, Jones's thesis is no longer defended by anyone today. In France, Max Sorre (on whose research Fernand Braudel based his work in 1966[21]) followed Jones and Celli only loosely; reluctant to adopt the causality thesis and likely influenced by the cautious approach of Maurice Le Lannou, Sorre preferred to talk of "*commune mesure*" (possible comparison) between the upsurge of the endemic disease and the decline of civilization.[22] Present-day research, from which the idea of decadence of the ancient world is now absent, questions the fact of the depopulation of mainland Greece after the classical period.[23]

The fate of Angelo Celli's theory, after its author's death, was very different. Changes to the landscape made by humans, the development of rural areas, the emergence of densely populated countries, and the permanence of people's relations with the land were all dimensions of the malaria-civilization concept that remained entrenched in the epidemiological analyses of writers of the 1930s and 1940s (in France, Le Lannou and Sorre). Twenty years after Celli's death (in 1914) and two years after the English translation of his *Storia della malaria nell'agro romano* (1933), the geohistory of diseases related to the climate and to archaeological remains was already a well-established research focus.[24]

Hackett and the "Ecological" Model of Malaria

When Lewis Hackett put forward his stronger version of the link between malaria and rural development in 1934, Celli's model was in the process of being firmly established. Hackett's *Malaria in Europe: An Ecological Study* highlighted three points: the absence of a direct link between agricultural productivity and malaria; the specific nature of interaction between milieu and behaviors, depending on locality; and the key role of the vector, whose particular sensitivity to alterations in the environment made the anopheles mosquito the strategic variable of any public health intervention.

Lewis Wendell Hackett (1884–1962) was no newcomer to international public health. He was sent to Rome in January 1924 by the Rockefeller Foundation, which had received an invitation from the Italian government to cooperate in combating malaria. Trained at Harvard as a doctor and hygienist, Hackett (who wrote his doctoral thesis under the direction of M. J. Rosenau, at that time head of the public health section of Harvard Medical School) joined the International Health Commission in April 1914, becoming one of its first staff members. After leading the struggle against hookworm disease in Central America, he ran the International Health Board's public health programs in Brazil. Rapidly converted, as he put it, from a helminthologist to a malariologist at the training station set up by the board in Leesburg, Georgia, he came to the malaria experimental station in Italy and served as its director until shortly before World War II.[25] The station hosted malariologists from all over the world, sent by Geneva or the Rockefeller Foundation for two-week or two-month periods to study the latest scientific and operational developments.[26]

The strong version of the linkage between malaria and agriculture was characterized by the view that the relationship between malaria and underdevelopment was only indirect. In practice, this view separated the struggle against the vector from the care of patients. Its origins are unclear. The first evidences may be found at the beginning of the century in the writings of some American entomologists such as L. O. Howard, who in 1901 advocated using oil as a larvicide because it could be employed by small teams and at little expense.[27] Although the handful of experiments in protecting villages against malaria that began in Arkansas and Mississippi in 1916 under the direction of U.S. Public Health Service engineers and at the expense of the Rockefeller Foundation provided important experience, Hackett credited Ronald Ross with inspiring his thinking. Apparently (as the American would recount forty years later), at a meeting with Wickliffe Rose in London in 1914, Ross vented his rage at the stubbornness of malariologists who stuck to quinine therapy and rejected the antianopheline drive. Rose would pass this view on to his young "malariologists."[28] Ross's approach, which underlay policies implemented by the Rockefeller Foundation in Macedonia between the two world wars and in Greece immediately after World War II, and then in the 1950s by the WHO, prompted the divorce between malariology and social medicine that the "weaker" version sought to unite in an effort to educate and "civilize" rural society.

It was above all the causal relationship between malaria and agricultural productivity that Hackett seriously questioned. On the one hand, "skilful engineering and free labour" (more on this later) could eliminate important mosquito-breeding places and so control malaria transmission. A poor country would thus be able to expand cultivable land, which conferred a benefit to both health and agriculture.[29] On the other hand, reclamation did not necessarily lead to a takeoff for the rural economy. "In East Macedonia," wrote Hackett, "the most malaria-ridden region, the Plain of Chrysoupolis, is probably the most prosperous of the rural areas. A wet season produces a good crop, an inflow of money, and a high malaria intensity; but a dry year reduces malaria and prosperity at the same time."[30] The experience of eradication in Sardinia after World War II provided further evidence of this pattern. Although the decline in mortality was beneficial to the growth of the local population, there was no proof that the control (or eradication) of malaria had any real influence on peasant productivity on the island.[31]

More radically, the very idea of malaria as the cause of the decline of rural civilization was challenged. With that challenge, the features of the malarial landscape underwent a complete transformation.

Hackett believed that even if the presence of malaria precluded the recolonization of abandoned lands, it could not have been responsible for people's abandoning crops and land. In this respect Hackett's thesis differs from that of Celli, who posited that by encouraging extensive agriculture and by moving livestock away in the malaria season (therefore turning mosquitoes toward humans[32]) the *latifundia* system facilitated contamination. In contrast to Celli, Hackett believed that the prevalence of latifundia was not enough to explain malaria. Otherwise, he reasoned, why would malaria persist in Yugoslavia or Bulgaria, where even between the world wars great landed estates were virtually nonexistent?[33] He insisted that other factors were in play, not least of which was war, which generated the instability of populations and the destruction of agriculture, thus prompting the disruption of both the geographic distribution of the gametocyte carriers and the vector's food habits.[34] In Hackett's hands, the causal arrows were inverted: malaria was not the cause, but the effect, of social crisis, which facilitated prevalence and contamination. This thesis has generally been accepted by malariologists and historians from Maurice Le Lannou to Salvatore Collari.[35] Far from being the cause, epidemic or hyperendemic outbreaks are rather an associated effect of political factors (war) and social factors (displacement of populations); in other words, malaria is a condition contributing to social and economic disorder but whose action can and must be considered secondary. It is not malaria that destroys economic life, but the destruction of economic life due to war and insecurity that promotes the propagation of malaria.

What about the inverse relationship? Does the disease recede as the rural world is civilized, as Le Lannou, Émile Brumpt, and Collari maintained?[36] By comparing the proportion of anopheles infected in the Val di Chiana, on the border between Tuscany and Umbria, and in Fiumicino in the Latium, Missiroli and Hackett noted that the relationship of the dwellings—the sign of civilization par excellence[37]—to the level of infection did not correspond with expectations. The dwellings tended to be insalubrious and badly protected in Val di Chiana villages uninfected by malaria, and well built and mosquito proofed in the malaria-infected region of Fiumicino.[38] According to Hackett and Missiroli, the solution to this riddle was not social but entomological: the key lay not in the level of hygiene in houses—as was believed by the League of Nations Malaria Commission, which was quick to classify malaria, typhus, and the plague as diseases of the poor—but rather in the diurnal or nocturnal, anthropophilic or zoophilic habits of the vector.[39]

To sum up, for the direct link between malaria and depopulation posited by Jones and Celli, Hackett substituted not so much an efficient as a contributory cause. Without being the sole cause of underdevelopment, malaria worsened the devastating impact of insecurity and war. The debate here reflects the tribulations of epidemiological concepts. From 1900 to 1937, malaria ceased to be associated with marshes and ponds, that is, with humid areas; it became seen as a product of anophelism, that is, of the mosquito's biology. Hence, far from being governed by the hydraulic, urban, and agricultural improvements that Celli systematically studied, malaria-related morbidity and mortality seemed to be the outcome of a local context that was not only ecological (climate, relief, hydrology, population density) and entomological (geographic distribution and behavior of vectors), but also related to the socioeconomic and land structure of each locality.[40]

Historical inquiry partially refuted Hackett's thesis.[41] Anophelism without malaria was considered a combined effect of rural modernization, drainage, and the distribution of quinine to the population: could it be then proof of the validity of the socioeconomic model? In any case, the reduction of the insect population was not enough to explain the decline of malaria.[42]

The fact remains that from Celli to Hackett, the concept of a milieu changed substantially. For the Italian, milieu was an external frame, foreign to life: towers covered in water, abandoned farms, deserted countryside. In contrast, the American conceived of the environment as a relationship between one living being and others. Mosquitoes, livestock whose role as a screen (Brumpt would say "deviating" role) was highlighted by Roubaud and Wesenberg-Lund in the early 1920s, were, so to speak, either enemies or allies of the organism.[43] The milieu was a "set of living beings"[44] and malaria was "an independent factor"[45] whose impact on civilization remained indirect and depended on secondary causes that included eminently local factors such as war, insecurity, colonization of lowlands, or stagnation in an extensive agriculture. The logical implication of this view was a microhistory or microsociology of rural life that gave pride of place to the march of malariology toward an ecology of the vector, an "epidemiology of minutiae."[46]

The League of Nations Health Committee and Rural Life

Whereas American malariologists were more inclined to take the ecological view or perhaps a mixture of the ecological and socioeconomic models, within the League of Nations Malaria Commission, there was a strong argument in favor of the socioeconomic model. But the malaria issue was only one element in a broader discussion about rural hygiene and rural reconstruction that took place at the same time within the Health Committee.

"Rural hygiene [is] a big problem . . . in most countries," commented Ludwik Rajchman, the medical director of the Health Section of the League of Nations Health Organization, in 1928.[47] The endeavor to modernize agricultural areas required a number of conditions: stability of rural populations, a switch to intensive agriculture, and agrarian reform, all of which depended on the reduction of mortality rates. Malaria was one of the principal infectious diseases responsible for these populations' poor health. It plagued low-lying areas and marshlands, which were also the most fertile. It was a far greater problem than its highly localized geographical distribution suggested, especially in the less-developed agricultural countries of eastern Europe, which was the hardest-hit area on the continent. Anticipating the Agrarian Bloc's program of 1933,[48] the May 1927 International Economic Conference in Geneva highlighted in its final report the necessity to "put . . . agriculture on an equal footing with industry" and to enable farmers to have satisfactory living conditions by introducing social laws and technical measures (animal and plant health) or administrative measures (improvements of agrarian statistics, world agricultural census).[49] In tandem, in October of the same year the Health Committee put the question of rural hygiene on its agenda. In October 1927, a few months before the Geneva conference on malaria to which we will turn shortly, Rajchman suggested forming a group of hygienist-doctors and health engineers to "study the problem of health engineering in rural towns and small villages" in cooperation with the countries participating in the Agrarian Bloc and Russia.[50] From then on, issues of rural hygiene were to play a crucial part in the Health Organization's "general activity" and "future."[51] The eradication or the control of malaria in particular seemed to be decisive factors in rural development. It is little wonder that the dispute about malaria was as much about social engineering as about epidemiology.

The first Intergovernmental Conference on Rural Health, which opened on June 29, 1931 in Geneva, at the initiative of Spain, did not result in an immediate watershed.[52] The real turning point occurred at a meeting held in June 1936 in Moscow, at which the officers of the Health Committee heard the report of Jacques Parisot, professor of hygiene at the Medical Faculty of Nancy, on "the work to be continued in the rural health field by the League of Nations Health Organization." After noting that the 1931 conference had "marked an era," he rapidly highlighted its conceptual limits.[53] The "vast domain" laid out by the conference had covered "the medico-hygiene field in particular," but it had become important to move beyond that stage to "link more closely" the health and social points of view, to consider the issue of "repopulating the countryside," and to guarantee farmers living conditions that would stem the tide of the exodus from the rural sector. To this end, hygienists were to work "in close coordination" with other specialists in the areas of food, labor relations, rural economics, and agriculture.[54] Rajchman told the committee that "Professor Parisot conceives of rural hygiene as part of a mechanism designed to raise the general economic and social level of rural areas" and suggested extending the mandate of the future European conference "to make it a conference of rural improvement."[55] The idea was not only to guarantee the access of the rural populations to medical care and health services, but also to consider problems of rural hygiene "in a more general framework" that took into account "all kinds of factors concerning health in the countryside."[56]

Lacking substantial appreciation of the jumble of reforms envisioned by the advocates of change, the British and Americans were not inclined to think that certain diseases were not only induced by poverty but might also contribute to it. In contrast, protecting rural populations from the burden of infectious diseases and thereby giving decisive impetus to development was the idea endorsed by the Russian Volf Bronner, the Pole Witold Chodzko and, last but not least, the Yugoslav Andrija Štampar (all members of the Health Committee).[57] An old hand at "enlargement" in his own country, Štampar was to assist the Health Organization in setting up a "rural reconstruction plan" in 1934–35 in China, in the former communist province of Jiangxi. The program, which called for abolishing sharecropping, limiting the number of large landowners, and "rural protection" (education, agriculture, public hygiene, social issues), seemed radical.[58] Indeed, Štampar informed the Health Committee that "radical changes of an economic and social order were necessary."[59] Between 1930 and 1933, the Balkan Conferences (Yugoslavia, Albania, Romania, Bulgaria, Greece, and Turkey) pushed in the same direction, at least on paper.[60] Anticipating the malaria and smallpox strategy that the WHO would implement in the first thirty years of its existence, the Health Committee of the League of Nations and agrarian populism converged in supporting the same program: cooperatives, small farms, technical assistance, and the organization of educational and social services in rural areas.[61]

Hackett versus the League of Nations

The portrait painted thus far is one of two opposing schools, with the Americans' technological optimism confronting the Malaria Commission's scientific pessimism. Whereas the former celebrated research efforts, the latter publicized its disappointment regarding the dashed hopes of science and technology. The reality was, of course, less clear cut.

It took a couple of years and two Malaria Commission reports for the dispute to ripen. Since "miserable living conditions, insalubrious housing and lack of hygiene" were seen as the underlying causes of the propagation and gravity of the disease, the first report of the League of Nations Malaria Commission in 1925 had concluded that "it is essentially with welfare that malaria is transformed and disappears."[62] There was some dissent, but nothing serious. Still, all of a sudden, a war of words started when the Health Committee brought rural hygiene into focus. The Malaria Commission's second report, submitted in 1927 after a research trip to the United States, was the spark that ignited a crisis. The report was rather harsh regarding U.S. malariology.[63] Hackett criticized it severely—indeed, when he recalled it in 1960, his voice still trembled with anger. During the 1920s, the production and distribution of quinine received the lion's share of budgets for combating malaria.[64] A symbol of a benevolent government, this distribution of resources conferred on states prestige and authority that derived from a monopoly on the manufacturing and free (or cost-price) distribution of drugs to their populations.[65] In the Pontine Marshes (Lazio), on the Tavoliere in Apulia, in the Maremma (Etruria) and the Po delta, social improvement and agrarian development were combined with control over malaria through the use of quinine.[66] Since it was said to have allowed production and agricultural outputs to increase substantially,[67] the *bonifica integrale* (limited chemotherapy associated with land reclamation, agricultural improvement, and housing reform) made it tempting to conclude that malaria was linked to socioeconomic conditions.[68] During the 1930s, the Tennessee Valley Authority (TVA), which showed what intensive farming can do for eradicating malaria, enjoyed the same luster as the Pontine swamps experiment. In 1952, Charles-Edward Winslow would call once more on the WHO General Assembly to adopt the antimalaria policy of the New Deal: the key to getting the world's agriculture off the ground and one of the solutions to Europe's food crisis was to replicate the TVA experiment.[69] Briefly, the League of Nations Malaria Commission wanted to believe in the impact of state "civilization"—in the sense of state administrative action being at the service of individuals—if not on the issue of prevalence, at least on the level of malaria mortality. Even so, by rejecting the anophelism thesis and favoring social reforms, Geneva hardly encouraged future progress in entomology or parasitology.

The Americans were so annoyed about the 1927 commission's report that they managed to bar its publication.[70] In 1925, through the efforts of Nikolas H. Swellengrebel, a Dutch malariologist and a member of the Malaria Commission, the commission had decisively tilted against Hackett's method. The first report pointed out the dangers of the chemical Paris green for the health of livestock. It also refused to acknowledge the difference in the impact of the antianophelic struggle compared with quinine, for it was often difficult to distinguish between the reduction in the number of vectors and that of gametocytes in the population under treatment.[71] In fact, the author of the first report, Price James of the Ministry of Health in London, seemed to have lost all reason. He went so far as to claim that, apart from quinine, nothing could be done except wait patiently for public health as a whole to improve.[72] According to Rajchman the report was "a hopeless document," the adoption of which would have led to the complete cessation of malaria campaigns in Europe.[73] After long and laborious discussions, this risible diatribe was taken up anew. In 1926, following the commission's study trip to Palestine, Rajchman thought he perceived a convergence between the thinking of the commission members and that of the American scientists.[74] In fact, the Malaria Commission's June 1928 meeting (held in Geneva with a view to putting together the pieces) revealed trench warfare, and this but a year after it had submitted its second and problematical report.

Lewis Hackett, who participated in the meeting, noted that there was no possibility of convergence.[75] There was a gulf between the Europeans and the Americans. The Americans seemed horrified by the Europeans' attitude of resignation; it seemed their only hope for salvation lay in the—necessarily slow—advance of civilization. The Europeans barely hid their contempt for the idea of eradication and their surprise at the Americans' obvious condescension on the use of quinine. Hackett, who had contracted a *vivax* infection in Leesburg and a *falciparum* infection in Panama and had thus "been afforded a splendid opportunity to study at first hand . . . standard quinine treatment,"[76] rightly retorted that administration of the treatment tended to be inefficient, especially in the Balkans. "Assistance for patients is generally limited to recognizing the ailment of those people who consult of their own accord," Donato Ottolenghi, one of the Italian representatives in the League of Nations Malaria Commission, had written four years earlier. Medical surveillance was irregular, as was the taking of medication. In villages, screening was insufficient and quinine prophylaxis rare.[77]

Hackett effectively rejected any social approach to malaria. "The spleen rate is much more apt to vary with the numbers of anophelines than with economic status," he wrote.[78] No, the plough did not chase away malaria. He was prepared to admit that malaria death rates could be compounded by famine and other economic plagues and that an improvement in living standards was likely to lessen the severity of attacks. But the idea that social

reform could replace the fight against mosquitoes or, even more fantasti-
cally, that the reduction of contamination should wait until social problems
of poverty and ignorance had been solved, was for him surely based neither
on science nor on experience.

In reality, the Europeans were also less united than they appeared initially.
Irritated by Geneva's prevailing pessimism, which barely masked an excessive quiescence, Hackett tended to exaggerate the positions of both sides.
The Italians were divided between proquinine (Lutrario) and pro-American
(Missiroli) approaches; the British, between quietists (James) and eradicators
(Weynon[79]). Swellengrebel, the Dutchman, gradually shifted toward some
of the ideas defended by the American camp. Hackett wrongly thought that
the Germans were hostile to his method. Keenly interested in the economic
aspect of the "ecological" model during his visit to Yugoslavia for the commission two years earlier, Bernhard Nocht, a member of the commission from
its inception, had recommended the antilarvae measures (spraying with Paris
green) that Hackett proposed, measures that were already being applied in
Montenegro and Dalmatia.[80] Finally, the French summed up the Continent's
divisions in their own way. "A little civilization, a pinch of prosperity, and two
measures of quinine" was the recipe suggested by Émile Marchoux who had
his head constantly in the clouds, it seemed. Brumpt, more alert, showed
curiosity about everything concerning the struggle against the vector but was
strangely silent when it came to applications in the field. This can perhaps be
explained by the French administration's abiding distrust—despite bouts of
feigned cooperation—of Geneva's antimalaria initiatives.[81]

Whatever the balance of opinion among Europeans, the scales tipped
toward the socioeconomic model. Rajchman emphasized the extent to
which rural hygiene was addressed in Europe less from a strictly scientific
angle than from one of improving living standards.[82] The 1928 conference
spawned a method that summed up the principles that the commission
stated and that was to serve as a guideline to the health administration of
Greek Macedonia in the early 1930s.[83] As Hackett wrote, "The 'mitigators'
had been there before and staked out the ground; and the general lines had
to be respected."[84] The positions seemed so entrenched that one of the participants sarcastically commented that only the abolition of the age difference between the "eradicators" (mostly young) and the "mitigators" (mostly
older) would enable everyone eventually to agree.

Hence, American ideas had less of a rapid impact in Europe than some
observers have claimed.[85] If Frank Boudreau, former director of the Ohio
health services and deputy medical director of the League's Health Section
is to be believed, around 1930 U.S. public health, which had a firm grip on
the new countries of central and eastern Europe as the result in particular
of the deep and wide-ranging influence of American private philanthropy
(see Paul Weindling's contribution to this volume), had only a very limited

impact on the old European countries (Great Britain, Germany, the Netherlands, and Scandinavia).[86]

The contradiction between the two models was not obvious. Neither Maurice Le Lannou nor Max Sorre saw any problem in picking up elements here and there; at the end of World War II, Brumpt elegantly combined the two approaches.[87] He was able to do so because malariology was not yet divorced from social medicine.[88] Of course, in Hackett's view the struggle against mosquitoes started off outside the health care system. Not that he denied the advantages of a system of primary care and prevention, but he insisted that the struggle against mosquitoes had to fit into the existing public health system by proceeding in three steps: the destruction of anopheles, the multiplication of malaria stations and, finally, the transformation of the stations into health centers.[89] Although they praised Hackett's work, Selskar Gunn and Charles-Edward Winslow, respectively vice president of the Rockefeller Foundation and a professor of public health at Yale,[90] were by no means critical of Andrija Stampar 's more medical orientation in Yugoslavia. F. F. Russell, director of the Rockefeller Foundation International Health Board, was also far from considering outrageous the idea that social medical services might be able to "stimulate" the struggle against malaria.[91]

Like its European counterpart, American malariology was in no way monolithic. Paul F. Russell, of the Office of the Surgeon General (not to be confused with F. F. Russell), was himself an advocate of "control" comprising mechanical protection, spraying, destruction of breeding places, drainage, treatment, and education. He entertained the reconciliation of the two schools as Hackett envisioned. Paul Russell explained the retreat of the disease in the United States in the 1940s by the combined action of technical methods (drainage, spraying, and so on), agricultural methods (destruction of pools and dams, orientation toward intensive livestock farming in the Old South), cultural methods (spread of mechanical protection of homes, more compliance in treatment), and social methods (exodus of carriers toward the large cities of the North, urbanization of the South).[92] In France, a few years earlier, Brumpt had put forward the same explanation for the spontaneous downturn (determined by entomological and socioeconomic factors) of malaria in the temperate zone. According to him, the interaction among rural civilization, welfare, and quinine prophylaxis was conditioned by the relations among certain biotypes and humans; in areas where the malaria season was short and the rural exodus reduced the number of reservoir subjects, these relations were limited. As a result, during the 1940s the initially antagonistic Hackett doctrine became compatible with the principles of the League of Nations Malaria Commission, which itself had been amended.[93]

In reality, the scientific discussion masked an underlying political debate. The issue turned on the regime of authority of health campaigns or, in other words, both the method (education or constraint) and the legitimacy (population's welfare or productivity gains) through which and in the name of which malaria campaigns were conducted. Could the population be engaged in the struggle against mosquitoes and against the disease or not? Could malariology incorporate the peasant masses? Could the peasant masses accept and support the aims and methods of hygienists? These issues were part and parcel of the democratization of public health.

The Anophele and the *Corvée*

The answers were not self-evident. All too often populations resigned themselves to their misery. "There is hail," said Carlo Levi's Basilicate peasants, "mud slides, droughts and malaria, and there is also the State. They are inevitable evils, they have always existed and they will always exist."[94] For those who had survived infantile episodes, hyperendimicity no longer seemed to be a major problem.[95] And if the educated officers of the armies on the Eastern Front, decimated by malaria, neglected the recommendations of the health service in time of war (as they did during World War I),[96] what could be expected of the backward populations of rural areas in the Balkans? Was it at least possible to force them to take their medication? Were they able to implement the techniques of the mosquito campaign on their own, with the required consistency and permanence? Certainly not.[97]

Today even hygienists rely only partially on the commitment and perseverance of populations that are often too poor to support effectively a combat that sometimes distracts them from the more urgent struggle of subsistence.[98] Eighty years ago, even such a moderate will to engage populations in the malaria campaigns hardly existed. Local people counted for nothing: the experts ran the show. In 1927, when the "social disease" approach prevailed in the fight against malaria, a hygienist was in charge of the work with the assistance of an engineer and (sometimes) a malariologist. In Italy, for example, the medicosocial team (doctors and nurses) were usually the first ones on site.[99] Hackett radically changed this system of action. Not that he would have turned back the clock—rather, it was the hierarchy he overturned, so that a malariologist (doctor) ran the operation, with a hygienist and an engineer working under his orders.[100]

Yet the struggle against mosquitoes required work (draining, clearing rivers and streams, building dykes, spraying), and therefore humanpower. Hackett, who was not afraid to call a spade a spade, commented that in the Balkans malaria control "does not cost money, it costs labor." In Albania the war on mosquitoes was based on *corvée* (compulsory, unpaid labor).[101] Like its Albanian counterpart, which used young recruits and even women's battalions, the Bulgarian government also understood the importance of labor. In 1931, some thirty thousand families were resettled on 120,000 hectares, primarily around Bourgas and Yambol in southern Bulgaria, after the drying out of the swamps and the draining of the polders on the bed of the Danube by compulsory labor service.[102] In 1928–29, the Rockefeller Foundation employed the same methods in Kriva Palanka in Yugoslavian Macedonia, and in the same period in Petrich on the other side of the border.[103]

Today, it seems strange that the Rockefeller Foundation was apparently as willing as it was to cooperate with the Mussolini regime.[104] Indeed, the fascist policy of *bonifica integrale* had much in common with Hackett's demonstrations, for example, a shared antipathy toward gratuitous distribution of quinine (once a powerful spur to popular mobilization, and the *bête noire* of doctors and pharmacists as well as the landowners who paid for it).[105] Even more important is the relationship between the system Hackett proposed and a certain type of social structure, especially land structure. Because he denied any role to the population in the war on mosquitoes apart from being available for "free labor," Hackett could pride himself on the appeal to the state and to leading citizens in Italy, where land reform, especially in the center and the south, was very limited.[106] Besides, had he not succeeded in capturing Mussolini's personal support?[107] Moreover, was it not symptomatic that the example considered in greatest detail in *Malaria in Europe* was Albania, a country dear to Hackett's heart,[108] and where the government was simply the creature of the large landowners and the influence of Italy was preponderant? (It would also be fair to ask what sort of connection with terrorist groups the Rockefeller officers had in Petrich, Bulgarian Macedonia, the site of one of their greatest achievements, but where the local paramilitary organization, which was effectively a state within the state, was responsible for a reign of terror.[109])

"Of course I believe in sanitation through evolution, education and prosperity," wrote Hackett in 1925. "But with a backward people, I believe in a preliminary cleaning up through strict enforcement of a sanitary code, whether the people thoroughly understand it or not! This is easier in a colony or under a mandate than in a democracy."[110] Education needed time; governments wanted more or less immediate results. In such a situation, action could only be independent of the villagers' good will.[111] As James Scott put it, "the peasants are the problem to which the experts are the solution."[112] A doctrine more opposed to the ideas of the Malaria Commission and, more generally, to those of the Health Section of the League of Nations could hardly be imagined.

The Malaria Commission was surely not so blind that it failed to notice in Yugoslavia, for example, "the ignorance and indolence of the population" regarding the use of mosquito nets or the cleanliness of houses, "even in the vicinity of large health stations."[113] Nor was it so credulous that it failed to notice that the peasants "quite frequently destroy . . . [the collectors and systems of draining the land] or change them to suit their own convenience and thus render them useless . . . when they obstruct their crops."[114] Had the commission been more familiar with popular habits it would also have noticed that some peasants happily fished gambusiae (top minnows) that were deliberately introduced into rivers to destroy mosquito larvae.[115]

Yet those same populations gradually abandoned their passive attitude. Although the draining of marshes sometimes ran counter to "the agronomic interests of the population," which often opposed the health measures in place, the destruction of larvae did not preclude the cultivation of rice.[116] In Montenegro, Bernhard Nocht noted that villagers accepted the malaria campaign with interest.[117] Frank Boudreau marveled at the sight of Dalmatian peasants "building and farming: all due, in my opinion, to the [antimalarial] work."[118] Two years earlier, Donato Ottolenghi had already noted that, when questioned, children in Dalmatian and Macedonian schools "indicated with exactitude the main characteristics of anophele larvae and showed that they had clearly understood the essential role of mosquitoes in the transmission of malaria."[119]

The villagers' participation in antimalarial work was therefore not doomed to failure. Was it not in 1938—the same year that Hackett's book was published—that, following the intergovernmental conference of Far Eastern countries on rural hygiene, Ludwik Rajchman declared that "cooperation with the people" in rural improvement and public health had been "the keystone of the conference"? The opinion of the League of Nations Health Section's medical director was that "total cooperation of the village population," through "village committees," was required for "supplying water, sanitizing [and] improving dwellings."[120] Could the ideological divide between Hackett and the League of Nations have been wider? Behind Rajchman's oration lingered the "rural reconstruction" idea. Launched in Bengal in around 1912 by Rabindranath Tagore's Institute of Rural Reconstruction, the idea was fleshed out in the late 1920s. "Reconstructed" villages would be given an administrative body that would manage funds, cooperatives, schools, and health centers semi-autonomously.[121] Štampar, as we have seen, made much fuss over this theme at the Health Committee. But Hackett had not had his final say.

Miniature Utopia: Two Antagonistic Concepts of the "Local"

"Malaria," Lewis Hackett claimed, "[is] an entomological rather than a social problem."[122] He had not always thought so.[123] The Porto Torres demonstration he conducted in Sardinia seems to have changed his mind. Set up in March 1925, this experimental deployment of the means for combating malaria mosquitoes enabled Hackett and Missiroli to show that it was possible to reduce the incidence of malaria substantially by means of the spectacular decrease in the insect population in dwellings and in their immediate surroundings. In contrast, in two control villages treated with quinine, the prevalence of malaria hardly declined.[124] With Paris green, used first here (in 1930, twenty sites were treated in Italy with surprising success[125]), the Rockefeller Foundation ensured that antianophele technology was within the financial and technical reach of rural authorities, the very goal that Wickliffe Rose had set himself from the beginning.[126] Spraying by rapidly trained locals was to remain the only permanent element of antimalaria programs.[127]

In Hackett's mind, the "competition between quinine and Paris green" would inevitably push "quinine out of the running as an antimalaria measure."[128] As we saw, the Malaria Commission was initially sceptical. If antilarvae measures were applied in a limited radius around villages, was there not a risk of excluding dispersed dwellings from the preventive campaign? Was this type of strategy—well suited to southern Italy where dwellings were usually grouped together—not likely "to result in a deplorable waste of money, energy and time in other countries"?[129] Hackett's answer was that in the Balkans the struggle against mosquitoes depended on two chief peculiarities of the anophele population: its endophily and its flying power. "Control" measures had to be carried out in a radius of four to five kilometers around dwellings, in an area five times larger than in the tropics.[130] Thus, even if disinfestation did not cover the entire area of the most exposed dispersed dwellings,[131] it would nevertheless treat a large portion of the roads and fields (external areas of activity) in addition to villages (peridomestic areas), and thus would protect both men and women.

Above all, the problem could be treated only by proceeding "locality by locality"—a logical follow-up to an approach that defined the risk in relation to the dispersion of the vector.[132] This was the point on which the entire debate turned. To the social, sociological, and ethnographic doctrine of the commission, Hackett opposed a medical geography; to an approach framed in terms of the people, he opposed an approach that relied on space, place, and milieu. But what did this concept of locality mean?

The concept related above all to a particularity, a specific characteristic. The importance of "eminently local epidemiology," and of the "particular character of malaria in a given locality" was the subject of broad agreement among malariologists, from Lewis Hackett to Paul F. Russell. It was also the crux of the dominant lesson of the struggle against malaria, according to the authors of the first volume of *Global Epidemiology*, published in 1944 by the Medical Intelligence Division (created in 1941 by the U.S. surgeon general). A product of the ecosystem and local society, malaria was an unstable and diverse evil, an epidemiological and demographic Proteus that made a mockery of the ready-made schemas so dear to Geneva. Hygienists were aware of the close relationship between health and environmental conditions. For Hackett, each malaria-infected village was a center that took in elements from its environment in order to build up its own unique milieu, a milieu centered on the village and created by the village. Each paludal village was its own norm, a norm that differed from any uniform model or centralizing tendency. From Hackett's point of view, normalization was based on diversity, difference, and singularity, rather than on a political norm (read: central norm, like Mussolini's *bonifiche*).

Hence, "locality" meant "normalized locality," a normalization captured in the fifteen maps drawn between 1925 and 1927 by Nelson Rector, an engineer at the International Health Division and Hackett's assistant in Rome. In the Rockefeller Foundation's arsenal, these maps were at the summit of a triangle, the other two corners consisting of surveys (epidemiological and entomological) and the training of staff in spraying and drainage techniques. These rare examples of detailed local maps of medical geography resembled the map of cholera deaths in Aubing, a village close to Munich, that Max von Pettenkofer drew in 1854 for the Bavarian Cholera Commission.[133] A map was a model, a tool, a "mediating" institution among the different specialists, engineers, hygienists, and administrators who had set out to give a health demonstration—in short, an incentive for the interdisciplinarity called for by Rajchman and Parisot.[134] In Rector's hands, the map was a mosaic of networks on which the American engineer represented the network of water mains, wells, and cisterns; the distribution of breeding places (larvae and adult mosquitoes) and cases of disease; and the locations of points to be treated with Paris green. In a word, Rector's maps fit what present-day epistemologists would call a network of networks.[135] They were both technical and conceptual (epidemiological, entomological, ethnographic) but oriented in relation to a particular goal and specific needs, all related to the singularity of a place, a landscape, and a population.

For several reasons, the conceptual normalization of the locality in the Porto Torres demonstration represented a quantum leap forward in Hackett's political methodology. Faced with the all too apparent disparity between this miniexperiment, with its 3-kilometer radius, and the gigantic scale of malaria problems in the Mediterranean, Hackett feared that the experiment would "fail to convince an incredulous Europe."[136] But the Porto Torres experiment achieved its objective fully. It won over leading citizens, becoming the Rockefeller Foundation's trademark, its "fetish." Hackett himself was appointed vice president of the League of Nations Malaria Commission (a position he occupied from 1935 to 1946).[137] It was a shining result in a country (Italy) in which he constantly heard the rumblings of nationalist discontent.[138]

Hackett had counted on fieldwork far more than on planning in the ministries. His method had two real advantages. First, the cost of antilarvae operations was far lower than that of quininization.[139] The average cost of protecting a Calabrian village with larvicidal spraying, including the inspection of the work, was half that of treating patients.[140] The cost was incomparably lower than the huge investments required by the *grande bonifica*.[141] Because their action was cumulative and allowed the increase in the surface area of cultivable land, larvae-control measures (destruction of breeding places), which mobilized only the simplest means, proved to be twice as profitable from both the agricultural and the sanitary points of view. And this is why, according to Hackett, antilarvae measures would be the method used most in the Mediterranean basin.[142]

Second, by counting mosquitoes rather than cases, Hackett was evaluating the antimosquito strategy rather than measuring the prevalence of the disease. This technique had a twofold advantage: it was feasible in areas with no statistical apparatus worthy of the name, such as Yugoslavia or Greece (no worse than the United States in the same period),[143] and it produced results fast. These were crucial concerns, the alpha and the omega for the empire of American philanthropy, in a hurry to hand the country back to its natives before packing its bags.[144]

It was for the purposes of demonstration that the Yugoslav, Bulgarian, and Greek authorities had to host this miniature utopia. The scale of the operations was variable, from the small locality (the Mezzogiorno), to "covering a whole drainage area" (Kriva Palanka).[145] The appeal of the health demonstration lay in its ability to increase or decrease the scale of parameters almost at will, in relation to needs and local usage. Their maps enabled Rector and Hackett to slice up the health campaign into the exact measures of a technically masterable microenvironment. Public health measures thus appeared as a perfect form of rationality, an island of order and modernity.[146]

Conclusion

During more than half of the twentieth century, and certainly during the interwar period, two models of antimalaria struggle competed for the allegiance of malariologists. The socioeconomic, or social medicine, model was aimed at national revival on a populist basis, by means of the village "civilization." Proponents of this model distrusted the state but thought to reform village life through the activity of the state.[147] In contrast, the ecological, or public health, model focused on the complex interactions among biological factors, the environment, and social behaviors. Its proponents aimed to reconcile state authority with local self-determination, seeking above all rapid, economical, results. Between the partisans of public health (the reduction of the anophele population) and those of social medicine (the treatment of the human population), the conception of the "local" differed. An ecological-technological conception (such as Hackett's) based on the American methodology of health demonstration, in which the village was conceived of as a functional unit contributing to the maintenance of a risk through biophysical factors (ecology of the vector) and biosocial factors (lifestyles), was contrasted with a cultural and political conception (such as that of the Health Committee of the League of Nations) that was close to the idea of the peasant parties, which identified the "local" with the cooperative and the economic village unit with self-government.[148] It can certainly be said here that politics were at the center of expertise. Lewis Hackett thought he could conquer popular opinion because he had first convinced governments and leading citizens. Ludwik Rajchman, Jacques Parisot, and Andrija Štampar , on the other hand, believed that they could not convince the authorities without first having gained the people's support and participation.[149]

Notes

1. "A House Divided" was the title of the first chapter of L. W. Hackett, *Malaria in Europe: An Ecological Study* (London: Oxford University Press, 1937). The volume was the edition of the Heath Clark Lectures that Hackett delivered in London in 1934. In 1925, N. H. Swellengrebel had already used this metaphor to qualify the state of malariology in relation to the *bonifica integrale*. See N. H. Swellengrebel, "Some aspects of the malaria problem in Italy," Commission du paludisme, *Rapport sur son voyage d'étude dans certains pays d'Europe en 1924*, March 26, 1925, C.H. 273, Annex 11, 171, League of Nations Archives, Geneva (hereafter LNA).

2. Hackett, *Malaria in Europe*, xvi; E. Sergent, "L'Oeuvre de la commission du paludisme de la Société des Nations depuis 1930," in *Acta Conventus tertii de malariæ morbis*, vol. 2 (Amsterdam: Spin & Zoon, 1938), 27.

3. Swellengrebel, cited in Hackett, *Malaria in Europe*, 283; see also R. H. Hazemann, "Les Tendances récentes de la politique médico-sociale en Europe," *Bulletin de l'Organisation d'Hygiène* 8 (1939): 720 (epigraph), 721, note 1.

4. H. Haskell Ziperman, "A Medical History of the Panama Canal," *Surgery, Gynecology & Obstetrics* 137 (1973): 111; G. Harrison, *Mosquitoes, Malaria and Man: A History of the Hostilities Since 1880* (London: John Murray, 1978), 162–67; L. W. Hackett, "Once Upon a Time," *American Journal of Tropical Medicine and Hygiene* 9 (1960): 109; M. Humphreys, "Water Won't Run Uphill: The New Deal and Malaria Control in the American South, 1933–1940," *Parassitologia* 40 (1998): 184; M. Humphreys, "Kicking a Dying Dog: DDT and the Demise of Malaria in the American South, 1942–1950," *Isis* 87 (1996): 10–11; G. Corbellini and L. Merzagora, *La Malaria tra passato e presente. Storia e luoghi della malaria in Italia* (Rome: Museo di Storia della Medicina, Università La Sapienza, 1998), 95–99; G. Livadas and D. Athanassatos, "The Economic Benefits of Malaria Eradication in Greece," *Rivista di Malariologia* 42 (1963): 179–80; J. Siddiqi, *World Health and World Politics: The World Health Organization and the UN System* (London: Hurst, 1995), 146–51.

5. On the role of technology, see J. Farley, "Mosquitoes or Malaria? Rockefeller Campaigns in the American South and Sardinia," *Parassitologia* 36 (1994): 167. For

a far more balanced treatment, see P. F. Russell, *Malaria: Basic Principles Briefly Stated* (Oxford: Blackwell, 1952), 169.

6. Close relations between malaria and agriculture have been perceived since antiquity. See J. A. Najera, "The Control of Tropical Diseases and Socioeconomic Development (With Special Reference to Malaria and Its Control)," *Parassitologia* 36 (1994): 19; R. Sallares, *Malaria and Rome: A History of Malaria in Ancient Italy* (Oxford: Oxford University Press, 2002), 179.

7. M. A. Barber, "History of Malaria in the United States," *Public Health Report* 44 (1929), cited by Najera, "Control of Tropical Diseases," 22.

8. Hackett, *Malaria in Europe*, 262.

9. P. J. Brown, "Malaria, Miseria, and Underpopulation in Sardinia: The 'Malaria Blocks Development' Cultural Model," *Medical Anthropology* 17 (1997): 242, 248–49.

10. M. N. Cohen, *Health and the Rise of Civilization* (New Haven: Yale University Press, 1989), 42.

11. Harrison, *Mosquitoes*, 184–86; H. Evans, "European Malaria Policy in the 1920s and 1930s: The Epidemiology of Minutiæ," *Isis* 80 (1989): 40–59.

12. J. Farley, *To Cast Out Disease: A History of the International Health Division of the Rockefeller Foundation, 1913–1951* (New York: Oxford University Press, 2004), 113.

13. G. Donelli and E. Serinaldi, *Dalla lotta alla malaria alla nascita dell'Istituto di Sanità Pubblica. Il ruolo della Rockefeller Foundation in Italia: 1922–1934* (Rome and Bari: Laterza, 2003).

14. Harrison, *Mosquitoes*, 269, note 15.

15. In fact, Jones excludes all monocausal explanation. W. H. S. Jones, *Malaria and Greek History* (New York: AMS Press, 1977), 88, note 2. We omit consideration here of the first thesis that Jones developed concerning the debate between the "eternal presence" of malaria in Greece and its introduction *ex novo*. M. Grmek, *Les Maladies à l'aube de la civilisation occidentale* (Paris: Payot, 1994), 397–407.

16. A. Momigliano, *Problèmes d'historiographie ancienne et moderne* (Paris: Gallimard, 1983), 344–48.

17. W. H. S. Jones, "Malaria and History," *Annals of Tropical Medicine and Parasitology* 1 (1908): 539.

18. On Celli, see G. Feligioni, "Angelo Celli, medico e deputato. Dalla malaria all'agitazione pro Marche, Umbria e Lazio," *Quaderni del Consiglio Regionale delle Marche* 6 (2001): 166.

19. Jones, "Malaria and History," 540.

20. A. Celli, *The History of Malaria in the Roman Campagna from Ancient Times* (New York: AMS Press, 1977), 4–5, 8, 10. On this hypothesis, see Sallares, *Malaria and Rome*, 256–61; Y.-M. Bercé, "Influence de la malaria sur l'histoire événementielle du Latium (XVIe–XIXe siècles)," in *Maladies et société (XIIe–XVIIIe siècles)*, ed. N. Bulst and R. Delort, 235–45 (Paris: Éditions du CNRS, 1989). Today, variations of endemism and the severity of the disease are related more to the selective adaptation of the different anophele species due to changes in their habitat.

21. Braudel serves as a historical guarantee to J. de Zulueta, "Malaria and Mediterranean History," *Parassitologia* 15 (1973): 2.

22. M. Sorre, *Les fondements de la géographie humaine*, vol. 1, *Les fondements biologiques* (Paris: Colin, 1947), 398–400; M. Le Lannou, "Le rôle géographique de la malaria,"

Annales de géographie 45 (1936): 113–35. It is true that Sorre also seemed to acknowledge a "relationship of cause and effect" between malaria and the "civilization curve." Sorre, *Fondements*, 397.

23. J.-N. Corvisier, "Eau, paludisme et démographie en Grèce péninsulaire," *Bulletin de correspondance hellénique* 28 (1994, supplement): 316. But depopulation resulting from endemic malaria was not questioned in Italy: Sallares, *Malaria and Rome*, 167.

24. F. A. Barrett, *Disease and Geography: The History of an Idea* (Toronto: Becker, 2000), 425.

25. Hackett, "Once Upon a Time"; Donelli and Serinaldi, *Lotta*, 18–19.

26. Société des Nations, Organisation d'hygiène, Procès-verbal de la session du Bureau du Comité d'hygiène, 1st session, April 29, 1936, 5 (L. Rajchman), Jacques Parisot Papers, Office d'hygiène sociale, Vandoeuvres-lès-Nancy; D. H. Stapleton, "Internationalism and Nationalism: The Rockefeller Foundation, Public Health, and Malaria in Italy, 1923–1951," *Parassitologia* 42 (2000): 129–30; Donelli and Serinaldi, *Lotta*, 110–50.

27. U. Kitron, "Malaria, Agriculture, and Development: Lessons from Past Campaigns," *International Journal of Health Services* 17 (1987): 305; Farley, *To Cast Out Disease*, 108–13.

28. Hackett, "Once Upon a Time," 109–10.

29. Hackett, *Malaria in Europe*, 319; I. T. Berend, *Decades of Crisis: Central and Eastern Europe Before World War II* (Berkeley: University of California Press, 1998), 256–57; F. M. Snowden, "'Fields of Death': Malaria in Italy, 1861–1962," *Modern Italy* 4 (1999): 45.

30. Hackett, *Malaria in Europe*, 263.

31. P. J. Brown, "Socioeconomic and Demographic Effects of Malaria Eradication: A Comparison of Sri Lanka and Sardinia," *Social Science & Medicine* 22 (1986): 856–57; Farley, "Mosquitoes or Malaria?" 171–73.

32. According to the hygienists, the keeping of livestock in stables, favoring the zoophilic orientation of the mosquito, satisfactorily explained the disappearance of malaria in areas with intensive agriculture such as Denmark or the American Midwest. C.-E. A. Winslow, "Malaria Control in Italy, Albania, and Macedonia," 1929, 5, 2/stack 1929/554/3729, Rockefeller Archive Center, Tarrytown, NY (hereafter RAC). Hackett applied the same reasoning to southern Europe. Harrison, *Mosquitoes*, 197.

33. Hackett, *Malaria in Europe*, xiii–xv. On the problem of *latifundia*, see Sallares, *Malaria and Rome*, 239–46.

34. Hackett, *Malaria in Europe*, xii, 1–3.

35. Hackett, *Malaria in Europe*, xii, 8. E. Brumpt, "Anophélisme sans paludisme et régression spontanée du paludisme," *Annales de parasitologie* 20 (1944–45): 83; S. Collari, "L'Agro Pontino e la bonifica antimalarica," *Rivista di Malariologia* 28 (1949): 300–301; M. I. Rostovtseff, *Histoire économique et sociale de l'Empire romain* (Paris: Laffont, 1988), 348–49, 615; Le Lannou, "Rôle," 121–25.

36. And today, H. K. Heggenhougen, V. Hackethal, and P. Vivek, *The Behavioural and Social Aspects of Malaria and its Control* (Geneva: World Health Organization on behalf of the Special Programme for Research and Training in Tropical Diseases, 2003), 23.

37. Le Lannou, "Rôle," 133.

38. B. Fantini, "Anophelism Without Malaria: An Ecological and Epidemiological Puzzle," *Parassitologia* 36 (1994): 97.

39. Hackett, *Malaria in Europe*, 291–92.

40. M. Sorre, "Complexes pathogènes et géographie médicale," *Annales de géographie* 42 (1933): 1–18. At the same time as Hackett, Sorre had established this line of thinking. Barrett, *Disease and Geography*, 430–32.

41. Sallares, *Malaria and Rome*, 260–61.

42. H. Cumming, U.S. Surgeon General, cited in Hackett, *Malaria in Europe*, 264. This doctrine was to become, in the late 1940s, the official doctrine of the WHO's Malaria Commission; see the WHO declaration of 1950, reproduced in Russell, *Principles*, 175–78.

43. Hackett, *Malaria in Europe*, 10–11.

44. This expression is borrowed from G. Canguilhem, *La connaissance de la vie* (Paris: Vrin, 1971), 136–37.

45. Hackett, *Malaria in Europe*, 265.

46. Evans, "European Malaria Policy."

47. Selskar Gunn's diary, March 14, 1928, RG 12.1, RAC.

48. A. Bussot, "Le Bloc des Etats agricoles de l'Europe centrale et orientale et son programme," *Revue d'économie politique* 47 (1933): 1544–58. The Agrarian Bloc consisted of the countries of the Little Entente (Yugoslavia, Romania, and Czechoslovakia), as well as Bulgaria, Greece, Hungary, and Poland. It called for coordinating commercial policies among the countries of the bloc, lifting industrial nations' trade barriers in order to favor agricultural exports, and relieving state finances through loans.

49. M. Augé-Laribé, *La politique agricole de la France de 1880 à 1940* (Paris: PUF, 1950), 402–4.

50. L. Rajchman, Procès-verbal de la 11e session du Comité d'hygiène, 3rd meeting, October 30, 1927, 17, C.579.M.205.1927.III, December 15, 1927, LNA.

51. J. Parisot, L'Oeuvre poursuivie et à poursuivre dans le domaine de l'hygiène rurale, Report to the Health Committee Bureau, Moscow, June 1936; C.H. 1218, LNA; L. Rajchman, Procès-verbal de la session du Bureau du Comité d'hygiène tenue à Moscou du 22 au 28 juin 1936, meeting of June 22, C.H./Bureau/IV/Procès-verbal, January 1937, LNA.

52. See L. Murard, "Health Policy Between the International and the Local: Jacques Parisot in Nancy and Geneva," in *Facing Illness in Troubled Times: Health in Europe in the Interwar Years 1918–1939*, ed. I. Borowy and W. D. Gruner, 207–45 (Frankfurt am Main: Peter Lang, 2005).

53. On the 1931 conference, see Hazemann, "Tendances," 717–19.

54. J. Parisot, Œuvre, C.H. 1218, LNA; J. Parisot and L. Rajchman, Note du Prof. Parisot et du Directeur médical [L. Rajchman] au sujet des études ultérieures sur l'hygiène rurale, Paris, October 8, 1936, 5e Réunion du Bureau du Comité d'hygiène, October 29, 1936, C.H./Bureau/6, LNA. For recent developments in this pluridisciplinary concern, see D. Brewster, "Environmental management for vector control," *British Medical Journal* 319 (1999): 651.

55. Bureau du Comité d'hygiène, Geneva, January 1937, meeting of June 25, 1936, C.H./Bureau/IV/Procès-verbal, LNA. The European conference "on rural life" was unable to meet as scheduled in 1939.

56. Minutes of the 5e Réunion du Bureau du Comité d'hygiène, Paris, October 30, 1936, afternoon session, C.H./Bureau/6, LNA; J. Parisot and L. Rajchman, Note du Prof. Parisot et du Directeur médical, October 8, 1936; Hazemann, "Tendances," 786, 718.

57. N. M. J. Jitta, the Dutch representative and vice president of the executive board, seemed to approve, whereas G. Pittaluga, the Spanish representative, on whose initiative the conference had met in 1931, demonstrated excessive moderation regarding the new course. For his part, Bonner gave his "complete approbation" to the proposal tabled by Parisot and Rajchman.

58. Minutes of the 5e Réunion du Bureau du Comité d'hygiène, Paris, October 29, 1936, 2nd session, Rapport du Dr Štampar sur ses missions en Chine, 1–9, C.H./1220, LNA. For the reforms implemented in Jiangxi, see F.-L. Chang, *When East Met West: A Personal Story of Rural Reconstruction in China* (New Haven: Yale University Press, 1972), 41–72.

59. Bureau du Comité d'hygiène, Moscow, session of June 25, 1936 C.H./Bureau/IV/Procès-verbal, January 1937, LNA.

60. R. J. Kerner and H. N. Howard, *The Balkan Conferences and the Balkan Entente 1930–1935* (Berkeley: University of California Press, 1936), 159. In the wake of the Locarno Treaty (1925) and Aristide Briand's speech on the United States of Europe (1930), cooperation in health was discussed at a series of conferences. A Balkan medical union was formed in Belgrade in September 1933. However, the animosity between Belgrade and Sofia precluded any concrete results of this goodwill.

61. D. Mitrany, *Marx Against the Peasant: A Study in Social Dogmatism* (Chapel Hill: University of North Carolina Press, 1951), 39; K. Lee, S. Collinson, G. Walt, et al., "Who Should Be Doing What in International Health: A Confusion of Mandates in the United Nations?" *British Medical Journal* 312 (1996): 302–7.

62. D. Ottolenghi, "Rapport sur le voyage de la commission du paludisme en Yougoslavie," 1924, 41, C.H./Malaria/19, LNA; L. Raynaud, "Rapport provisoire sur la visite en Italie de la commission du paludisme," in Société des Nations, Organisation d'hygiène, Commission du paludisme, *Rapport sur son voyage d'étude dans certains pays d'Europe en 1924*, March 26, 1925, C.H. 273, LNA. The commission, set up in 1924, was composed of Alberto Lutrario, former director general of health in Rome, president Price James (Indian Medical Service), L. Bernard (Paris), E. Marchoux (Institut Pasteur), B. Nocht (Hamburg), L. Raynaud (Algiers), D. Ottolenghi (Bologna), G. Pittaluga (Madrid). Also members of the commission were N. H. Swellengrebel and W. A. P. Schüffner (the Hague), E. Marcinowski (Moscow), A. Sfarcic (Belgrade), M. Ciuca (Bucharest), L. Anigstein (Warsaw). See S. Gunn to F. F. Russell, May 2, 1924, 1.1/100 International/20/167, RAC; and L. Raynaud, "Rapport provisoire sur la visite en Italie de la commission du paludisme," March 26, 1925, preface, C.H. 273, LNA. In 1938, apart from Nocht, Marchoux, James, Schüffner, Swellengrebel, and Sfarcic, the commission included G. A. Alfaro and S. Mazza (Argentina); W. G. MacCallum (U.S.), E. Sergent (France), who replaced L. Bernard, who had died four years earlier; G. Bastianelli (Italy) who replaced Ottolenghi (racial laws); and H. Kural (Turkey). See *Acta Conventus tertii de malariæ morbis*, vol. 2, 11. The commission's work was interrupted in 1939.

63. S. P. James and N. H. Swellengrebel, "Principles and Methods of Antimalarial Measures in Europe," 1927, C.H./M.A.L./73, Malaria Commission, LNA. See Harrison, *Mosquitoes*, 185, and Evans, "European Malaria Policy," 48–49. Ten years later,

the controversy had died down, but the doctrine remained unchanged. See Sergent, "Commission du paludisme depuis 1930," 27–31, and Hackett, "Once Upon a Time," 111.

64. For Bulgaria, see W. Mollow, "Ueber Malaria in Bulgarien," *Acta Conventus tertii de malariæ morbis*, vol. 2, 243.

65. Quinine was followed later by plasmoquine and atabrine (not forgetting medicinal chocolate for children). See C. Levi, *Le Christ s'est arrêté à Eboli* (Paris: Gallimard, 1948), 202. Atabrine was not without danger. See R. S. Desowitz, *The Malaria Capers: Tales of Parasites and People* (New York: Norton, 1991), 204–5. See also W. U. Eckart and H. Vondra, "Malaria and World War II: German Malaria Experiments 1939–45," *Parassitologia* 42 (2000): 53–58. (I owe this reference to Iris Borowy.)

66. See, among others, J. Parisot, *Le projet d'équipement national et les assurances sociales* (Paris: Berger-Levrault, 1937), 17–21; Le Lannou, "Rôle," 125–26.

67. Review of "Travaux publics exécutés en Italie pendant les dix premières années du régime fasciste, Ministère des Travaux publics du Royaume d'Italie (Rome, 1934)," *Bulletin mensuel de l'Office international d'hygiène publique* 27 (1935): 612. This picture was fairly distant from reality, according to P. Ginsborg, *A History of Contemporary Italy: Society and Politics, 1943–1988* (London: Penguin Books, 1990), 26, 30; Swellengrebel, "Some aspects," 171. Swellengrebel, in reality, saw *bonifiche* as a method to improve agricultural productivity rather than as malaria prevention. This idea still held sway in the 1960s. See Livadas and Athanassatos, "Benefits," 184.

68. Evans, "European Malaria Policy," 45–47; Brumpt, "Anophélisme," 85, accepted the thesis of the influence of welfare, but only for the temperate zone.

69. S. Litsios, "Malaria Control, the Cold War, and the Postwar Reorganization of International Assistance," *Medical Anthropology* 17 (1997): 267. For the TVA and the struggle against malaria, see Kitron, "Malaria," 308–14. For the depth of the TVA's influence on subsequent reflection by experts at both the WHO and the FAO, see J. C. Scott, *Seeing Like a State: How Certain Schemes to Improve the Human Condition Have Failed* (New Haven: Yale University Press, 1998), 224, 404.

70. Hackett, *Malaria in Europe*, 16; Harrison, *Mosquitoes*, 185; L. J. Bruce-Chwatt and J. de Zulueta, *The Rise and Fall of Malaria in Europe: A Historico-epidemiological Study* (Oxford: Oxford University Press, 1980), 170.

71. Swellengrebel, "Some aspects," 171. Paris green is an arsenical component, invented in 1814, whose larvicidal properties were discovered in 1921. When spread on the surface of water, its fine particles are ingested by the insect, which dies from arsenic and copper acetate poisoning. However, it has no effect on eggs and pupae. In the 1950s, it had not yet been identified as dangerous for human health. See Russell, *Principles*, 133–35. Its use today is extremely limited.

72. James remained marked by the serious failure in the Punjab in 1901 to 1909. See Harrison, *Mosquitoes*, 131–35, 184–85. Some thirteen years later, Sergent's report on the Malaria Commission's work during the 1930s was hardly any better. See Sergent, "Commission du paludisme depuis 1930," 38.

73. S. Gunn to F. F. Russell, March 30, 1925, 1.1/100/20/169, RAC.

74. L. Rajchman to H. Cumming, March 8, 1926, 1.1/100/20/170, RAC. The 1925 report did not minimize the antilarvae measures any less.

75. L. W. Hackett, Comments on the conference held by the Malaria Commission of the League of Nations at Geneva, June 25–29, 1928, 1.1/100/21/173, RAC.

76. Hackett, "Once Upon a Time," 110.

77. Ottolenghi, "Yougoslavie," 34–36. Born in 1874, director (1929–32), then president, of the Bologna School of Pharmacy (1932–35), Donato Ottolenghi was a professor of hygiene at the Naples faculty of medicine when he was dismissed due to the 1938 racial laws. He was a member of the League's Malaria Commission and editor in chief of the publication *Problemi igienici della bonifica integrale* (Florence: Berbera, 1936).

78. Hackett, *Malaria in Europe*, 263.

79. Wenyon, who had led the health service in Macedonia, remained affected by the failure of the quinine campaign in the British expeditionary corps. See C. M. Wenyon, A. G. Enderson, K. McLay, et al., "Malaria in Macedonia, 1915–1919," *Journal of the Royal Army Medical Corps* 37 (1921), no. 2: 81–108; no. 3: 172–80; no. 4: 264–68.

80. B. Nocht, Report of a journey undertaken by Professor Nocht in Jugoslavia at the request of the Malaria Commission and upon the invitation of Professor Štampar from June 25th to July 26th, 1926, for the purpose of investigating the campaign against malaria, September 18, 1926, C.H./Malaria/63, LNA. Bernhard Nocht was the founder (1901) and the director of the Hamburg Institute of Tropical Medicine.

81. Le Haut-Commissaire de la République française à Beyrouth à M. le ministre des Affaires étrangères, Enquête de la S.D.N. sur les besoins en quinine pour le traitement du paludisme, dossier Paludisme et malariologie (1924–1938), SDN/IL/Hygiène/1588, Ministère des Affaires étrangères (hereafter MAE).

82. G. K. Strode's diary, August 2, 1928, RAC. See also L. Rajchman, Sténogramme de son intervention devant l'assemblée annuelle du Conseil général consultatif, Paris, May 19, 1938, 2nd session, 56, 8A/33354/28671, LNA; R. H. Hazemann, "Aperçu général sur la politique médico-sociale à la campagne," *Bulletin de l'Organisation d'Hygiène* 7 (1938): 1009.

83. Z. Fierlinger, Travaux de l'Organisation d'Hygiène, Rapport présenté par la deuxième commission à l'Assemblée, A/67/1929/III, 19–20, SDN/IL/Hygiène/1583, MAE.

84. Hackett, Comments, 6.

85. U. P. Hubbard, "The Cooperation of the United States with the League of Nations and with the International Labour Organization," *International Conciliation* (1931): 725.

86. F. G. Boudreau, The European Conference on Rural Hygiene, memorandum clipped on Sweetser to Fosdick, February 24, 1931, 1.1/100/21/176, RAC. F. G. Boudreau was deputy medical director of the Health Section from March 1925 to June 1937.

87. Le Lannou, "Rôle" was based on the book A. Missiroli, *Lezioni di epidemiologia e profilassi della malaria* (Rome: Armani, 1934). Sorre, *Fondements*, which ignored Hackett, drew on Marchoux and Brumpt.

88. Kitron, "Malaria," 318.

89. Hackett, *Malaria in Europe*, 279–80. It was the idea of Ross. See M. Worboys, "Tropical Diseases," in *Companion Encyclopedia of the History of Medicine*, ed. W. F. Bynum and R. Porter, 524–25 (London: Routledge, 1993).

90. Winslow, "Malaria Control," 3.

91. J. Ferrell to H. Cumming, March 12, 1926, 1.1/100/20/170, RAC. Farley supported the existence of identical views between Hackett and the International Health Board. See Farley, *To Cast Out Disease*, 117–18. In the mid-1930s, that is, at the time that Hackett gave the speeches in London that would form the material for his book, the thing seemed obvious; at the time of the 1928 Geneva meeting, it was not so sure.

92. Russell, *Principles*, 91–92, 123; Hackett, *Malaria in Europe*, xvi. The decline of the endemic disease in the United States has still not been satisfactorily explained. See Humphreys, "Dying Dog," 15–16.

93. Brumpt, "Anophélisme," 77–78, 85–87.

94. Levi, 73.

95. Sallares, *Malaria and Rome*, 83, 198–99.

96. The Bulgarian army met with similar defeat in Macedonia, where in 1918 von Mühlens substituted the war on mosquitoes for quinine treatment. See Mollow, "Malaria in Bulgarien," 241.

97. Hackett, *Malaria in Europe*, 276, 302; Russell, *Principles*, 172.

98. Heggenhougen, Hackethal, and Vivek, *Aspects*, 141.

99. Celli, *History of Malaria*, 173; and, more generally, Hazemann, "Tendances," 777–78.

100. Hackett, *Malaria in Europe*, 269. This was the prevalent idea in the experimental station in Rome. Similar institutions were created along the same lines shortly afterwards in Bulgaria, Greece, and Spain.

101. Hackett, *Malaria in Europe*, 305.

102. H. Prost, *La Bulgarie de 1912 à 1930: Contribution à l'histoire économique et financière de la guerre et de ses conséquences* (Paris: Pierre Roger, 1932), 189–90, 195. A similar operation was also implemented in the Strumica Valley (Petrich).

103. Hackett, *Malaria in Europe*, 318–19. On Petrich, see Mollow, "Malaria in Bulgarien," 243, and D. H. Stapleton, "Technology and Malaria Control, 1930–1960: The Career of Rockefeller Foundation Engineer Frederick W. Knipe," *Parassitologia* 42 (2000): 59–68.

104. Stapleton, "Internationalism," 133.

105. Snowden, "Fields," 46; Ginsborg, *Contemporary Italy*, 132, 138; Brown, "Cultural Model," 244; G. Vicarelli, *Alle Radici della Politica sanitaria in Italia. Società e salute da Crispi al fascismo* (Bologna: il Mulino, 1997), 268–74.

106. Hackett, *Malaria in Europe*, 280. This was one of the intangible principles of the Rockefeller Foundation's strategy that Hackett often had occasion to implement in Central America and Brazil. See S. C. Williams, "Nationalism and Public Health: The Convergence of Rockefeller Foundation Technique and Brazilian Federal Authority During the Time of Yellow Fever, 1925–30," in *Missionaries of Science: The Rockefeller Foundation and Latin America*, ed. M. Cueto (Bloomington: Indiana University Press, 1994), 29.

107. Stapleton, "Internationalism," 133. Hackett gave credit to Missiroli for having been able to obtain Mussolini's support. See Hackett, "Once Upon a Time," 111. Yet, as the director of the *stazione*, he could not have been completely foreign to this tactical move, however discreet a Rockefeller officer should have been when he was on mission. In 1925, when Hackett started to work with the Italian authorities, Mussolini was both head of the government and minister of the interior, with authority over the Health Department. Il Duce personally took the initiative of the *grande*

bonifica of the Pontine marshes and the Agro Romano in 1928. Mussolini was not only considered with great favor in the United States, he himself was, according to Selskar Gunn, known to be pro-American. See Donelli and Serinaldi, *Lotta*, 123–24, 140.

108. J. Viggiano, "Lewis Hackett Photograph Collection," *Rockefeller Archive Center Newsletter*, spring 2004, 9.

109. The Inner Macedonian Revolutionary Organization (VMRO), founded in Thessaloniki in 1893, called for a "Macedonia for the Macedonians." With its nine thousand paramilitaries, it managed, in the Petrich area, to secure all the powers of a government after the assassination of Stamboliiski, the Bulgarian prime minister, in 1923. See H. Poulton, *Who Are the Macedonians?* (London: Hurst & Company, 1995), 80–84.

110. L. Hackett to S. Gunn, March 25, 1925, 710 Public Health, RAC, cited by L. Killen, "The Rockefeller Foundation in the First Yugoslavia," *East European Quarterly* 24 (1990): 353. At the experimental station, Hackett willingly submitted to the authorities' witch-hunt. See Donelli and Serinaldi, *Lotta*, 116–18. See also his comments on the rapid spread of protective screens on the windows of houses, owing to the government's efforts, in Harrison, *Mosquitoes*, 189.

111. Hackett, *Malaria in Europe*, 264, 275.

112. Scott, *Seeing Like a State*, 241.

113. Ottolenghi, "Yougoslavie," 36.

114. Nocht, Journey (1926), 18.

115. Levi, *Christ*, 161.

116. A. Štampar to L. Rajchman, March 10, 1924, C.H./S.C./Malaria/2, LNA.

117. Nocht, Journey (1926), 12.

118. F. G. Boudreau to F. F. Russell, October 14, 1927, 1.1/100/20/171, RAC.

119. Ottolenghi, "Yougoslavie," 42.

120. L. Rajchman, Sténogramme de son intervention devant l'assemblée annuelle du Conseil général consultatif, Paris, May 19, 1938, 2nd session, 62, 65, 8A/33354/28671, LNA.

121. L. S. Hsu, Reconstruction rurale et réorganisation sociale, note personnelle adressée à la Conférence intergouvernementale d'hygiène rurale pour les pays d'Orient, May 11, 1937, 8A/26764/88573 bis, LNA.

122. Hackett, *Malaria in Europe*, 107.

123. Harrison, *Mosquitoes*, 176.

124. Hackett, *Malaria in Europe*, 17–18; C.-E. A. Winslow, "Malaria Control," 4. Alberto Missiroli, who had a degree in bacteriology from the University of Bologna, was attached to the central hygiene laboratory in Rome in 1914 before becoming codirector of the experimental station with Hackett. It was under Missiroli's direction that the plan to eradicate malaria in the *Mezzogiorno* was devised in 1947.

125. D. H. Stapleton, "A Success for Science or Technology? The Rockefeller Foundation's Role in Malaria Eradication in Italy, 1924–35," *Medicina nei Secoli* 6 (1994): 219–20; Winslow, "Malaria Control," 3–4.

126. Winslow, "Malaria Control," 5. See also Hackett, *Malaria in Europe*, 318.

127. Stapleton, "Success," 224–25. After World War II, aerosol sprays (which eradicated adult mosquitoes) often made the spreading of larvicidal products unnecessary.

128. Hackett, "Once Upon a Time," 111.

129. Swellengrebel, "Some aspects," 170.

130. Hackett, *Malaria in Europe*, 205–6.

131. Hackett, *Malaria in Europe*, 318.

132. Hackett, *Malaria in Europe*, 274.

133. Barrett, *Disease and Geography*, 500–501. The Aubing map remained unpublished until 1927, when it was published in E. E. Hume, *Max von Pettenkofer* (New York: Hoeber, 1927). Stapleton, "Success," 221–23.

134. Stapleton, "Success," 222.

135. J. Ziman, *Real Science: What It Is, and What It Means* (Cambridge: Cambridge University Press, 2000), 126–32.

136. Hackett, *Malaria in Europe*, 19; and his letter to F. F. Russell of October 18, 1924, cited by Harrison, *Mosquitoes*, 287, note 16.

137. Hackett, "Once Upon a Time," 111. For the word *fetish*, see E. Embree, untitled manuscript, ca. 1930, Embree Papers, AC 9/1, RAC. Harrison, *Mosquitoes*, 187.

138. Donelli and Serinaldi, *Lotta*, 89–90.

139. Hackett, *Malaria in Europe*, 289–90.

140. Hackett, *Malaria in Europe*, 300.

141. According to the Italian Ministry for Public Works, between 1924 and 1932 the state spent 24 billion lira on all development works in malaria areas (close to 2.5 million hectares), of which 1.5 billion was for *bonifiche* (3 billion if we add the expenses of private individuals) and 692 million for sanitary works as such, "Travaux publics (1935)," 611. The work in the Pontine marshes should not cause us to forget that other infested areas were completely overlooked in the same period, such as the Basilicate. See Levi, *Christ*, 165.

142. Hackett, *Malaria in Europe*, 300, 303, 319.

143. M. C. Balfour, "Malaria Studies in Greece: Measurements of Malaria, 1930–1933," *American Journal of Tropical Medicine* 15 (1935): 302; K. Gardikas, "History of Malaria in Modern Greece," *Research Reports from the Rockefeller Archive Center*, winter 2004/2005, 14–18. For the United States, see Humphreys, "Dying Dog," 3–5.

144. "Interview de L. W. Hackett," *New York Herald*, July 4, 1925, European edition, cited by Donelli and Serinaldi, *Lotta*, 92.

145. Hackett, *Malaria in Europe*, 318.

146. Scott, *Seeing Like a State*, 257–58. On the point that the preliminary mapping of the habitat of *A. labranchiæ* was held partly responsible for the failure to eradicate the vector in Sardinia, see Harrison, *Mosquitoes*, 224.

147. P. Zylberman, "Fewer Parallels than Antitheses: René Sand and Andrija Štampar on Social Medicine, 1919–1955," *Social History of Medicine* 17 (2004): 77–92.

148. The public health model is still that of current epidemiology. See A. Prost, "Environnement, comportements et épidémiologie des maladies," in *Planifier, gérer, évaluer la santé en pays tropicaux*, ed. A. Rougemont and J. Brunet-Jailly (Paris: Doin, 1989); Mitrany, *Marx Against the Peasant*, 114–17, 66.

149. J. Parisot, Oeuvre, f. 14; 5e Réunion du Bureau du Comité d'hygiène, Paris, 29/10/1936, Rapport du Dr Štampar sur ses missions en Chine, 2nd session, 6, C.H./1220, Organisation d'hygiène, LNA.

Selected Bibliography

This bibliography includes a selection of secondary sources on medical history (monographs and journal articles) referred to in the chapters. Full citations for primary sources are provided in the endnotes.

Acheson, Roy. *Wickliffe Rose of the Rockefeller Foundation, 1862–1942*. Cambridge: Cambridge University Press, 1992.

Ackerknecht, Erwin H. "Anticontagionism between 1821 and 1867." *Bulletin of the History of Medicine* 22, no. 5 (1948): 562–93.

———. "Recollections of a Former Leipzig Student." *Journal of the History of Medicine and Allied Sciences* 13 (1958): 147–50.

———. *Medicine at the Paris Hospital 1794–1848*. Baltimore: Johns Hopkins University Press, 1967.

Aly, Götz, Peter Chroust, and Christian Pross. *Cleansing the Fatherland: Nazi Medicine and Racial Hygiene*. Baltimore: Johns Hopkins University Press, 1994.

American Committee on the Costs of Health Care. *Medical Care for the American People: The Final Report*. Chicago: University of Chicago Press, 1932.

Amrith, Sunil. "Development and Disease: Public Health and the United Nations, c. 1945–55." In *Worlds of Political Economy*, edited by M. J. Daunton and F. Trentmann, 217–40. Basingstoke: Palgrave, 2004.

———. *Decolonizing International Health: India and Southeast Asia, 1930–1965*. London: Palgrave, 2006.

Amsterdamska, Olga. "Standardizing Epidemics: Infection, Inheritance, and Environment in Pre-War Experimental Epidemiology." In *Heredity and Infection: The History of Disease Transmission*, edited by J.-P. Gaudillière and I. Löwy, 135–79. London: Routledge, 2001.

Armstrong, David. "Public Health Spaces and the Fabrication of Identity." *Sociology* 27 (1993): 393–410.

Ashton, John, and Howard Seymour. *The New Public Health*. Milton Keynes: Open University Press, 1988.

Auerbach, W. "Gedanken zum Neuaufbau der Niedersächsischen Gesundheitsverwaltung." *Mitteilungen des Niedersächsischen Landesgesundheitsrates*, Heft 1 (1948): 11–22.

Aykroyd, Wallace R. "International Health. A Retrospective Memoir." *Perspectives in Biology and Medecine* 11, no. 1 (1967): 273–85.

Baader, Gerhard. "Politisch motivierte Emigration deutscher Ärzte." *Berichte zur Wissenschaftsgeschichte* 7 (1984): 67–84.

Baldwin, Peter. *Contagion and the State in Europe, 1830–1930*. Cambridge: Cambridge University Press, 1999.

————. *Disease and Democracy: The Industrialized World Faces AIDS.* Berkeley and New York: University of California Press, 2005.

Balfour, M. C. "Malaria Studies in Greece: Measurements of Malaria, 1930–1933." *American Journal of Tropical Medicine* 15, no. 3 (1935): 301–30.

Balinska, Marta. "Assistance and Not Mere Relief: The Epidemic Commission of the League of Nations, 1920–1923." In *International Health Organizations and Movements, 1918–1939,* edited by P. Weindling, 81–108. Cambridge: Cambridge University Press, 1995.

————. *Une vie pour l'humanitaire: Ludwik Rajchman 1881–1965.* Paris: La Découverte, 1995; English edition: 1998.

Ball, M. "Brownell Calls for Food Tax to Fight Epidemic." *Yale Herald,* February 13, 1998.

Balter, Michael. "Europe: AIDS Research on a Budget." *Science* 280 (1998): 1856–59.

Banks, Stanley H. "Discussion of the Present Status of Infectious Disease Control in Continental Europe." *Proceedings of the Royal Society of Medicine* 40 (28 February 1947): 627–29.

Barrett, Frank. *Disease and Geography: The History of an Idea.* Toronto: York University Press, Becker, 2000.

Bashford, Alison. *Imperial Hygiene: A Critical History of Colonialism, Nationalism, and Public Health.* London: Palgrave Macmillan, 2004.

Bayer, Ronald. "AIDS Prevention and Cultural Sensitivity: Are They Compatible?" *American Journal of Public Health* 84, no. 6 (1994): 895–98.

Beatty, T. J. "Soziale Sicherheit in Großbritannien." *Arbeitsblatt für die britische Zone* 2 (1949): 338–40, 419–22.

Bercé, Yves-Marie. "Influence de la malaria sur l'histoire événementielle du Latium (XVIe–XIXe siècles)." In *Maladies et société (XIIe–XVIIIe siècles),* edited by N. Bulst and R. Delort, 235–45. Paris: Éditions du CNRS, 1989.

Berridge, Virginia. "Morality and Medical Science: Concepts of Narcotic Addiction in Britain." *Annals of Science* 36 (1979): 67–85.

————. "Science and Policy: The Case of Post-War British Smoking Policy." In *Ashes to Ashes: The History of Smoking and Health,* edited by S. Lock, L. Reynolds, and E. M. Tansey, 143–63. Amsterdam and Atlanta: Rodopi, 1998.

Beyer, Alfred, and Kurt Winter. *Lehrbuch der Sozialhygiene.* Berlin: Verlag Volk und Gesundheit, 1953.

Birn, Anne-Emanuelle. "Local Health and Foreign Wealth: The Rockefeller Foundation's Public Health Programs in Mexico, 1924–1951." ScD diss., Johns Hopkins University, 1993.

————. "Eradication Control or Neither? Hookworm vs. Malaria Strategies and Rockefeller Public Health in Mexico." *Parassitologia* 40 (1998): 137–48.

————. "A Revolution in Rural Health? The Struggle over Local Health Units in Mexico, 1928–1940." *Journal of the History of Medicine* 53 (1998): 43–76.

————. *Marriage of Convenience. Rockefeller International Health and Revolutionary Mexico.* Rochester, NY: University of Rochester Press, 2006.

Bishop, Eugene L. "The TVA's New Deal in Health." *American Journal of Public Health* 24 (1934): 1023–27.

————. "Consideration of the Malaria Problem in the Tennessee Valley." *Southern Medical Journal* 30, no. 8 (1937): 858–61.

Borowy, Iris, and Wolf D. Gruner, eds. *Facing Illness in Troubled Times: Health in Europe in the Interwar Years, 1918–1939.* Frankfurt am Main and Bern: Peter Lang, 2005.

Bösche, J. W. "Die Reichärztekammer im Lichte von Gesetzgebung und Rechtssprechung der Bundesrepublik Deutschland." *Deutsches Ärzteblatt* 94 (1997): A 1406–10.

Brand, Jane L. "The United States Public Health Service and International Health, 1945–1950." *Bulletin of the History of Medicine* 63 (1989): 579–99.

Brandt, Allan. "Public Health and the Heterogeneous State." Paper presented at Public Health and the State: Yesterday, Today and Tomorrow, Columbia University, NY, October 17–18, 2005.

Brenko, Aida, Zeljko Dugac, and Mirjana Randic. *Narodna Medicina* [Folk Medicine]. Zagreb: Ethnographic Museum, 2001.

Brewster, David. "Environmental Management for Vector Control." *British Medical Journal* 319, no. 11 (September 1999): 651–52.

Broberg, G., and N. Roll-Hansen, eds. *Eugenics and the Welfare State: Sterilization Policy in Denmark, Sweden, Norway, and Finland.* East Lansing: Michigan State University Press, 1996.

Broquet, Charles. "Le Bureau d'hygiène de la Société des Nations." *Revue d'hygiène et de police sanitaire* 48, no. 2 (1921): 124–31.

Brown, Peter J. "Socioeconomic and Demographic Effects of Malaria Eradication: A Comparison of Sri Lanka and Sardinia." *Social Science and Medicine* 22, no. 8 (1986): 847–59.

————. "Malaria, Miseria, and Underpopulation in Sardinia: The 'Malaria Blocks Development' Cultural Model." *Medical Anthropology* 17 (1997): 239–54.

Brown, Richard E. "Public Health and American Imperialism: Early Rockefeller Programs at Home and Abroad." *American Journal of Public Health* 66 (1976): 897–903.

————. *Rockefeller Medicine Men: Medicine and Capitalism in America.* Berkeley: University of California Press, 1979.

Browning, Christopher R. "Genocide and Public Health: German Doctors and Polish Jews, 1939–1941." In *The Path to Genocide: Essays on Launching the Final Solution,* 145–68. Cambridge: Cambridge University Press, 1992.

Bruce-Chwatt, Leonard J., and Julian de Zulueta. *The Rise and Fall of Malaria in Europe: A Historico-Epidemiological Study.* Oxford: Oxford University Press, 1980.

Brumpt, Émile. "Anophélisme sans paludisme et régression spontanée du paludisme." *Annales de parasitologie* 20, no. 1–2 (1944–45): 67–91.

Bruno, Alexander. "Contre la tuberculose: La Mission américaine Rockefeller en France et l'effort français, 1917–1925." Med. diss., Faculté de Médecine, Paris, 1925.

Bucur, Maria. *Eugenics and Modernization in Interwar Romania.* Pittsburgh: Pittsburgh University Press, 2002.

Bullock, Mary B. *An American Transplant: The Rockefeller Foundation and the Peking Union Medical College.* Berkeley: University of California Press, 1980.

Burleigh, Michael. *Death and Deliverance: 'Euthanasia in Germany' c. 1900–1945.* Cambridge: Cambridge University Press, 1994.

Burnet, Etienne, and Wallace R. Aykroyd. "L'alimentation et l'hygiène publique." *Bulletin de l'Organisation d'hygiène de la Société des Nations* 5, no. 2 (1935): 330–481.

Büttner, Lothar, and Bernhard Meyer. "Gesundheitspolitik der revolutionären deutschen Arbeiterbewegung. Vom Bund der Kommunisten bis zum Thälmannschen ZK der KPD." In *Medizin und Gesellschaft*, vol. 25, 82–84. Berlin: Verlag Volk und Gesundheit, 1984.

Buurman, Otto. *Gesundheitspolitik*, rev. enl. ed. Stuttgart: Thieme, 1953.

Carrier, Joseph. "Miguel: Sexual Life History of a Gay Mexican American." In *Gay Culture in America: Essays from the Field*, edited by G. Herdt, 202–24. Boston: Beacon Press, 1992.

Carrier, Joseph M., and J. Raul Magana. "Use of Ethnosexual Data on Men of Mexican Origin for HIV/AIDS Prevention Programs." In *The Time of AIDS: Social Analysis, Theory, and Method*, edited by G. Herdt and S. Lindenbaum, 243–58. Newbury Park, CA: Sage Publications, 1992.

Caumanns, U., and M. G. Esch. "Fleckfieber und Fleckfieberbekämpfung im Warschauer Getto und die Tätigkeit der deutschen Gesundheitsverwaltung 1941/42." In *Geschichte der Gesundheitspolitik in Deutschland Von der Weimarer Republik bis in die Frühgeschichte der „doppelten Staatsgründung,"* edited by W. Woelk and J. Vögele, 225–62. Berlin: Duncker and Humblot, 2002.

Cavailhès, Jean, and Pierre Dutey. *Rapport gai: Enquête sur les modes de vie homosexuels en France.* Paris: Persona, 1984.

Celli, Angelo. *The History of Malaria in the Roman Campagna from Ancient Times.* London: John Bale Sons & Danielsson, 1933. Reprint, New York: AMS Press, 1977.

Chen, C. C. "State Medicine and Medical Education." *Chinese Medical Journal* 49 (1935): 951–54.

———. "Some Problems of Medical Organization in Rural China." *Chinese Medical Journal* 51 (1937): 803–14.

———. *Medicine in Rural China: A Personal Account.* Berkeley: University of California Press, 1989.

Chodzko, Witold. "L'Assainissement de la campagne et l'organisation du service de la santé publique dans les campagnes." *Bulletin de l'Office international d'hygiène publique* 20, no. 8 (1928): 1261–82.

Closen, Michael L. *AIDS: Cases and Materials.* Houston: John Marshall, 1989.

Cohen, Mark N. *Health and the Rise of Civilization.* New Haven: Yale University Press, 1989.

Colla, Piero S. *Per la Nazione e per la Razza. Citadini ed esclusi nel "modello svedese."* Rome: Carocci, 2000.

Collari, Salvatore. "L'Agro Pontino e la bonifica antimalarica." *Rivista di Malariologia* 28 (1949): 299–322.

Colombain, Maurice. "L'hygiène rurale et les coopérative sanitaires en Yougoslavie." *Revue internationale du travail* 32 (1935): 21–41.

Cooper, Richard N. "International Cooperation in Public Health as a Prologue to Macroeconomic Cooperation." In *Can Nations Agree? Issues in International Economic Cooperation*, 178–254. Washington, DC: Brookings Institution, 1989.

Cooter, Roger, Mark Harrison, and Steve Sturdy, eds. *War, Medicine and Modernity.* Stroud, GLS: Sutton, 1998.

Corbellini, Gilberto, and Lorenza Merzagora. *La Malaria tra passato e presente. Storia e luoghi della malaria in Italia.* Rome: Museo di Storia della Medicina, Università La Sapienza, 1998.

Corner, George W. *A History of the Rockefeller Institute, 1901–1953: Origins and Growth.* New York: Rockefeller Institute Press, 1965.

Corvisier, Jean-Nicolas. "Eau, paludisme et démographie en Grèce péninsulaire." *Bulletin de correspondance hellénique,* Supplt 28 (1994): 297–19.

Coxon, Anthony P. M. "Sex Role Separation in Sexual Diaries of Homosexual Men." *AIDS* 7 (1993): 877–82.

Crosby, Alfred W. *America's Forgotten Pandemic: The Influenza of* 1918. Cambridge: Cambridge University Press, 1990.

Cueto, Marcos. "Visions of Science and Development: The Rockefeller Foundation's Latin American Surveys of the 1920s." In *Missionaries of Science: The Rockefeller Foundation and Latin America,* 1–22. Bloomington: Indiana University Press, 1994.

———. "The Cycles of Eradication and Latin America Public Health, 1918–1940." In *International Health Organizations and Movements, 1918–1939,* edited by P. Weindling, 222–43. Cambridge: Cambridge University Press, 1995.

———. "Science Under Adversity: Latin American Medical Research and American Private Philanthropy, 1920–1960." *Minerva* 35 (1997): 233–45.

———. "The Origins of Primary Health Care and Selective Primary Health Care." *American Journal of Public Health* 94 (2004): 1864–74.

Dahlgren, G., and M. Whitehead. *Policies and Strategies to Promote Social Equity in Health.* Stockholm: Institute of Futures Studies, 1991.

Davies, Stephen. *The Historical Origins of Health Fascism.* London: Forest, 1991.

Desowitz, Robert S. *The Malaria Capers: Tales of Parasites and People.* New York: Norton, 1991.

Digby, Anne. "Medicine and the English State, 1901–1948." In *The Boundaries of the State in Modern Britain,* edited by S. J. D. Green and R. C. Whiting, 213–30. Cambridge: Cambridge University Press, 1996.

Doll, Richard, and Austin B. Hill. "Smoking and Carcinoma of the Lung." *British Medical Journal* 2 (1950): 739–48.

———. "Lung Cancer and Other Causes of Death in Relation to Smoking." *British Medical Journal* 2 (1956): 1071–81.

Domeinski, Heinz. "Zur Entnazifizierung der Ärzteschaft im Lande Thüringen." In *Medizin im Faschismus Symposium über das Schicksal der Medizin in der Zeit des Faschismus in Deutschland* 1933-1945, edited by A. Thom and H. Spaar, 320–27. Berlin: Akad. für Ärztl. Fortbildung d. DDR, Arbeitsgruppe Gesundheitspolitik im Kapitalismus, 1983.

Domergue-Cloarec, Danielle. "Les Problèmes de santé à la Conférence de Brazzaville." In *Brazzaville: janvier–février* 1944: *Aux sources de la décolonisation,* edited by Institut Charles de Gaulle and Institut d'Histoire du Temps Présent, 157–69. Paris: Plon, 1988.

Donelli, Gianfranco, and Enrica Serinaldi. *Dalla lotta alla malaria alla nascita dell'Istituto di Sanità Pubblica. Il ruolo della Rockefeller Foundation in Italia: 1922–1934.* Rome and Bari: Laterza, 2003.

Dorolle, Pierre-Marie. "Commentaire sur l'oeuvre d'hygiène rurale intensive à Java." In *Hygiène rurale intensive,* edited by J. L. Hydrick, 66–80. Hanoi: Gouvernement général de l'Indochine, 1938.

Dressen, W., and Volker Rieß. "Ausbeutung und Vernichtung. Gesundheitspolitik im Generalgouvernement." In *Vierteljahreshefte für Zeitgeschichte. Medizin und Gesundheitspolitik in der NS-Zeit,* edited by N. Frei, 157–71. Munich: Oldenbourg, 1991.

Druten, Hans A. M. von. "Homosexual Role Behavior and the Spread of HIV." In *Aids in Europe—The Behavioural Aspect,* edited by D. Friedrich and W. Heckmann, vol. 4, 259–67. Berlin: Sigma, 1995.

Dubin, Martin David. "The League of Nations Health Organization." In *International Health Organizations and Movements, 1918–1939,* edited by P. Weindling, 56–81. Cambridge: Cambridge University Press, 1995.

Dublin, Louis I. "Mortality of Overweights According to Spine Length." Paper read at the annual meeting of the Association of Life Insurance Medical Directors. Newark: Committee on Dryer Measurements in Relation to Life Insurance Underwriting Practice, 1924.

———. "The Relation between Overweight and Cancer: A Preliminary Examination of Evidence from Insurance Statistics." In *Proceedings of the Association of Life Insurance Medical Directors of America,* vol. 15. New York: Association of Life Insurance Medical Directors of America, 1929.

———. "The American People: Studies in Population." *Annals of the American Academy of Political and Social Science* 188 (1936).

———. *A 40-Year Campaign Against Tuberculosis.* New York: Metropolitan Life Insurance Company, 1952.

Dublin, Louis I., and H. H. Marks. "Mortality Risks with Asthma." Paper read at the forty-fourth annual meeting of the Association of Life Insurance Medical Directors of America, October 1933. New York: Press of the Recording and Statistical Corporation, 1934.

———. "Mortality amongst Insured Overweights in Recent Years." Paper read at the sixtieth annual meeting of the Association of Life Insurance Medical Directors of America, October 11–12, 1951. New York: Association of Life Insurance Medical Directors of America, 1952.

Duffy, John. *The Sanitarians: A History of American Public Health.* Chicago: University of Illinois Press, 1990.

Dugac, Zeljko. "New Public Health for a New State: Interwar Public Health in the Kingdom of Serbs, Croats, and Slovenes (Kingdom of Yugoslavia) and the Rockefeller Foundation." In *Facing Illness in Troubled Times: Health in Europe in the Interwar Years, 1918–1939,* edited by Iris Borowy and Wolf D. Gruner, 277–304. Frankfurt am Main: Peter Lang, 2005.

Eckart, Wolfgang U., and Hana Vondra. "Malaria and World War II—German Malaria Experiments 1939–45." *Parassitologia* 42 (2000): 53–58.

Ernst, Anna-Sabine. "Die beste Prophylaxe ist der Sozialismus." *Ärzte und medizinische Hochschullehrer in der SBZ/DDR 1945–1961.* Münster and New York: Waxmann, 1997.

Ettling, John. *The Germ of Laziness: Rockefeller Philanthropy and Public Health in the New South.* Cambridge, MA: Harvard University Press, 1981.

Evans, Hughes. "European Malaria Policy in the 1920s and 1930s: The Epidemiology of Minutiae." *Isis* 80 (1989): 40–59.

Eyler, John. *Victorian Social Medicine: The Ideas and Methods of William Farr.* Baltimore: Johns Hopkins University Press, 1979.

———. *Sir Arthur Newsholme and State Medicine, 1885–1935.* Cambridge: Cambridge University Press, 1997.

Fantini, Bernardino. "Anophelism without Malaria: An Ecological and Epidemiological Puzzle." *Parassitologia* 36 (1994): 83–106.

Farley, John. "Mosquitoes or Malaria? Rockefeller Campaigns in the American South and Sardinia." *Parassitologia* 36, no. 1–2 (1994): 165–73.

———. "The International Health Division of the Rockefeller Foundation: The Russell Years, 1920–1934." In *International Health Organisations and Movements, 1918–1939,* edited by P. Weindling, 203–21. Cambridge: Cambridge University Press, 1995.

———. *To Cast Out Disease: A History of the International Health Division of the Rockefeller Foundation, 1913–1951.* Oxford: Oxford University Press, 2004.

Farrand, Livingston. "The Philosophy of Health Demonstrations." *American Journal of Public Health* Supplt 17 (February 1927): 1–4.

Favez, Jean-Claude. *Une mission impossible? Le CICR, les déportations et les camps de concentration nazis.* Paris: Payot, 1988; English edition, 1999.

Federhen, Ludwig. "Eugenik." In *Der Arzt des öffentlichen Gesundheitsdienstes,* 479–98. Stuttgart: Thieme, 1950.

Fee, Elizabeth. *Disease and Discovery: A History of the Johns Hopkins School of Hygiene and Public Health, 1916–1939.* Baltimore: Johns Hopkins University Press, 1987.

———. "Designing Schools of Public Health for the United States." In *A History of Education in Public Health: Health That Mocks the Doctors' Rules,* edited by E. Fee and R. M. Acheson, 155–94. Oxford: Oxford University Press, 1991.

———. "Public Health and the State: The United States." In *The History of Public Health and the Modern State,* edited by D. Porter, 224–75. Amsterdam: Rodopi, 1994.

Fee, E., and T. M. Brown, eds. *Making Medical History: The Life and Times of Henry E. Sigerist.* Baltimore and London: Johns Hopkins University Press, 1997.

Feligioni, Gianpaolo. "Angelo Celli, medico e deputato. Dalla malaria all'agitazione pro Marche, Umbria e Lazio." *Quaderni del Consiglio Regionale delle Marche* 6, no. 35 (2001): 15–166.

Ferguson, Mary E. *China Medical Board and Peking Union Medical College: A Chronicle of Fruitful Collaboration, 1914–1951.* New York: China Medical Board of New York, 1970.

Fidler, David P. *International Law and Infectious Diseases.* Oxford: Clarendon Press, 1999.

———. *SARS, Governance and the Globalization of Disease.* London: Palgrave, 2004.

Fisher, D. "Rockefeller Philanthropy and the British Empire: The Creation of the London School of Hygiene and Tropical Medicine." *History of Education* 7 (1978): 129–43.

Fitzpatrick, Michael. *The Tyranny of Health: Doctors and the Regulation of Lifestyle.* London: Routledge, 2001.

Flexner, Abraham. *Medical Education in the United States and Canada: A Report to the Carnegie Foundation for the Advancement of Teaching.* New York: Carnegie Foundation for the Advancement of Teaching, 1910.

——. *Medical Education in Europe: A Report to the Carnegie Foundation for the Advancement of Teaching.* New York: Carnegie Foundation for the Advancement of Teaching, 1912.

Fosdick, Raymond. *The Story of the Rockefeller Foundation.* New York: Harper & Bros., 1952.

Fox, Daniel M. *Health Policies, Health Politics: The British and American Experiences, 1911–1965.* Princeton, NJ: Princeton University Press, 1986.

——. "The Administration of the Marshall Plan and British Health Policy." *Journal of Policy History* 16 (2004): 191–211.

Freeburg, Victor O. "Yugoslavia Leads in Rural Health Centers." *Milbank Memorial Fund Quarterly* 12 (1934): 15–27.

Gardikas, Katerina. "History of Malaria in Modern Greece." *Research Reports from the Rockefeller Archive Center* (winter 2004/2005): 14–18.

Garrison, Fielding. "Medical Geography and Geographic Medicine." *Bulletin of the New York Academy of Medicine* 8 (1933): 39–58.

Gaudillière, Jean-Paul. "Rockefeller Strategies for Scientific Medicine: Molecular Machines, Virus and Vaccines." *Studies in History and Philosophy of Biology and Biomedical Sciences* 31C (2000): 491–509.

Giannuli, Dimitra. "'Repeated Disappointment': The Rockefeller Foundation and the Reform of the Greek Public Health System, 1929–1940." *Bulletin of the History of Medicine* 72 (1998): 47–72.

Gillespie, James A. "The Rockefeller Foundation, the Hookworm Campaign and a National Health Policy in Australia, 1911–1930." In *Health and Healing in Tropical Australia and Papua New Guinea,* edited by R. M. MacLeod and D. Denoon, 5–87. Townsville: James Cook University, 1991.

——. "The Rockefeller Foundation and Colonial Medicine in the Pacific, 1911–1929." In *New Countries and Old Medicine,* edited by L. Bryder and D. A. Dow, 380–86. Auckland: Pyramid Press, 1995.

——. "Social Medicine, Social Security and International Health, 1940–60." In *The Politics of the Healthy Life: An International Perspective,* edited by E. Rodríguez-Ocaña, 219–39. Sheffield: EAHMH, 2002.

Girard, Jacques. *Le mouvement homosexuel en France: 1945–1980.* Paris: Syros, 1981.

Goldenberg, J. "Wege und Ausblick der Zusammenarbeit Deutschlands und Sowjetrusslands auf dem Gebiete der Gesundheitspflege." *Osteuropa* 2 (1926/1927): 474–81.

——. "Zusammenarbeit der deutschen und sowjetischen Medizin." *Deutsch-Russische Medizinsche Zeitschrift* 4, no. 1 (1928): 562–64.

Goodman, Neville M. *International Health Organizations and Their Work.* London: J. and A. Churchill, 1952.

Gosse, Louis André. *Rapport sur l'épidémie de choléra en Prusse, en Russie et en Pologne.* Geneva: Bonnaud, 1833.

Goudsblom, Johan. "Zivilisation, Ansteckungsangst und Hygiene: Betrachtungen über ein Aspekt des europäischen Zivilisationsprozesses." In *Materialen zu Norbert Elias' Zivilisationstheorie,* edited by P. Gleichmann, J. Goudsblom, and H. Korte, 215–53. Frankfurt am Main: Suhrkamp, 1979.

Grant, John B. "Public Health as a Social Service [1940]." In *Health Care for the Community: Selected Papers of Dr John B. Grant,* edited by C. Seipp, 14–20. Baltimore: Johns Hopkins University Press, 1963.

———. "Philosophy of Rural Reconstruction in China." *Journal of the Royal Asiatic Society of Bengal Letters* 6 (1940): 119–38.

———. "The Reminiscences of Doctor John B. Grant" [1961]. Glen Rock, NJ: Microfilming Corporation of America, 1976.

Gregg, Alan. "Report on Medical Education in Russia." In *Medical Education in Russia,* vol. 1. 1927.

Grmek, Mirko D. "Géographie médicale et histoire des civilisations." *Annales ESC* 18, no. 6 (1963): 1071–97.

———. *Serving the Cause of Public Health: Selected Papers of Andrija Štampar* . Zagreb: University of Zagreb Press, 1966.

———. *Histoire du SIDA: Début et origine d'une pandémic actuelle.* Paris: Payot, 1989; English edition: 1990.

———. *Les Maladies à l'aube de la civilisation occidentale.* Paris: Payot, 1994.

Hacker, Jacob. *The Divided Welfare State: The Battle over Public and Private Social Benefits in the United States.* Cambridge: Cambridge University Press, 2002.

Hackett, Lewis W. *Malaria in Europe: An Ecological Study.* London: Oxford University Press, 1937.

———. "Once Upon a Time." *American Journal of Tropical Medicine* 9, no. 2 (1960): 105–15.

Hansen, Bent Sigurd. "Something Rotten in the State of Denmark: Eugenics and the Ascent of the Welfare State." In *Eugenics and the Welfare State Sterilization Policy in Denmark, Sweden, Norway, and Finland,* edited by G. Broberg and N. Roll-Hansen, 9–76. East Lansing: Michigan State University Press, 1996.

Hansen, Eckhard, and Paul Klein. *Seit über einem Jahrhundert . . . : Verschüttete Alternativen in der Sozialpolitik. Sozialer Fortschritt, organisierte Dienstleistermacht und nationalsozialistische Machtergreifung: Der Fall der Ambulatorien in den Unterweserstädten und Berlin.* Cologne: Bund-Verlag, 1981.

Hardy, Anne. *The Epidemic Streets: Infectious Disease and the Rise of Preventive Medicine, 1856–1900.* Oxford: Clarendon Press, 1994.

———. *Health and Medicine in Britain since 1860.* Basingstoke: Palgrave, 2001.

Hardy, Anne, and Lise Wilkinson. *Prevention and Cure: From Tropical Medicine to Global Public Health.* London: Kegan Paul, 2000.

Harrison, Gordon. *Mosquitoes, Malaria and Man: A History of the Hostilities since 1880.* London: John Murray, 1978.

Harrison, Mark. *Disease and the Modern World: 1500 to the Present Day.* Cambridge: Polity, 2004.

Harvey, Abner McGee, and Susan Abrams. *"For the Welfare of Mankind": The Commonwealth Fund and American Medicine.* Baltimore: Johns Hopkins University Press, 1986.

Hayry, Matti, and Heta Hayry. "AIDS and a Small North European Country: A Study in Applied Ethics." *International Journal of Applied Philosophy* 3, no. 3 (1987): 51–61.

Hazemann, Robert H. "Aperçu général sur la politique médico-sociale à la campagne." *Bulletin de l'Organisation d'hygiène de la Société des Nations* 7 (1938): 971–1014.

———. "Les Tendances récentes de la politique médico-sociale en Europe." *Bulletin de l'Organisation d'hygiène de la Société des Nations* 8, no. 4–5 (1939): 715–88.

Hellmich, N. "Obesity is the Target." *USA Today,* July 5, 2003.

Henriksson, Benny. *Social Democracy or Societal Control? A Critical Analysis of Swedish AIDS Policy.* Berlin: WZB, Forschungsgruppe Gesundheitsrisiken u. Präventionspolitik, 1988.

Henriksson, Benny, and Hasse Ytterberg. "Sweden: The Power of the Moral(istic) Left." In *AIDS in the Industrialized Democracies: Passions, Politics, and Policies,* edited by D. L. Kirp and R. Bayer, 317–38. New Brunswick, NJ: Rutgers University Press, 1992.

Higgs, Edward. "A Cuckoo in the Nest? The Origins of Civil Registration and State Medical Statistics in England and Wales." *Continuity and Change* 11 (1996): 115–34.

———. "The Statistical Big Bang of 1911: Ideology, Technological Innovation, and the Production of Medical Statistics." *Social History of Medicine* 9, no. 3 (1996): 409–26.

Himes, Norman E. *Medical History of Contraception.* New York: Schocken Books, 1970.

Hirshfield, Daniel. *The Lost Reform: The Campaign for Compulsory Health Insurance in the United States from 1932 to 1943.* Cambridge, MA: Harvard University Press, 1970.

Hockerts, H. G. "Deutsche Nachkriegssozialpolitik vor dem Hintergrund des Beveridge-Plans. Einige Beobachtungen zur Vorbereitung einer vergleichenden Analyse." In *Die Entstehung des Wohlfahrtsstaats in Großbritannien und Deutschland 1850–1950,* edited by W. J. Mommsen, 325–50. Stuttgart: Klett Cotta Verlag, 1982.

Hoffman, Beatrix. *The Wages of Sickness: The Politics of Health Insurance in Progressive America.* Chapel Hill: University of North Carolina Press, 2001.

Howard-Jones, Norman. *The Scientific Background of the International Sanitary Conferences, 1851–1938.* Geneva: WHO, 1975.

———. *International Public Health between the Two World Wars: The Organizational Problems.* Geneva: WHO, 1978.

Huisman, Frank and John Harley Warner, eds. *Locating Medical History: The Stories and their Meanings.* Baltimore and London: Johns Hopkins University Press, 2004.

Humphreys, Margaret. "Kicking a Dying Dog: DDT and the Demise of Malaria in the American South, 1942–1950." *Isis* 87 (1996): 1–17.

———. "Water Won't Run Uphill: The New Deal and Malaria Control in the American South, 1933–1940." *Parassitologia* 40 (1998): 183–91.

Humphreys, Noel A. "The Value of Death-Rates as a Test of Sanitary Condition." *Journal of the Royal Statistical Society* (1874): 437–77.

Hutchinson, John F. *Politics and Public Health in Revolutionary Russia, 1890–1918.* Baltimore: Johns Hopkins University Press, 1990.

———. "'Who Killed Cock Robin?': An Enquiry into the Death of Zemstvo Medicine." In *Health and Society in Revolutionary Russia,* edited by S. G. Solomon and J. F. Hutchinson, 3–26. Bloomington: Indiana University Press, 1990.

———. "'Custodians of the Sacred Fire': The ICRC and the Post-War Reorganisation of the International Red Cross." In *International Health Organizations and Movements, 1918–1939,* edited by P. Weindling, 17–35. Cambridge: Cambridge University Press, 1995.

————. *Champions of Charity: War and the Rise of the Red Cross.* Boulder and London: Westview, 1996.

————. "'Dances with Commissars': Sigerist and Soviet Medicine." In *Making Medical History: The Life and Times of Henry E Sigerist,* edited by E. Fee and T. Brown, 229–58. Baltimore: Johns Hopkins University Press, 1997.

Hydrick, John L. *Intensive Rural Hygiene Work and Public Health Education of the Public Health Service of Netherlands India.* Batavia-Centrum: [Public Health Service of Netherlands India], 1937.

"Hygiène publique et problèmes sociaux aux États-Unis. Rapport élaboré par les médecins hygiénistes qui ont pris part au voyage d'études préparé sous les auspices de l'Organisation d'Hygiène de la Societé des Nations et du Science fédéral d'hygiène publique des États-Unis d'Amérique (4 novembre–7 décembre 1935)." *Bulletin de l'Organisation d'hygiène de la Société des Nations* 5, no. 4 (1936): 811–989.

Illich, Ivan. *Limits to Medicine: Medical Nemesis, the Expropriation of Health.* London: Marion Boyars, 1976.

Illingworth, Patricia. *AIDS and the Good Society.* London: Routledge, 1990.

Immergut, Ellen M. *Health Politics: Interests and Institutions in Western Europe.* Cambridge: Cambridge University Press, 1992.

————. "The Rules of the Game: The Logic of Health Policy-Making in France, Switzerland, and Sweden." In *Structuring Politics: Historical Institutionalism in Comparative Perspective,* edited by S. Steinmo, K. Thelen and F. Longstreth, 57–89. Cambridge: Cambridge University Press, 1992.

Isbell, Michael T. "AIDS and Public Health: The Enduring Relevance of a Communitarian Approach to Disease Prevention." *AIDS and Public Policy Journal* 8, no. 4 (1993): 157–77.

Jacobs, Lawrence. *The Health of Nations: Public Opinion and the Making of American and British Health Policy.* Cambridge: Cambridge University Press, 1993.

Jacobson, Michael F. "Obesity in America: Inevitable?" *Nutrition Action Healthletter,* March 2000: 2.

————. "FDA: Gutless Tiger." *Nutrition Action Healthletter,* July/August 2003: 2.

————. "Big Problem, Small Solution." *Nutrition Action Healthletter,* May 2004: 2.

Janssens, J. G. "Comparative Aspects: I—the Belgian Congo." In *Health in Tropical Africa During the Colonial Period,* edited by E. E. Sabben, D. J. Bradley, and K. Kirkwood. Oxford: Clarendon Press, 1980.

Jeanselme, Édouard. *Traité de la syphilis,* vol. 1. Paris: Doin, 1931.

Jones, Helen. *Health and Society in Twentieth-Century Britain.* Harlow: Longman, 1994.

Jones, W. H. S. "Malaria and History." *Annals of Tropical Medicine and Parasitology* 1, no. 4 (1908): 529–46.

————. *Malaria and Greek History.* Manchester: at the University Press, 1909. Reprint, New York: AMS Press, 1977.

Jordanova, Ludmilla. "Guarding the Body Politic: Volney's Catechism of 1793." In *1789: Reading Writing Revolution—Proceedings of the Essex Conference on the Sociology of Literature, July 1981,* edited by F. Barker, 12–21. Colchester: University of Essex, 1982.

Jorland, Gérard, Annick Opinel, and George Weisz, eds. *Body Counts: Medical Quantification in Historical and Sociological Perspectives.* Montreal: McGill-Queen's University Press, 2005.

Kamminga, Harmke. "'Axes to Grind': Popularising the Science of Vitamins, 1920s and 1930s." In *Food, Science, Policy and Regulation in the Twentieth Century*, edited by D. F. Smith and J. Phillips, 83–100. London: Routledge, 2000.

Kane, Stephanie C. *AIDS Alibis: Sex, Drugs and Crime in the Americas.* Philadelphia: Temple University Press, 1998.

Kater, Hermann. *Politiker und Ärzte. 600 Kurzbiographien und Porträts.* Hameln: Ostertorwall 21 [author's publication], 1968.

Kater, Michael H. *The Nazi Party: A Social Profile of Members and Leaders, 1919–1945.* Cambridge, MA: Harvard University Press, 1983.

———. "Professionalization and Socialization of Physicians in Wilhelmine and Weimar Germany." *Journal of the Contemporary History* 20 (1985): 677–701.

———. *Doctors under Hitler.* Chapel Hill: University of North Carolina Press, 1989.

Kayal, Philip M. *Bearing Witness: Gay Men's Health Crisis and the Politics of AIDS.* Boulder: Westview Press, 1993.

Kearns, Robin, and Alun E. Joseph. "Space in its Place: Developing the Link with Medical Geography." *Social Science and Medicine* 37, no. 6 (1993): 711–17.

Killen, Linda. "The Rockefeller Foundation in the First Yugoslavia." *East European Quarterly* 24, no. 3 (1990): 349–72.

Kingsbury, John. *Health in Handcuffs: The National Health Crisis—and What Can Be Done.* New York: Modern Age Books, 1939.

Kirp, David. "The Politics of Blood: Hemophilia Activism in the AIDS Crisis." In *Blood Feuds: AIDS, Blood and the Politics of Medical Disaster,* edited by E. A. Feldman and R. Bayer, 293–321. New York: Oxford University Press, 1999.

Kitron, Uriel. "Malaria, Agriculture, and Development: Lessons from Past Campaigns." *International Journal of Health Services* 17, no. 2 (1987): 295–326.

Klose, F. "Die Krise des deutschen öffentlichen Gesundheitswesens." *Ärztliche Mitteilungen* 2 (1948): 287–93.

Knopf, Sigard A. *A History of the National Tuberculosis Association: The Anti-Tuberculosis Movement in the United States.* New York: The National Tuberculosis Association, 1922.

Kohler, Robert E. "Science and Philanthropy: Wickliffe Rose and the International Education Board." *Minerva* 23 (1985): 75–95.

Konstantinovitch, B., and K. Schneider. *Principles of Rural Hygiene and Health Cooperatives.* Beograd: Union of Health Cooperatives, 1931.

Krieger, Nancy. "Introduction." In *AIDS: The Politics of Survival,* edited by N. Krieger and G. Margo, vii–xiii. Amityville, NY: Baywood, 1994.

Labisch, Alfons. "Alfred Grotjahn (1869–1931) und das gesundheitspolitische Programm der Mehrheitssozialdemokraten von 1922." *Medizin, Mensch, Gesellschaft* 8 (1983): 192–97.

Labisch, Alfons, and Florian Tennstedt. *Der Weg zum 'Gesetz über die Vereinheitlichung des Gesundheitswesens' vom 3. Juli 1934.* Düsseldorf: Akademie für öffentliches Gesundheitswesen, 1985.

Lafosse, Georges. "Le Centre d'hygiène et d'assistance médico-sociale de Vanves." *Revue philanthropique* (1929): 842–65.

Lauritsen, John. *The AIDS War: Propaganda, Profiteering and Genocide from the Medical-Industrial Complex.* New York: Asklepios, 1993.

Lawrence, Christopher. *Rockefeller Money, the Laboratory, and Medicine in Edinburgh.* Rochester, NY: University of Rochester Press, 2005.

Leavitt, Judith Walzer. *Typhoid Mary, Captive to the Public's Health*. Boston: Beacon Press, 1996.

Lee, Kelley, S. Collinson, and Gill Walt. "Who Should Be Doing What in International Health: A Confusion of Mandates in the United Nations?" *British Medical Journal* 312 (1996): 302–7.

Le Fanu, James. *The Rise and Fall of Modern Medicine*. London: Little Brown, 1999.

Leibfried, Stephan, and Florian Tennstedt. *Berufsverbote und Sozialpolitik 1933. Die Auswirkungen der nationalsozialistischen Machtergreifung auf die Krankenkassenverwaltung und die Kassenärzte*. Bremen: Universität, Forschungsschwerpunktes Reproduktionsrisiken, Soziale Bewegungen u. Sozialpolitik, 1979.

Le Lannou, Maurice. "Le rôle géographique de la malaria." *Annales de géographie* 45, no. 254 (1936): 113–35.

Leroy, Edgar. "Prophylaxie de la tuberculose à la campagne." *Le Mouvement Sanitaire* 5, no. 9 (1929): 552–57.

Levy, B. K. "Dimensions of Personality as Related to Obesity in Women." PhD diss., University of California Berkeley, 1955.

Lewis, G. A. *Your Weight and Your Life: A Scientific Guide to Weight Reduction and Control*. New York: Norton, 1951.

Lewis, Jane. *What Price Community Medicine? The Philosophy, Practice and Politics of Public Health since 1919*. Brighton: Wheatsheaf Books, 1986.

Liebman, B., and J. Hurley. "Beyond Fast Food: 'Fast Casuals' Come of Age." *Nutrition Action* (April 2003): 10–16.

Litsios, Socrates. "Malaria Control, the Cold War, and the Postwar Reorganization of International Assistance." *Medical Anthropology* 17 (1997): 255–78.

———. "The Long and Difficult Road to Alma Ata: A Personal Reflection." *International Journal of Health Services* 32, no. 4 (2002): 709–32.

———. "Selskar Gunn and China: The Rockefeller Foundation's 'Other' Approach to Public Health." *Bulletin of the History of Medicine* 79 (2005): 295–318.

Liubina, G. I. "Osnovnye napravleniia sotrudnichestva sovetskikh i frantsuzskikh uchenykh v 20–30-khgg. XX v. (tochnye i estestvennye nauki)." *Voprosy istorii estestvoznaniia i tekhniki* 3 (1985): 120–27.

Livadas, Gregory, and Demetrios Athanassatos. "The Economics Benefits of Malaria Eradication in Greece." *Rivista di Malariologia* 42 (1963): 177–87.

Logan, John. *The Sardinian Project: An Experiment in the Eradication of an Indigenous Malarious Vector*. Baltimore: Johns Hopkins University Press, 1953.

Ma, Qiusha. "The Rockefeller Foundation and Modern Medical Education in China." PhD diss., Case Western Reserve University, 1995.

———. "The Peking Union College and the Rockefeller Foundation's Medical Programs in China." In *Rockefeller Philanthropy and Modern Biomedicine: International Initiatives from World War I to the Cold War*, edited by W. Schneider, 159–83. Bloomington: Indiana University Press, 2002.

Manderson, Lenore. "Wireless Wars in the Eastern Arena: Epidemiological Surveillance, Disease Prevention and the Work of the Eastern Bureau of the League of Nations Health Organisation, 1924–1942." In *International Health Organizations and Movements 1918–1939*, edited by P. Weindling, 109–33. Cambridge: Cambridge University Press, 1995.

Mann, Jonathan M., and Daniel J. M. Tarantola, eds. *AIDS in the World II: Global Dimensions, Social Roots, and Responses.* The Global AIDS Policy Coalition. New York: Oxford University Press, 1996.

Marcusson, Erwin. *Sozialhygiene. Grundlagen und Organisation des Gesundheitsschutzes.* Leipzig: Thieme, 1954.

Markowitz, Gerald, and David Rosner. *Deceit and Denial: The Deadly Politics of Industrial Pollution.* Berkeley and Los Angeles: University of California Press, 2002.

Marks, Shula. "South Africa's Early Experiment in Social Medicine: Its Pioneers and Politics." *American Journal of Public Health* 87 (1997): 452–59.

Marshall, Tom, Eileen Kennedy, and Susan Offutt. "Exploring a Fiscal Food Policy: The Case of Diet and Ischaemic Heart Disease." *British Medical Journal* 320 (2000): 301–5.

Martet, Christophe. *Les combattants du sida.* Paris: Flammarion, 1993.

Ministerium für Arbeit und Gesundheitswesen der DDR, Hauptabteilung Gesundheitswesen, ed. *Das demokratische Gesundheitswesen in der Deutschen Demokratischen Republik.* Berlin: Arbeitsgemeinschaft medizinischer Verlag, 1950.

Mollow, W. "Ueber Malaria in Bulgarien." In *Acta Conventus Tertii de Malariæ Morbis,* vol. II, 240–49. Amsterdam: Spin & Zoon, 1938.

Montagnier, Luc. *Vaincre le SIDA: entretiens avec Pierre Bourget.* Paris: Fondation internationale pour l'information scientifique: Cana, 1986.

Mooney, Graham. "Professionalisation in Public Health and the Measurement of Sanitary Progress in Nineteenth-Century England and Wales." *Social History of Medicine* 10, no. 1 (1997): 53–78.

Mooney, Graham, Bill Luckin, and Andrea Tanner. "Patient Pathways: Solving the Problem of Institutional Mortality in London during the Later Nineteenth Century." *Social History of Medicine* 12, no. 2 (1999): 227–69.

Moriyama, I. M. "Statistical Studies of Heart Disease 1–9." *Public Health Reports* 1. 63 (1948) no 16: 537–45; 2. 63 (1949) no. 39: 1247–69; 3. 64 (1949) no. 4: 104–9; 4. 64 (1949), no. 14: 439–56; 5. 64 (1949), no. 46: 1439–92; 6. 65 (1950), no. 17: 555–71; 7. 65 (1950), no. 26: 819–38; 8. 66 (1951), no. 3: 57–80; 9. 66 (1951), no. 12: 355–68.

Morris, J. N. "Coronary Heart-Disease and Physical Activity of Work." *Lancet* 257 (1953): 1053–57.

Morrison, L. M. *The Low-Fat Way to Health and Longer Life: The Complete Guide to Better Health Through Automatic Weight Control, Modern Nutritional Supplements, and Low-Fat Diet.* Englewood Cliffs, NJ: Prentice-Hall, 1958.

Moser, Gabriele. *"Im Interesse der Volksgesundheit . . ." Sozialhygiene und öffentliches Gesundheitswesen in der Weimarer Republik und der frühen SBZ/DDR. Ein Beitrag zur Sozialgeschichte des deutschen Gesundheitswesens im 20. Jahrhunderts.* Basel: VAS Verlag, 1999.

Mosse, Max, and Gustav Tugendreich, eds. *Krankheit und soziale Lage.* Munich: Lehmann, 1913.

München, Rolf Schuster, ed. *Deutsche Verfassungen.* rev. enl. ed. Munich: Goldmann Verlag, 1992.

Münchow, S. "Über die Gründung der Akademie für Staatsmedizin in Hamburg." *Hamburger Ärzteblatt* 21 (1967): 302–5.

Murard, Lion. "Atlantic Crossings in the Measurement of Health: From the US Appraisal Forms to the League of Nations's Health Indices." In *Medicine, the Market and the Mass Media*, edited by V. Berridge and K. Loughlin, 19–54. London: Routledge, 2005.

———. "Health Policy between the International and the Local: Jacques Parisot in Nancy and Geneva." In *Facing Illness in Troubled Times: Health in Europe in the Interwar Years, 1918–1939*, edited by Iris Borowy and Wolf D. Gruner, 207–45. Frankfurt am Main and Bern: Peter Lang, 2005.

Murard, Lion, and Patrick Zylberman. "La Mission Rockefeller en France et la création du Comité national de défense contre la tuberculose, 1917–1923." *Revue d'histoire moderne et contemporaine* 34 (1987): 257–81.

———. "French Social Medicine on the Map of International Public Health in the 1930s." In *The Politics of the Healthy Life: An International Perspective*, edited by E. Rodríguez-Ocaña, 197–218. Sheffield: EAHMH, 2002.

Najera, J. A. "The Control of Tropical Diseases and Socioeconomic Development (with Special Reference to Malaria and its Control)." *Parassitologia* 36 (1994): 17–33.

Newsholme, Arthur. "The New York State Health Demonstrations in Syracuse and in Cattaraugus County." *Milbank Memorial Fund Quarterly Bulletin* 4 (1926): 49–66.

———. *International Studies in the Relation between the Private and Official Practice of Medicine, with Special Reference to the Prevention of Disease*. London: Allen & Unwin, 1931.

———. *Medicine and the State. The Relation between the Private and Official Practice of Medicine, With Special Reference to Public Health*. London: George Allen & Unwin, 1932.

Newsholme, Arthur, and John Adams Kingsbury. *Red Medicine: Socialized Health Care in Soviet Russia*. New York: Doubleday, 1933.

Niehoff, Jens-Uwe, and Thomas Röding. "Steuerung und Regulierung von Prävention in der Deutschen Demokratischen Republik." In *Prävention und Prophylaxe Theorie und Praxis eines gesundheitspolitischen Grundmotivs in zwei deutschen Staaten 1949–1990*, edited by T. Elkeles, J.-U. Niehoff, R. Rosenbrock, et al., 159–67. Berlin: Sigma, 1991.

Oppenheimer, Gerald M. "Becoming the Framingham Study 1947–1950." *American Journal of Public Health* 95 (2005): 602–10.

Osborne, Michael. "The Geographical Imperative in Nineteenth-Century French Medicine." In *Medical Geography in Historical Perpective*, edited by N. Rupke, 31–50. London: Wellcome Institute for the History of Medicine, 2000.

"Overeating, Overweight, and Obesity." Paper read at proceedings of the Nutrition Symposium, Harvard School of Public Health, Boston, Massachusetts, October 29, 1952. Nutrition Symposium Series. New York: National Vitamin Foundation, 1953.

Packard, Randall. "Visions of Post-War Health and Development and Their Impact on Public Health Interventions in the Developing World." In *International Development and the Social Sciences*, edited by R. Packard and F. Cooper, 96–113. Berkeley: University of California Press, 1997.

Page, Benjamin B. "First Steps: The Rockefeller Foundation in Early Czechoslovakia." *East European Quarterly* 35 (2001): 259–308.

———. "The Rockefeller Foundation and Central Europe: A Reconsideration." *Minerva* 40 (2002): 265–87.

Parisot, Jacques. "Les Assurances sociales en France. Les enseignements de l'étranger." *Revue d'hygiène et de prophylaxie sociales* 9 (1930): 14–18, 51–57, 74–93, 113–29.

———. *Le projet d'équipement national et les assurances sociales.* Paris: Berger-Levrault, 1937.

Paz Soldan, Carlos Enrique. *La OMS y la Soberanía Sanitaria de las Américas.* Lima: Instituto de Medicina Social de la Universidad Mayor de San Marcos, 1949.

Petersen, Alan, and Deborah Lupton. *The New Public Health: Health and Self in the Age of Risk.* London and Thousand Oaks, CA: Sage, 1996.

Pollak, Michael. *The Second Plague of Europe: AIDS Prevention and Sexual Transmission among Men in Western Europe.* New York: Haworth Press, 1994.

Porter, Dorothy. "John Ryle: Doctor of Revolution?" In *Doctors, Politics and Society: Historical Essays*, 247–74. Amsterdam: Rodopi, 1993.

———, ed. *The History of Public Health and the Modern State.* Amsterdam and Atlanta: Rodopi, 1994.

———. "Public Health and Centralisation: The Victorian State." In *Oxford Text Book of Public Health*, vol. 1: *The Scope of Public Health*, edited by R. Detels and W. W. Holland, 19–34. Oxford: Oxford University Press, 1997.

———. *Health, Civilization and the State: A History of Public Health from Ancient Times to Modern Times.* London: Routledge, 1999.

———. "Eugenics and the Sterilization Debate in Sweden and Britain Before World War II." *Scandinavian Journal of History* 24 (2000): 145–62.

———. "The Healthy Body in the Twentieth Century." In *Medicine in the Twentieth Century*, edited by R. Cooter and J. Pickstone, 201–16. Amsterdam: Harwood Academic Publications, 2000.

Prausnitz, Carl. "L'enseignement de l'hygiène en Yougoslavie." *Rapport sur les travaux des Conférences des Directeurs d'Écoles d'hygiène tenues à Paris, du 20 au 23 mai 1930 et à Dresde du 14 au 17 juillet 1930*, 117–22. Geneva: Société des Nations, 1930.

———. *The Teaching of Preventive Medicine in Europe.* London: Humphrey Milford, Oxford University Press, 1933.

Pressman, J. "Human Understanding: Psychosomatic Medicine and the Mission of the Rockefeller Foundation." In *Greater than the Parts: Holism in Biomedicine, 1920–1950*, edited by C. Lawrence and George Weisz, 189–208. New York: Oxford University Press, 1998.

Preußer/Landesgesundheitsrat, Die Eugenik im Dienste der Volkswohlfahrt. *Bericht über die Verhandlungen eines zusammengesetzten Ausschusses des Preußischen Landesgesundheitsrats vom 2. Juli 1932.* Veröffentlichungen aus dem Gebiet der Medizinalverwaltung. Vol. 38, Heft 5. Berlin: 1932.

Proctor, Robert N. *The Nazi War on Cancer.* Princeton, NJ: Princeton University Press, 1999.

Prost, André. "Environnement, comportements et épidémiologie des maladies." In *Planifier, gérer, évaluer la santé en pays tropicaux*, edited by A. Rougemont and J. Brunet-Jailly, 65–90. Paris: Doin, 1989.

Rafferty, Anne Marie. "Internationalising Nursing Education during the Interwar Period." In *International Health Organisations and Movements, 1918–1939*, edited by P. Weindling, 266–82. Cambridge: Cambridge University Press, 1995.

"Rapport sur la réunion des directeurs d'instituts et d'écoles d'hygiène tenue à Genève du 22 au 27 novembre 1937." *Bulletin de l'Organisation d'hygiène de la Société des Nations* 7, no. 2 (1938): 180–383.

Rechy, John. *The Sexual Outlaw: A Documentary; A Non-fiction Account, with Commentaries, of Three Days and Nights in the Sexual Underground.* New York: Grove Press, 1977.

Registrar-General. *Standardization of Mortality Comparisons—New Procedure.* Statistical Review of England and Wales for the year 1941 (New Annual Series, no. 21), Tables, Part I, Medical Appendix. London: HMSO, 1945.

Renker, Karlheinz, and Kurt Winter. "Sozialhygiene und Gesundheitsschutz im Sozialismus am Beispiel der DDR. Zur gesellschaftlichen Bedingtheit der Medizin in der Geschichte." In *Medizin und Gesellschaft Beihefte zur Zeitschrift für ärztliche Fortbildung,* vol. 10, edited by D. Tutzke, 200–212. Jena: Gustav Fischer Verlag, 1981.

"Report of the Subcommittee on Policies with Respect to Health and Medical Care. 1st Session of Council, Atlantic City, 10 November to 1 December 1943." *UNRRA Journal* (1947).

"Résolutions de la Conférence intergouvernementale des pays d'Orient sur l'hygiène rurale." *Journal officiel de la Société des Nations* (December 1937): 1311.

Reverby, Susan. *Tuskegee's Truths: Rethinking the Tuskegee Syphilis Study.* Chapel Hill: University of North Carolina Press, 2000.

Rodríguez-Ocaña, Esteban, ed. *The Politics of the Healthy Life: An International Perspective.* Sheffield: EAHMH, 2002.

Rodríguez-Ocaña, E., J. Bernabeu-Mestre, and J. L. Barona. "La Fundación Rockefeller y Espana, 1914–1936. Un acuerdo para la modernización cientifica y sanitaria." In *Estudios de historia de las tecnicas, la arqueologia industrial y las ciencias,* vol. II, edited by J. L. Garcia, J. M. Moreno, and G. Ruiz, 531–39. Valladolid: Consejería de Educación y Cultura, 1998.

Rosen, George. *From Medical Police to Social Medicine: Essays on the History of Health Care.* New York: Science History Publications, 1974.

Rosenberg, W. "The Zemstvo in 1917." In *The Zemstvo in Russia: An Experiment in Local Self-Government,* edited by T. Emmons and W. Vuchinich, 383–421. Cambridge: Cambridge University Press, 1982.

Rotello, Gabriel. *Sexual Ecology: AIDS and the Destiny of Gay Men.* New York: Dutton, 1997.

Rothstein, William G. *Public Health and the Risk Factor: A History of an Uneven Medical Revolution.* Rochester, NY: University of Rochester Press, 2003.

Roubakine, Alexandre N. "Avortement, problème social, et sa solution dans l'Union des Républiques socialistes soviétiques." *Annales d'hygiène publique et de médecine légale* 9 (1929): 153–68.

———. "La réforme de l'enseignement de la médecine dans l'Union des Républiques socialistes soviétiques." *Revue d'hygiène et de médecine sociales* (1931): 69–80.

———. *La Protection de la santé publique dans l'URSS, principes et résultats.* Paris: Bureau d'éditions, 1933.

Rubakin, Alexander N. *Frantsuzskie zapisi, 1939–1943.* Moscow: Sov. Pisatel,' 1947.

Rubenstein, William. "Law and Empowerment: The Idea of Order in the Time of AIDS." *Yale Law Journal* 98 (1989): 975–97.

Rupke, Nicolaas A., and Karen E. Wonders. "Humboldtian Representations in Medical Cartography." In *Medical Geography in Historical Perpective*, edited by N. Rupke, 163–77. London: Wellcome Institute for the History of Medicine, 2000.

Russell, Paul F. *Malaria: Basic Principles Briefly Stated.* Oxford: Blackwell, 1952.

Rüther, M. "Ärztliches Standeswesen im Nationalsozialismus 1933–1945." In *Geschichte der deutschen Ärzteschaft Organisierte Berufs- und Gesundheitspolitik im 19 und 20 Jahrhundert*, edited by R. Jütte, 143–93. Cologne: Dt. Ärzte-Verlag, 1997.

Ruzheinikov, I. S. "Reforma vysshego meditsinskogo obrazovaniia." *Biulleten' Narkomzdrava*, 1924, no. 11: 27.

Sachße, Christoph. *Mütterlichkeit als Beruf. Sozialarbeit, Sozialreform und Frauenbewegung 1871–1929.* Frankfurt am Main: Suhrkamp, 1986.

Sachße, Christoph, and Florian Tennstedt. *Geschichte der Armenfürsorge in Deutschland*, vol. 2: *Fürsorge und Wohlfahrtspflege 1871–1929*. Berlin and Cologne: 1988.

Sallares, Robert. *Malaria and Rome: A History of Malaria in Ancient Italy.* Oxford: Oxford University Press, 2002.

Sand, René. *The Advance to Social Medicine.* London: Staples, 1952.

Savigny, Jean de. *Le Sida et les fragilités françaises: Nos réactions face à l'épidémie.* Paris: Albin Michel, 1995.

Sawyer, Wilbur A. "Achievements of UNRRA as an International Health Organization." *American Journal of Public Health* 37 (1947): 41–58.

Schagen, Udo. "Kongruenz der Gesundheitspolitik von Arbeiterparteien, Militäradministration und der Zentralverwaltung für das Gesundheitswesen in der Sowjetischen Besatzungszone." In *Geschichte der Gesundheitspolitik in Deutschland Von der Weimarer Republik bis in die Frühgeschichte der "doppelten Staatsgründung,"* edited by W. Woelk and J. Vögele, 379–404. Berlin: Duncker and Humblot, 2002.

Schagen, Udo, and Sabine Schleiermacher. "Gesundheitswesen und Sicherung bei Krankheit und im Pflegefall. Einleitung: Rahmenbedingung für die Reorganisation des Gesundheitswesens. Die Sowjetische Besatzungszone und Berlin." In *Geschichte der Sozialpolitik in Deutschland seit 1945*, vol. 2/1: *1945–1949, Die Zeit der Besatzungszonen*, edited by the Bundesarchiv, Bundesministerium für Arbeit und Sozialordnung, 464–528. Baden-Baden: Nomos Verlag, 2001.

Schleiermacher, Sabine. "Experte und Lobbyist für Bevölkerungspolitik. Hans Harmsen inder Weimarer Republik, nationalsozialismus und Bevölkerungspolitik." In *Experten und Politik: Wissenschaftliche Politikberatung in geschichtlicher Perspektive*, edited by S. Fisch and W. Rudloff, 211–38. Berlin: Duncker und Humblot, 2004.

Schneider, William H. "The Men Who Followed Flexner: Richard Pearce, Alan Gregg and the Rockefeller Foundation Medical Divisions, 1919–1951." In *Rockefeller Philanthropy and Modern Biomedicine*, edited by W. Schneider, 7–60. Bloomington: Indiana University Press, 2002.

———. "War, Philanthropy, and the Creation of the French National Institute of Hygiene." *Minerva* 41 (2003): 1–23.

Schröder, E. "Gesundheitspflege als Aufgabe von Gesetzgebung und Verwaltung." *Der öffentliche Gesundheitsdienst* 12, no. 9 (1950): 317–36.

Schünemann, Bernd. "Die Rechtsprobleme der AIDS-Eindämmung." In *Die Rechtsprobleme von AIDS*, edited by B. Schünemann and G. Pfeiffer, 373–509. Baden-Baden: Nomos, 1988.

Schütt, Eduard, and Nathanael Wollenweber, eds. *Der Arzt des öffentlichen Gesundheitswesens* 1941. Leipzig: G. Thieme, 1941.

Schwoch, R. "Ärztliche Standespolitik im Nationalsozialismus. Julius Hadrich und Karl Haedenkamp als Beispiele." Diss. phil. Fachbereich Geschichts- und Kulturwissenschaften, Freie Universität Berlin, 1999.

Sealander, Judith. *Private Wealth and Public Life: Foundation Philanthropy and the Reshaping of American Social Policy from the Progressive Era to the New Deal.* Baltimore: Johns Hopkins University Press, 1997.

Semachko, Nikolai A. "Das Gesundheitswesen in Sowjetrussland." *Deutsche medizinische Wochenschrift* 4 (1924): 117–19.

———. "L'hygiène en Russie soviétique." *Revue franco-russe de médecine et de biologie,* 1924, no. 2: 10–16.Semashko, Nikolai A. *Nauka o zdorov'e obshchestva.* Moscow: 1921.

———. "L'hygiène en Russie soviétique II." *Revue franco-russe de médecine et de biologie,* 1925, no. 2: 9–15.

———. "Quelques aperçus de l'hygiène soviétique." *Revue franco-russe de médecine et de biologie,* 1926, no. 1: 1–13.

Sergent, Edmond. "L'oeuvre de la commission du paludisme de la Société des Nations depuis 1930." In *Acta Conventus Tertii de Malariae Morbis,* vol. 2, 25–48. Amsterdam: Spin & Zoon, 1938.

Shorter, Edward. *From Paralysis to Fatigue: A History of Psychosomatic Illness in the Modern Era.* New York: Free Press, 1993.

Shryock, Richard H. *National Tuberculosis Association 1904–1954: A Study of the Voluntary Health Movement in the United States.* New York: National Tuberculosis Association, 1957.

———. *The Development of Modern Medicine: An Interpretation of the Social and Scientific Factors Involved.* Madison: University of Wisconsin Press, 1979.

Siddiqi, Javed. *World Health and World Politics: The World Health Organization and the UN System.* London: Hurst, 1995.

Sigerist, Henry E. *Civilization and Disease.* Ithaca, NY: Cornell University Press, 1943.

"Sitzung des Interkommunalen Ausschusses für das Gesundheitswesen am 8. Dezember 1930 in Berlin." *Zeitschrift für Gesundheitsverwaltung und Gesundheitsfürsorge* 2 (1931): 185–91.

Snowden, Frank M. "'Fields of Death': Malaria in Italy 1861–1962." *Modern Italy* 4, no. 1 (1999): 25–57.

Solomon, Susan Gross. "Social Hygiene in Soviet Medical Schools, 1922–1930." *Journal of the History of Medicine and Allied Sciences,* October 1990: 153–221.

———. "The Soviet Legalization of Abortion in German Medical Discourse: A Study of the Use of Selective Perceptions in Cross-Cultural Scientific Relations." *Social Studies of Science* 22, no. 3 (1992): 455–87.

———. "Das Reisetagebuch als Quelle für die Analyse binationaler medizinischer Unternehmungen." In *Karl Wilmanns: Lues, Lamas, Leninisten Tagebuch einer Reise durch Russland in die Burjatische Republik im Sommer 1926,* edited by J. Richter, 1–41. Pfaffenweiler: Centaurus, 1995.

———. "Vergleichende Völkerpathologie auf unerforschtem Gebiet: Ludwig Aschoffs Reise nach Russland und in den Kaukasus im Jahre 1930." In *Vergleichende Völkerpathologie oder Rassenpathologie,* edited by S. G. Solomon and J. Richter, 1–50. Pfaffenweiler: Centaurus, 1998.

———. "Through a Glass Darkly: The Rockefeller Foundation's International Health Board and Soviet Public Health." *Studies in History and Philosophy of Biological and Biomedical Science* 31C, no. 3 (2000): 409–18.

———. "Fact Finding and Policy Making: The Rockefeller Foundation's Division of Medical Education and the 'Russian Matter,' 1925–1927." *Journal of Policy History* 14, no. 4 (2002): 384–417.

———. "Local Knowledge or Knowledge of the Local: Rockefeller Foundation Officers' Site Visits to Russia in the 1920s." *Slavic Review* 62 (2003): 710–33.

———, ed. *Doing Medicine Together: Germany and Russia between the Wars.* Toronto: University of Toronto Press, 2006.

———. "The Intermediary as Strategist: John A. Kingsbury, Soviet Socialized Medicine, and 1930s America." *Annales ESC* (forthcoming).

Solomon, Susan Gross, and Nikolai Krementsov. "Giving and Taking Across Borders: The Rockefeller Foundation and Russia, 1919–1928." *Minerva* 39 (2001): 265–98.

Sons, Hans-Ulrich. *Gesundheitspolitik während der Besatzungszeit. Das öffentliche Gesundheitswesen in Nordrhein-Westfalen 1945–1949.* Wuppertal: Hammer, 1983.

Soper, Fred L. *Building the Health Bridge: Selections from the Works of Fred L. Soper,* edited by J. A. Kerr. Bloomington: Indiana University Press, 1970.

Sorre, Max. "Complexes pathogènes et géographie médicale." *Annales de Géographie* 42 (1933): 1–18.

———. *Les Fondements de la géographie humaine,* vol. 1: *Les fondements biologiques.* Paris: Colin, 1947.

Srikameswaran, A. "WHO Wants 'Twinkie Tax' to Discourage Junk Foods." *Pittsburgh Post-Gazette,* December 6, 2003.

Stambolian, George. *Male Fantasies/Gay Realities: Interviews with Ten Men.* New York: SeaHorse Press, 1984.

Štampar, Andrija. "Méthodes les plus effectives pour organiser les services d'hygiène dans les régions rurales." In Société des Nations, Organisation d'Hygiène, *Conférence européanne sure l'Hygiène rurale (29 Juin–7 Juillet 1931),* vol. 1: *Recommendations sur les principes directeurs de l'Organisation de l'Assistance Médicale, des Sciences d'Hygiène et de l'assaissment dans les districts rureaux,* C.473. M.202, Geneva: Société des Nations, 1931, 24–41.

———. "Rapport du Dr. A. Štampar sur ses missions en Chine." *Bulletin de l'Organisation d'hygiène de la Société des Nations* 5 (1936): 1208–50.

———. *Public Health in Jugoslavia.* London: School of Slavonic and East European Studies in the University of London, 1938.

Stapleton, Darwin H. "A Success for Science or Technology? The Rockefeller Foundation's Role in Malaria Eradication in Italy, 1924–35." *Medicina nei Secoli* 6, no. 1 (1994): 213–28.

———. "Internationalism and Nationalism: The Rockefeller Foundation, Public Health, and Malaria in Italy, 1923–1951." *Parassitologia* 42, nos. 1–2 (2000): 127–34.

———. "Technology and Malaria Control, 1930–1960: The Career of Rockefeller Foundation Engineer Frederick W. Knipe." *Parassitologia* 42 (2000): 59–68.

Stewart, A. M., J. W. Webb, and D. Hewitt. "Observations on 1,078 Perinatal Deaths." *British Journal of Social Medicine* 9 (1955): 57–61.

Stone, Diane. "Learning Lessons and Transferring Policy across Time, Space and Disciplines." *Politics* 19, no. 1 (1999): 51–59.

Stouman, Knud, and Isidore S. Falk. "Health Indices: A Study of Objective Indices of Health in Relation to Environment and Sanitation." *Quarterly Bulletin of the Health Organisation* 5 (1936): 901–66.

Strickland, Stephen P. *Politics, Science, and Dread Disease: A Short History of United States Medical Research Policy.* Cambridge, MA: Harvard University Press, 1972.

Sydenstricker, Edgar. "The Incidence of Illness in a General Population Group: General Results of a Morbidity Study from December 1, 1921 through March 31, 1924, in Hagerstown, Maryland." *Public Health Reports*, 1925, no. 49: 271–91.

———. *Health and Environment.* New York: McGraw-Hill, 1933.

Szreter, Simon. "The Importance of Social Intervention in Britain's Mortality Decline c. 1850–1914: A Re-interpretation of the Role of Public Health." *Social History of Medicine* 1, no. 1 (1988): 1–37.

———. "Economic Growth, Disruption, Deprivation, Disease and Death: On the Importance of the Politics of Public Health for Development." In *Plagues and Politics: Infectious Disease and International Policy*, edited by A. T. Price-Smith, 76–116. London: Palgrave, 2001.

———. *Health and Wealth: Studies in History and Policy.* Rochester, NY: University of Rochester Press, 2005.

Tennstedt, Florian. "Sozialgeschichte der Sozialversicherung." In *Handbuch der Sozialmedizin*, vol. 3, edited by M. Blohmke, 385–492. Stuttgart: Enke Verlag, 1976.

———. *Geschichte der Selbstverwaltung in der Krankenversicherung von der Mitte des 19. Jahrhunderts bis zur Gründung der Bundesrepublik Deutschland.* Bonn: Verlag der Ortskrankenkassen, 1977.

Thomsen, Peter. *Ärzte auf dem Weg ins "Dritte Reich." Studien zur Arbeitsmarktsituation, zum Selbstverständnis und zur Standespolitik der Ärzteschaft gegenüber der staatlichen Sozialversicherung während der Weimarer Republik.* Husum: Matthiesen, 1996.

Tilley, Helen. "Ecologies of Complexity: Tropical Environments, African Trypanosomiasis, and the Science of Disease Control in British Colonial Africa, 1900–1940." *Osiris* 19 (2004): 21–38.

———. *Africa as a Living Laboratory: Science, Nature, and Imperial Development in the Tropics* (forthcoming).

Towers, Bridget. "Red Cross Organisational Politics, 1918–1922: Relations of Dominance and the Influence of the United States." In *International Health Organizations and Movements, 1918–1939*, edited by P. Weindling, 36–55. Cambridge: Cambridge University Press, 1995.

Tutzke, Dietrich. *Alfred Grotjahn. Biographien hervorragender Naturwissenschaftler, Techniker und Mediziner*, vol. 36. Leipzig: Teubner, 1979.

United Nations Relief and Rehabilitation Administration, Division of Operational Analysis, Paper no. 6. *UNRRA's Welfare Programme in Italy: Supplementary Feeding of Mothers and Children.* London: UNRRA, European Regional Office, 1946.

Vaughan, Henry F. "Local Health Services in the United States: The Story of the CAP." *American Journal of Public Health* 62 (1972): 95–111.

Venkataramani, M. S. *The Bengal Famine of 1943: The American Response.* Delhi: Vikas, 1973.

Vicarelli, Giovanna. *Alle Radici della Politica sanitaria in Italia. Società e salute da Crispi al fascismo.* Bologna: il Mulino, 1997.

Viggiano, Julie. "Lewis Hackett Photograph Collection." *Rockefeller Archive Center Newsletter*, spring 2004, 9.

Vine, J. Miller. "UNRRA's Health Campaign in Greece." *Lancet* 247 (May 25, 1946): 790.

———. "Malaria Control with DDT on a National Scale—Greece 1946." *Proceedings of the Royal Society of Medicine* 40 (1946–47): 841–48.

Vingt-Cinq ans d'activité de l'Office international d'hygiène publique. Paris: Office international d'hygiène publique, 1933.

Viseltear, Arthur J. "C.-E. A. Winslow: His Era and His Contribution to Medical Care." In *Healing and History*, edited by C. Rosenberg, 205–28. New York: Dawson, 1979.

———. "Compulsory Health Insurance and the Definition of Public Health." In *Compulsory Health Insurance: The Continuing American Debate*, edited by R. L. Numbers, 25–55. Westport, CT: Greenwood Press, 1982.

Warner, Michael. *The Trouble with Normal: Sex, Politics and the Ethics of Queer Life*. New York: Free Press, 1999.

Watts, Sheldon. *Epidemics and History. Disease, Power and Imperialism*. New Haven: Yale University Press, 1997.

Webster, Charles. "The Elderly and the Early National Health Service." In *Life, Death and the Elderly: Historical Perspectives*, edited by M. Pelling and R. M. Smith, 165–93. London: Routledge, 1991.

Weill, J. "La maladie de la faim et son traitement dans des camps d'internés." *Bulletin de l'Organisation d'hygiène de la Société des Nations* 10, no. 4 (1944): 730–80.

Weindling, Paul. "Public Health and Political Stabilization: Rockefeller Funding in Interwar Central/Eastern Europe." *Minerva* 31 (1993): 253–67.

———, ed. *International Health Organizations and Movements, 1918–1939*. Cambridge: Cambridge University Press, 1995.

———. "Philanthropy and World Health: The Rockefeller Foundation and the League of Nations Health Organisation." *Minerva* 35 (1997): 269–81.

———. *Epidemics and Genocide in Eastern Europe, 1890–1945*. Oxford: Oxford University Press, 2000.

———. "German Overtures to Russia, 1919–1925: Between Racial Expansion and National Co-existence." In *Doing Medicine Together: Germany and Russia between the Wars*, edited by S. G. Solomon, 35–60. Toronto: University of Toronto Press, 2006.

Weindling, Paul, and Marius Turda, eds. *"Blood and Homeland": Eugenics and Racial Nationalism in Central and Southeast Europe, 1900–1940*. Budapest: Central European University Press, 2006.

Weiner, Dora. "Le droit de l'homme à la santé: Une belle idée devant l'Assemblée constituante 1790–1791." *Clio Medica* 5 (1970): 208–23.

———. "Public Health under Napoleon: The Conseil de salubrité de Paris 1802–1815." *Clio Medica* 9 (1974): 271–84.

Welsh, H. A. "Deutsche Zentralverwaltung für das Gesundheitswesen (DZVG)." In *SBZ-Handbuch Staatliche Verwaltungen, Parteien, gesellschaftliche Organisationen und ihre Führungskräfte in der Sowjetischen Besatzungszone 1945–1949*, 2nd ed., edited by M. Broszat and H. Weber, 244–52, 294–95. Munich: Oldenbourg, 1993.

Welshman, John. *Municipal Medicine: Public Health in Twentieth-Century Britain*. Oxford: Lang, 2000.

Wenyon, C. M., A. G. Enderson, K. McLay, T. S. Hele, and J. Waterston. "Malaria in Macedonia, 1915–1919." *Journal of the Royal Army Medical Corps* 37 (1921) no. 2: 81–108; no. 3: 172–80; no. 4: 264–68.

Wheatley, Steven C. *The Politics of Philanthropy: Abraham Flexner and Medical Education.* Madison: University of Wisconsin Press, 1988.

Williams, Linsly R. "La Fondation Rockefeller pour la lutte contre la tuberculose en France. Son action pendant et depuis la guerre." *La Revue du Musée Social,* 1922, no. 2 (excerpt from): 3–31.

Williams, Steven C. "Nationalism and Public Health: The Convergence of Rockefeller Foundation Technique and Brazilian Federal Authority During the Time of Yellow Fever, 1925–30." In *Missionaries of Science: The Rockefeller Foundation and Latin America,* edited by Marcos Cueto, 23–51. Bloomington: Indiana University Press, 1994.

Willoughby, Edward F. *Handbook of Public Health and Demography.* London and New York: MacMillan, 1893.

Wilsch, R. "Die öffentliche Gesundheitspflege in Hannover." In *20 Jahre Gesundheitsamt Hannover,* 13–29. Hannover: Presseamt, 1955.

Wilson, Petra. "Colleague or Viral Vector? The Legal Construction of the HIV-Positive Worker." *Law and Policy* 16, no. 3 (1994): 299–321.

Winslow, Charles-Edward A. "Public Health Administration in Russia in 1917." *Public Health Reports,* no. 445 (December 28, 1917): 2191–2219.

———. *The Evolution and Significance of the Modern Public Health Campaign.* New Haven: Yale University Press, 1923.

———. *Health Survey of New Haven: Conducted Under the Auspices of the Community Chest.* New Haven: Yale School of Medicine, 1928.

———. *The Road to Health: The Jayne Foundation Lectures for 1929.* New York: Macmillan, 1929.

———. *Health on the Farm and in the Village: A Review and Evaluation of the Cattaraugus Health Demonstration with Special Reference to Its Lessons for Other Rural Areas.* New York: Macmillan, 1931.

———. *A City Set on a Hill: The Significance of the Health Demonstration of Syracuse, New York.* Garden City: Doubleday, Doran and Co., 1934.

———. "The International Appraisal of Local Health Programs." *Milbank Memorial Fund Quarterly* 15 (1937): 3–5.

———. *International Organization for Health.* New York: Commission to Study the Organization of Peace, 1944.

———. *The Price of Sickness and the Cost of Health.* Geneva: World Health Organization, 1951.

———. "The Economic Value of Preventive Medicine." *Chronicle of the World Health Organization* 6 (1952): 191–202.

Winslow, Charles-Edward A., and Savel Zimand. *Health under the "El": The Story of the Bellevue-Yorkville Health Demonstration in Midtown New York.* New York: Harper and Bros., 1937.

Winter, I. "Zur Geschichte der Gesundheitspolitik der KPD in der Weimarer Republik (Teil I)." *Zeitschrift für ärztliche Fortbildung* 67 (1973): 445–72.

———. "Begründer der Sowjet-Medizin. Zum 100 Geburtstag von N. A. Semaschko." *Humanitas* 14, no. 2 (November 1974).

Winter, Kurt. "Die Gestaltung der Fürsorge für Mutter und Kind im neuen demokratischen Gesundheitswesen." *Das deutsches Gesundheitswesen* 4 (1949): 526.

———. *Lehrbuch der Sozialhygiene*, 2nd ed. Berlin: Verlag Volk und Gesundheit, VEB, 1980.

Wohl, Anthony S. *Endangered Lives: Public Health in Victorian Britain.* London: Dent, 1983.

Wolfenden, Hugh H. "On the Methods of Comparing the Mortalities of Two or More Communities, and the Standardization of the Death-Rates." *Journal of the Royal Statistical Society* 86, no. 3 (1923): 399–411.

Wolff, E. "Mehr als nur materielle Interessen. Die organisierte Ärzteschaft im Ersten Weltkrieg und in der Weimarer Republik 1914–1933." In *Geschichte der deutschen Ärzteschaft Organisierte Berufs- und Gesundheitspolitik im 19 und 20 Jahrhundert*, edited by R. Jütte, 97–142. Cologne: Dt. Ärzte-Verlag, 1997.

Woodbridge, George. *UNRRA: The History of the United Nations Relief and Rehabilitation Administration.* New York: Columbia University Press, 1950.

Woods, Robert I. *The Demography of Victorian England and Wales.* Cambridge: Cambridge University Press, 2000.

Worboys, Michael. "Tropical Diseases." In *Companion Encyclopedia of the History of Medicine*, vol. 1, edited by W. F. Bynum and R. Porter, 511–35. London: Routledge, 1993.

Yankauer, Alfred. "Sexually Transmitted Diseases: A Neglected Public Health Priority." *American Journal of Public Health* 84, no. 12 (1994): 1894–97.

Yip, Ka-Che. *Health and National Reconstruction in Nationalist China: The Development of Modern Health Services, 1928–1937.* Ann Harbor: Association for Asian Studies, 1995.

Zank, W. "Wirtschaftliche Zentralverwaltungen und Deutsche Wirtschaftskommission." In *SBZ-Handbuch Staatliche Verwaltungen, Parteien, gesellschaftliche Organisationen und ihre Führungskräfte in der Sowjetischen Besatzungszone 1945–1949*, 2nd ed., edited by M. Broszat and H. Weber, 253–90. Munich: Oldenbourg, 1993.

Ziperman, H. Haskell. "A Medical History of the Panama Canal." *Surgery, Gynecology & Obstetrics* 137 (1973): 104–14.

Zulueta, Julian de. "Malaria and Mediterranean History." *Parassitologia* 15, nos. 1–2 (1973): 1–15.

Zylberman, Patrick. "Hereditary Disease and Environmental Factors in the 'Mixed Economy' of Public Health: René Sand and French Social Medicine, 1920–1934." In *Heredity and Infection: The History of Disease Transmission*, edited by J.-P. Gaudillière and I. Löwy, 261–81. London: Routledge, 2001.

———. "Fewer Parallels than Antitheses: René Sand and Andrija Štampar on Social Medicine (1919–1955)." *Social History of Medicine* 17, no. 1 (2004): 77–91.

———. "René Sand." In *Dictionary of Medical Biography*, edited by W. F. Bynum and Helen Bynum. Westport, CT: Greenwood (forthcoming).

Contributors

PETER BALDWIN is a professor of history at the University of California, Los Angeles. He is the author of *The Politics of Social Solidarity: Class Bases of the European Welfare State, 1875–1975* (Cambridge University Press, 1990); *Contagion and the State in Europe, 1830–1930* (Cambridge University Press, 1999); and *Disease and Democracy: The Industrialized World Faces AIDS* (University of California Press, 2005).

IRIS BOROWY is a researcher associated with the Historical Institute of the University of Rostock. She is the author of "Wissenschaft, Gesundheit, Politik. Das Verhältnis der Weimarer Republik zur Hygieneorganisation des Völkerbundes," *Sozial.Geschichte* 20 (2005) and "International Social Medicine between the Wars: Positioning a Volatile Concept," *Hygiea Internationalis*, 6 (2007). She is the coeditor (with Wolf D. Gruner) of *Facing Illness in Troubled Times: Health in Europe in the Interwar Years, 1918–1939* (Peter Lang, 2005).

JAMES A. GILLESPIE is a senior lecturer in health policy and deputy director of the School of Public Health and Menzies Centre for Health Policy at the University of Sydney. Among his publications are *The Price of Health: Australian Governments and Medical Politics, 1910–1960* (Cambridge University Press, 1991) and "The Rockefeller Foundation and Colonial Medicine in the Pacific, 1911–1929," in *New Countries and Old Medicine*, edited by L. Bryder (Pyramid Press, 1995).

GRAHAM MOONEY is an assistant professor at the Institute of the History of Medicine at Johns Hopkins University. He has published widely on the history of public health, historical demography, and historical epidemiology. He is coeditor with Jonathan Reinarz of *Permeable Walls: Historical Perspectives on Hospital and Asylum Visiting* (Clio Medica/Rodopi, forthcoming) and is writing a book on infectious disease surveillance in Victorian Britain.

LION MURARD is a senior researcher at CERMES (Centre de Recherche Médecine, Sciences, Santé et Société), CNRS-EHESS-INSERM, Paris. His recent publications include *L'Hygiène dans la République. La santé publique en France, ou l'utopie contrariée, 1870–1918* (Fayard, 1996), with Patrick Zylberman; and "Atlantic Crossings in the Measurement of Health: From American Appraisal Forms to the League of Nations' Health Indices," in *Medicine, the Market and the Mass Media: Producing Health in the 20th Century*, edited by V. Berridge and K. Loughlin (Routledge, 2005).

DOROTHY PORTER is a professor of the history of health sciences and chair of the Department of Anthropology, History and Social Medicine at the University of California, San Francisco. Her last monograph was *Health, Civilization and the State. A History of Public Health from Ancient to Modern Times* (Routledge 1999; 2005). She is currently writing a history of the relationship between the social sciences and medicine in twentieth-century Britain, focusing on postwar "lifestyle" medicine. Together with Brian Dolan, she is studying the development of medical humanism in twentieth-century American academic medical centers.

SABINE SCHLEIERMACHER is a research associate in the Department of Contemporary History, Institute of the History of Medicine, Center for Humanities and Health Sciences at the Free University and Humboldt University of Berlin. She is the author of *Sozialethik im Spannungsfeld von Sozial- und Rassenhygiene: der Mediziner Hans Harmsen im Centralausschuss für die Innere Mission* (Matthiessen, 1998) and coeditor (with Mechtild Rössler and Cordula Tollmien) of *Der "Generalplan Ost": Hauptlinien der nationalsozialistischen Planungs- und Vernichtungspolitik* (Akademie Verlag, 1993). She is currently working on public health and medical education in postwar Germany.

SUSAN GROSS SOLOMON is a professor of political science at the University of Toronto. Among her publications are an edited volume, *Doing Medicine Together: Germany and Russia between the Wars* (University of Toronto Press, 2006); *Vergleichende Völkerpathologie oder Rassenpathologie* (Pfaffenweiler, 1998), edited with J. Richter; and "Giving and Taking Across Borders: The Rockefeller Foundation and Russia, 1919–1928," *Minerva* 3 (2001), with N. Krementsov. She is currently writing a book entitled *Bringing Russia Home: American and German Health Experts and "Red" Medicine, 1923–1933*.

PAUL WEINDLING is a Wellcome Trust research professor in the history of medicine at the School of Humanities, Oxford Brookes University. Among his publications are *Health, Race and German Politics between National Unification and Nazism* (Cambridge University Press, 1989); *Epidemics and Genocide in Eastern Europe 1890–1945* (Oxford University Press, 2000); *Nazi Medicine and the Nuremberg Trials: From Medical War Crimes to Informed Consent* (Palgrave MacMillan, 2004); and an edited volume, *International Health Organisations and Movements 1918–1939* (Cambridge University Press, 1995).

PATRICK ZYLBERMAN is a senior researcher at CERMES (Centre de Recherche Médecine, Sciences, Santé et Société), CNRS-EHESS-INSERM, Paris. His publications include "Fewer Parallels than Antitheses: René Sand and Andrija Štampar on Social Medicine, 1919–1955," *Social History of Medicine*, 17 (2004); and *L'Hygiène dans la République. La santé publique en France ou l'utopie contrariée, 1870–1918* (Fayard, 1996), coauthored with Lion Murard. He is currently working on bioterror and antipandemic scenarios that have imposed new images of microbial threats that might affect the management of epidemic crises.

INDEX

An italicized page number indicates a figure.